BRAVE NEW WORLD?

BRAVE NEW WORLD?

THEOLOGY, ETHICS AND THE HUMAN GENOME

edited by

Celia Deane-Drummond

Foreword by Professor Ted Peters

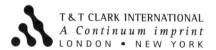

T & T CLARK INTERNATIONAL
A Continuum imprint
LONDON • NEW YORK

T & T CLARK LTD

A Continuum imprint

The Tower Building
11 York Road
London SE1 7NX

15 East 26th St
New York
NY 10010

www.continuumbooks.com

Copyright © T & T Clark Ltd, 2003

ISBN 0 567 08936 3 (paperback)
ISBN 0 567 08935 5 (hardback)

British Library Cataloguing-in-Publication Data
A catalogue record for this book is available from the British Library

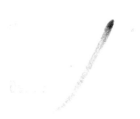

Typeset by Fakenham Photosetting Ltd, Fakenham, Norfolk NR21 8NN
Printed and bound in Great Britain by The Cromwell Press, Trowbridge, Wilts.

Crick, Watson and the Double Helix

A single insight made the Book of Life cohere,
Sent two men shouting into a Cambridge bar.
More slowly there steals upon us the power, the fear.

The X-ray from King's, and Chargaff's pairs,
Not one helix, but two, fugues on a common air;
A single insight made the Book of Life cohere.

An amazing future, suddenly laid bare –
New drugs, cheap insulin, strawberries all the year.
More slowly there steals upon us the power, the fear.

They were to find the grammar of genes trickier
Than expected, the syntax harder by far.
But a single insight had made the Book of Life cohere.

They could see the Nobel, and the patenting wars,
The complex hunger for profit, healing, honour.
More slowly there steals upon us the power, the fear.

It was all there, in the thin Cambridge beer,
The Text of Texts, laid ready for the sequencer,
A single insight made the Book of Life cohere.

Harder to take in the tears at the screening centre,
The many deaths of unborn others,
But slowly there steals upon us the power, the fear.

Now we face the uninsurable cancer,
Anticipate the repertoire of the baby-tweaker.
A single insight made the Book of Life cohere,
And slowly there steals upon us the power, the fear.

Christopher Southgate

Contents

Contributors

DR DONALD BRUCE spent fifteen years in chemistry research and risk assessment in nuclear energy. He holds doctorates in chemistry and theology. In 1992 he became Director of the Society, Religion and Technology Project (SRT) of the Church of Scotland. SRT was established in 1970 to address ethical and social issues arising out of modern technology. He chairs an interdisciplinary working group on genetic engineering and cloning, and has been at the forefront of the ethical debate on these issues and on gene patenting both in the UK and in Europe. He is a member of the bioethics working group of the Conference of European Churches, of the Scottish Science Advisory Committee, and the public issues advisory committee of the UK Biotechnology Research Council. He is an observer to the Global Summit of National Bioethics Committees. He is a frequent writer and broadcaster on bioethics issues.

PROFESSOR JOHN BRYANT is Professor of Cell and Molecular Biology at the University of Exeter, where, in addition to his research and teaching in molecular biology and biochemistry, he also runs a module on bioethics. He is President of the Society for Experimental Biology, Chair of Christians in Science and convenor of the Learning and Teaching Support Network's special interest group on Teaching Ethics to Bioscience Students. His next book (co-authored with Revd Dr John Searle) will be *Life in Our Hands*, to be published January 2004.

JULIE CLAGUE is Lecturer in Catholic Theology at the University of Glasgow. She has degrees in chemistry and theology and publishes in the fields of moral theology, bioethics and Catholic social thought. She co-edits the journal *Feminist Theology* and is a member of the editorial board of the journal *Political Theology*.

PROFESSOR CELIA DEANE-DRUMMOND trained originally as a plant scientist and has gained doctorates in plant physiology and theology. She currently holds a Chair in theology and the biological sciences at Chester College of Higher Education. In 2002 the Centre for Religion and the Biosciences at Chester College was formally launched, directed by Celia Deane-Drummond. Her most recently published books are *Creation Through Wisdom: Theology and the New Biology* (T & T Clark, 2000) and *Biology and Theology Today: Exploring the Boundaries* (SCM Press, 2001). She is also co-editor, with B. Szerszynski, of *Re-Ordering Nature: Theology, Society and the New Genetics* (T & T Clark, 2002).

DR MAUREEN JUNKER-KENNY is Associate Professor of Theology at Trinity College, Dublin where she teaches Christian ethics/practical theology. She gained a PhD in 1989, University of Münster, on F. Schleiermacher's theory of religion and Christology. *Habilitation* 1996, University of Tübingen, on J. Habermas's ethics of argumentation. Member of the Board of Directors of the international Catholic journal *Concilium*; co-editor of the *International Journal of Practical Theology*.

DR NEIL G. MESSER did research in molecular biology before being ordained as a minister of the United Reformed Church. He has taught Christian ethics in Oxford and Birmingham, and is now Lecturer in Christian Theology in the University of Wales, Lampeter. He is the author of a number of publications, including *The Therapeutic Covenant: Christian Ethics, Doctor–Patient Relationships and Informed Consent* (Grove, 1996) and *The Ethics of Human Cloning* (Grove, 2001), and the editor of *Theological Issues in Bioethics: An Introduction with Readings* (Darton, Longman & Todd, 2002).

DR RUTH PAGE taught theology in Dunedin, New Zealand, and in Edinburgh, her native Scotland. Impressed by change, diversity and variety of interpretation in the world and in theology, she wrote *Ambiguity and the Presence of God* (SCM Press, 1985). Her most recent book is *God With Us: Synergy in the Church* (SCM

Press, 2000). Having been Principal of New College, Edinburgh, she retired in 2000.

DR ESTHER D. REED is Lecturer in Theology and Christian Ethics at the University of St Andrews, Scotland. She has recently published *The Genesis of Ethics: On the Authority of God as the Origin of Christian Ethics* (Darton, Longman & Todd, 2000) and is editor of the journal *Studies in Christian Ethics* published by T & T Clark. She is currently working on selected topics concerning Christian ethics and the law.

THE REVEREND PROFESSOR MICHAEL J. REISS is Professor of Science Education and Head of the School of Science, Mathematics and Technology at the Institute of Education, University of London, and a priest – in charge of the parish of Toft. He currently directs the Salters-Nuffield Advanced Biology Project and is Visiting Honorary Professor at the University of York. His research, writing, teaching and consultancy expertise is in the fields of science education, bioethics and sex education. He was the specialist adviser to the House of Lords Select Committee into the use of animals in science, Chair of Europa Bio's External Advisory Group on Ethics and the ethicist on the UK Advisory Committee on Novel Foods and Processes. For further information see <www.reiss.tc>, email address <m.reiss@ioe.ac.uk>.

DR PETER SCOTT is Lecturer in Theology in the School of Humanities at the University of Gloucestershire. He is the author of *Theology, Ideology and Liberation* (Cambridge University Press, 1994), *A Political Theology of Nature* (Cambridge University Press, 2003) and co-editor of the *Blackwell Companion to Political Theology* (Blackwell, 2004). Email: <pscott@glos.ac.uk>

THE REVEREND PROFESSOR MARY J. SELLER gained a PhD in zoology and then a DSc, and her entire career has been spent in the Medical Genetics Department at Guy's Hospital, now the Division of Medical and Molecular Genetics, the Guy's, King's and St Thomas' Hospitals School of Medicine. She is Professor of Developmental Genetics and her main interest is in diagnosing and understanding the abnormalities of the body that some children are born with. She has an interest in medical ethics, is an Inspector for the Human Fertilisation and Embryology Authority, and has served on a number of government committees. She has been a Governor of the Royal Wanstead Foundation since 1988. She was ordained deacon in 1991 and priest in 1994, and she is a non-stipendiary curate of the parish church of Hurst Green near Oxted, Surrey.

DR ROBERT SONG is Lecturer in Christian Ethics at the University of Durham. He is author of *Christianity and Liberal Society* (Clarendon Press, 1997) and *Human Genetics: Fabricating the Future* (Darton, Longman & Todd, 2002), as well as several articles in the area of Christian ethics. He has also co-edited *A Royal Priesthood: The Use of the Bible Ethically and Politically* (Paternoster, 2002).

DR CHRISTOPHER SOUTHGATE trained originally in research biochemistry. He is now a poet and editor and part-time Lecturer in Theology at the University of Exeter. His previous books include *A Love and its Sounding* (University of Salzburg, 1997).

DR BRONISLAW SZERSZYNSKI is Lecturer in Environment and Culture at the Institute for Environment, Philosophy and Public Policy, Lancaster University. He is the author of a forthcoming Blackwell book on nature and the sacred, and co-editor of *Risk, Environment and Modernity: Towards a New Ecology* (Sage, 1996), *The Re-Ordering of Nature: Theology, Society and the New Genetics* (T & T Clark, 2002), and *Nature Performed: Environment, Culture and Performance* (Blackwell/Sociological Review, 2003). Email: <bron@lancaster.ac.uk>

DR PETER TURNPENNY has been Consultant Clinical Geneticist for Devon and Cornwall, based in Exeter, since 1993. His research interests include the genetic basis of congenital spinal deformities and foetal anticonvulsant syndromes. During the 1980s he worked as a paediatrician among the Arab population of Israel, which stimulated his interest in genetic medicine. He takes a keen interest in the ethical and social implications of the applications of new genetic technologies in medicine.

Foreword

All over the world governments are listening to questions about public policy formulation rising up from new discoveries in scientific laboratories combined with controversies in theological circles. Like liberated lab rats, agendas for genetic research have escaped the laboratories and are now running wildly through the churches as well as the wider society. During the year 2002 alone the United Nations along with national authorities in Singapore and the United States sponsored thorough studies of reproductive cloning and stem cell research. These study commissions invited scientists, ethicists and theologians from a variety of religious traditions to forecast the scientific future and to register their recommendations. What is important here for the guild of theologians is that the wider society now wants to hear what religious thinkers have to say.

Intuitively, our culture senses that something about our essential identity as human persons is at stake in genetic research. The euphoria over the prospect that gene manipulation will reap a harvest of medical advance clashes with a gut level repugnance at technologically remaking ourselves. Our ethical mandate to be stewards of our scientific resources to improve human health and well-being clashes with inchoate fears of human hubris and the risk of violating something sacred in nature. Our celebration of human engineering clashes with an anxious *sensus divinitatis* surrounding the nature we are engineering. Where is the wisdom? Is it in our scientific opportunity or in our intuitive repugnance?

As Celia Deane-Drummond suggests to us in the introduction to this book, we find ourselves at a critical point in setting a scientifically informed and ethically guided public policy. Options for further genetic research or even genetic technology compel us to ask about changes we might wish to avoid and changes we might wish to foster. We are confronted by choices; we did not invite them. What, now, is our responsibility?

To work toward defining that responsibility we need a team approach, one that elicits cooperation and shared understanding by scientists, ethicists and theologians. The scope of requisite knowledge exceeds what any individual can muster; so the expertise that each brings to the team is valuable to us all. Theologians informed by scientists have an opportunity to expand their horizon for understanding the world as God's creation and the factors entering into making human nature what it is. Ethicists and scientists informed by theologians can cultivate a more sophisticated apprehension of the sacred and gain from the cumulative wisdom of a long tradition regarding human nature. A dialogue with mutual interaction may lead to a broadening of everyone's horizon and perhaps even a fusion of horizons leading to insights beneficial for the wider society.

Like a ladder moving skyward, this collection of essays by expert authors builds from the ground up. It begins on the lower steps with a review of where the field of genetics is, scientifically. The next step is to consider existential questions raised by scientific contributions to our interpretation of life and death. Subsequent steps examine definitional issues surrounding human health and discerning historical trajectories with theological implications. The upper steps require rethinking bioethics and, finally, identifying social and political goods. At the top we emerge on a higher plateau.

This collection of essays is an indispensable aid to our religious communities and our wider society, relating as it does science to creation, genetics to theological anthropology, and ethics to wisdom at a singularly sophisticated level. I wish to commend Celia Deane-Drummond for her diligence in providing the reading audience with such a comprehensive treatment of this vital subject matter.

Ted Peters
Pacific Lutheran Theological Seminary
and Center for Theology and the Natural Sciences
at the Graduate Theological Union, Berkeley, California
1 January 2003

Acknowledgements

The original idea for this book emerged from a conversation that the editor had with Peter Francis, warden of St Deiniol's library in Hawarden, in the summer of 2001. The intention was to hold in this magnificent residential library a colloquium on the Human Genome Project (HGP), including those with particular scientific expertise in human genetics, along with ethicists, social scientists and theologians, in order to compile a book that would not only be of interest academically, but also help to foster public debate and discussion in the field. The enthusiastic response by everyone who was invited to this colloquium, generously supported by a grant to support research in science and religion at St Deiniol's library, was a promising start. As the book and discussions evolved it became clear that the book was not just about the HGP, but also about what might happen subsequently given the likely expansion in genetic knowledge. New chapters were added by participants to the original draft outline following a very fruitful colloquium at St Deiniol's library, 1–3 March 2002. Not all of those who attended the colloquium contributed specific chapters to the final book, but all served to stimulate discussion and offer constructive criticism on various draft chapters. Each chapter, then, was subject to far more scrutiny than is normally the case for an edited collection. The following were participants in the colloquium: Revd Stephen Bellamy, Dr Julie Clague, Professor Celia Deane-Drummond, Dr Lisa Goddard, Dr David Jones, Dr Neil Messer, Dr Ruth Page, Dr Esther Reed, Professor Michael

Reiss, Dr Peter Scott, Professor Mary Seller, Dr Robert Song, Dr Christopher Southgate, Dr Bronislaw Szerszynski. Unfortunately, due to personal circumstances, Dr Donald Bruce, Professor John Bryant and Professor Maureen Junker-Kenny were unable to attend the colloquium itself, but wanted to contribute to the final publication. The contributors are also grateful to Dr Lisa Goddard, currently studying for a doctorate at Chester College, who helped organize the colloquium, as well as acting as secretary during the discussions, which were also taped. Her work was generously supported by a grant given to the Centre for Religion and the Biosciences by the Christendom Trust. The editor is also grateful for valuable critical comments and feedback on the introduction, section introductions and postscript by Julie Clague, Peter Scott and Bronislaw Szerszynski. Overall the book emerged in the spirit of collaboration and exchange that many participants found particularly rewarding. Finally, all authors are indebted to Geoffrey Green of T & T Clark, who showed much enthusiasm for this book from the very early stages. We are also grateful to Fiona Murphy of Continuum for her helpful suggestions on the final text.

Abbreviations

AAS	*Acta Apostolicae Sedis*
AMA	American Medical Association
CSC-CEC	Church and Society Commission of the Conference of European Churches
EECCS	European Ecumenical Commission for Church and Society
ELSI	ethical, legal and social issues
EPO	European Patent Office
HFEA	Human Fertilisation and Embryology Authority
HGAC	Human Genetics Advisory Committee
HGP	Human Genome Project
HUGO	Human Genome Organization
IVF	*in-vitro* fertilization
PGD	pre-implantation genetic diagnosis
PND	pre-natal diagnosis
SNP	single nucleotide polymorphism
WMA	World Medical Association

Introduction

Celia Deane-Drummond

The Human Genome Project (HGP) achieved a breakthrough in June 2000 when the first draft sequence of the human genome was published amid a flurry of media excitement and political acclaim. Yet, perhaps in contrast to the wave of publicity following the announcement of the first mammalian clone, Dolly, the initial reaction to this announcement was one brimming with optimism, rather than fear. As Christopher Southgate reminds us in his poem at the start of this book, the real breakthrough in genetics happened when James Watson and Francis Crick discovered the way deoxyribonucleic acid (DNA) could replicate itself, and thus become what scientists somewhat mischievously called 'the Book of Life'. Indeed, as we probe deeper into the implications of the discovery of the genetic code for humans, it becomes clear that, like many scientific breakthroughs, it brings both power and promise, the possibility of both human misery and human liberation, and thus a need for reflection. In the aftermath of the announcement of mammalian cloning there are an increasing number of books available on religious and ethical responses, including reflection on human reproductive cloning.[1] By contrast, there is much less specific discussion on theological and ethical issues implicit in the human genome

---

[1] See, for example, R. Cole-Turner (ed.), *Human Cloning: Religious Responses* (Westminster: John Knox Press, 1997); and R. Cole-Turner (ed.), *Beyond Cloning* (Harrisburg: Trinity Press International, 2001).

project.[2] Phillip Sloan's monumental collection *Controlling Our Destinies* focused more specifically on eugenics and the immediate historical issues leading up to the completion of the first stage of the project.[3] It also raised general questions about whether scientific reductionism was compatible with humanistic and theological interpretations of human life. While timely, the book failed to consider in sufficient depth the theological and ethical questions arising out of the project.

One of the premises of the present book is that the discovery of the human gene sequence is the first stage in a much longer and more laborious unravelling of information about human genetics. Hence, the scientific research is still, relatively speaking, at an early stage in terms of its application. It therefore presents the possibility of a number of different available options. It is clear from Sloan's work that the social context in which the HGP was situated both influenced and informed the development of the science. Science, like any other research, is never conducted in a vacuum, but is dependent on funding, and the communities in which it is situated, as well as the motivation and creativity of the individual scientists themselves. It is therefore instructive to consider views in addition to those within the scientific contract. The research funded by the HGP into the ethical, legal and social issues (ELSI), for example, might be expected to take a particular stance given its source of funds. The validity of the project itself, for example, was never called into question.[4] Moreover, more broadly, the results of various committees in exploring applications of genetic science to human reproduction, including more recently the issue of cloning, can sometimes appear bland and more often than not written in a way which seems to favour particular scientific outcomes.[5]

[2] For an excellent discussion of general issues in genetics and ethics, see R. Song, *Human Genetics: Fabricating the Future* (London: Darton, Longman & Todd, 2002).

[3] Phillip R. Sloan (ed.), *Controlling Our Destinies: Historical, Philosophical, Ethical and Theological Perspectives on the Human Genome Project* (Notre Dame: University of Notre Dame Press, 2000).

[4] ELSI was awarded just 3 per cent, then 5 per cent, of the total funding for the HGP, which was enough to satisfy a public concerned that ethical issues were taken into account, but not sufficient to radically alter the direction of the research.

[5] The report of the Human Genetics Advisory Commission on Human and Reproductive Cloning falls into this category. While religious and ethical views

The question now arises, how might insights from science, ethics and theology mutually inform and enrich each other? Theological and ethical reflections are ways of thinking about religious belief and human practice. While it is possible to acknowledge the social conditioning of science, where there is a close correlation between scientific theory and application of that theory, then such statements can be considered to be 'robust' and useful for understanding, at least in a provisional sense, the way the world is.[6] An informed theology needs to take into account this particular way of understanding human existence, as well as other epistemologies emerging in other disciplines. The dialogue between science and religion has, at least in its more recent history, focused on this part of the conversation, that is in what way must theological faith become adjusted to the results of modern contemporary scientific insights. John Polkinghorne is one of the most prolific writers in this respect, arguing that in those cases where there is divergence then both science and religion offer complementary ways of knowing.[7] There can be little doubt that historically those prominent in science were also able to combine their scientific expertise with religious faith.[8] Yet, given the social and cultural rooting of science, is there any sense in which science, including genetics, might be influenced by voices outside its discipline, and by assumptions that it does not itself have the resources to examine? Those concerned with the public perception of science tend to see public science education as a primary goal, with scientists doing little more than allay the ignorance of a well-meaning populace. While it is important to dispel

---

were taken into account, when presented as just one of many concerns, the full weight of such arguments tends to become diffuse. See The Human Genetics Advisory Commission (HGAC) and The Human Fertilisation and Embryology Authority (HFEA) Report, *Cloning Issues in Reproduction, Science and Medicine* (London: HMSO, 1998).

[6] A. Peacocke, 'Relating Genetics to Theology on the Map of Scientific Knowledge', in Sloan, *Controlling Our Destinies*, pp. 343–66.

[7] See, for example, J. Polkinghorne, *One World: The Interaction of Science and Theology* (London: SPCK, 1986); *Belief in God in an Age of Science* (Newhaven: Yale University Press, 1998); *Science and Christian Belief: The Faith of a Physicist* (London: SPCK, 1994); *Scientists as Theologians* (London: SPCK, 1996); 'Kenotic Creation and Divine Action', in J. Polkinghorne (ed.), *The Work of Love: Creation as Kenosis* (London: SPCK, 2001).

[8] J. Hedley Brooke, *Science and Religion: Some Historical Perspectives* (Cambridge: Cambridge University Press, 1991); J. Brooke and G. Cantor, *Reconstructing Nature: The Engagement of Science and Religion* (Edinburgh: T & T Clark, 1998).

exaggerated misconceptions about science and its practice, equally it is important to allow issues of critical and public significance to become aired in a wider forum for debate. One of the purposes of this book is to facilitate this conversation between those of different disciplines, so that an enriching and informative way forward can be found amidst the challenges facing humanity arising out of genetic discoveries and possibilities. Once it is understood that science, at the limits of its knowing, reaches out into areas of ambiguity and uncertainty, and theology, also, is not just about doctrine, but also a delineation of what God is not through the apophatic tradition, then mutual appreciation can begin and the task of exploration can be facilitated through empathetic and careful conversations.

What might the role of theology become in conversations with genetic science? A theological approach is called for that is subtler than simply giving an outline of the dogmatic foundations of faith and asking whether science is compatible with this or not. Instead, theological threads that lend themselves to deeper reflection on the issues raised can begin the task of building a theological map superimposed, as it were, on the map of scientific knowing. The theological strands developed in this book do not presuppose a particular denominational tradition, but seek to gain insights from a number of different voices and contexts, and engage with, for example, liberal, evangelical, radical, Protestant and Roman Catholic traditions. Some of the contributors draw primarily from a particular theological tradition, all contributors are engaged in open conversation with those who are from different theological perspectives. Not all the contributors have a particular interest in theology as such; some are more concerned with social and political issues and the impact of scientific and religious understanding on the way we think about our place in the world. Over half the contributors either have had a formal training in science or are practising genetic scientists. That such a conversation is possible is a reminder that theology in the light of science indirectly achieves an ecumenical task, where respect for one another's traditions can become enlarged in the light of the particular problems and issues arising from a discussion of a particular controversial technology. In this book particular theological threads that became prominent in deliberation included, for example, questions about human identity and what it is to be made in God's image; eschatological questions on the limits of extending life, the relationship between theology and ethics, including virtue ethics; reflection on the common good and the significance of community and liturgy in building relationships. In addition, philosophical epistemology becomes crucial in the task of elaborating more fully the ethical questions arising out of the mutual conversation between theology and science.

The book begins (Part I: 'What is Genetic Science Doing?') with an exploration of scientific issues, from three well-established scientific practitioners, not thereby predicating the ontological priority of science, but in order to give some insights as to what genetic science is doing from the perspectives of scientists who are open-minded about the possibility of exploring other ways of knowing and understanding reality. John Bryant and Peter Turnpenny's chapter focuses on genetic modification of animals and humans, along with the possibilities of treatment of genetic disease. Mary Seller's chapter offers her own perspective on what genetic science is about and the possibilities for the future. Genetic science is a vast field and it would be impossible to cover all aspects of contemporary genetic science and practice. However, the issues raised in these chapters give a good flavour of what genetic science is like, as well as some indication of the way it might be used in applications in the future.

Part II ('Reinterpreting Life and Death') shifts to considering more speculative questions about what science might be like in the future, including the possibility of indefinitely extending life. What issues might this raise for our religious understanding of human identity and eschatology? Michael Reiss's chapter entitled '"And in the World to Come, Life Everlasting"', examines how this Christian hope might impinge on earthly reality in the future through genetic science. Or perhaps we should consider more fully the implication of the common genetic inheritance between animals and humans, thereby widening the theological concept of image-bearing? Ruth Page takes up this theme in her chapter entitled 'The Human Genome and the Image of God'.

Part III ('Questioning Implicit Norms') moves to consider the practical implementation of genetic science in the health professions and asks what are the specific implicit norms that are assumed in day-to-day medical practice. Neil Messer explores the theological implications of what is sometimes called the 'Tyranny of Normality'. What are the philosophical assumptions in such practice and how might this bear on a theological understanding of reality? Should a more philosophical approach to ethics be adopted, or one that is rooted more specifically in the Christian tradition? Maureen Junker-Kenny takes up these questions in relation to the development of a philosophical anthropology.

Part IV ('Discerning Historical Trajectories') invites the reader to step back and search the historical trends that led up to where genetic science is poised today. Is the Human Genome Project part of the cultural shift towards the development of a simplified reference language, one that by implication threatens to drown out other ways of knowing what it is to be human? Bronislaw Szerszynski takes up this theme in his chapter, asking if the Human Genome Project has led to what he calls the 'death of the human'. Or, again, is the HGP an extension of the cultural domination of nature in order to serve particular human ends? Robert Song takes up this thread in his chapter that explores the soteriological dimension of the Human Genome Project.

Part V ('Rethinking "Bioethics"') explores still further the theme of bioethics and asks questions about the way bioethical practice has developed from a Christian perspective. The authors ask whether traditional bioethical tools and frameworks are sufficient or adequate for tackling the socio/political effects of genetics. What are the particular issues arising out of the extensive literature on the morality of genetic practice? Julie Clague discusses this theme in her chapter entitled 'Beyond Beneficence: The Emergence of Genomorality and the Common Good'. Is it possible to take a rather different approach to genetics through development of a Christian appropriation of virtue ethics? I take up this idea in my chapter which focuses on the question: 'How Might A Virtue Ethic Frame Debates In Human Genetics?'.

Part VI ('Identifying Social and Political Goods') broadens the areas for debate. It considers, first of all, the specific legal and political issues associated with gene patenting. Donald Bruce writes out of his own experience working with the

European churches. Esther Reed then reflects in more detail on the significance of such a rendition in terms of Christian theology, ethics and liturgical practice. Peter Scott's chapter then invites readers to explore the nature of the good in a social, political and theological sense in the light of what is projected in the Human Genome Project.

While each of the chapters argue from particular viewpoints, some of the chapters emerged out of particular conversations between authors during and after the colloquium where the early drafts of some of the chapters represented here were discussed. The chapters by Mary Seller, Robert Song, Donald Bruce and Esther Reed, and the poems by Christopher Southgate, were all developed on this basis. Other chapters were subject to considerable revision and re-drafting as a result of these conversations. As such, this book represents both the way individuals can contribute to the debate, but also the value of conversation, of listening to a range of different perspectives in order to refine one's own. As will become apparent for those who read further, not all the authors agree on specific points, especially with respect to the philosophical framing of scientific knowing, the relationship between theology, ethics and philosophy, and the contribution of public understanding to debates in genetics. In addition, those who participated in the colloquium, but who did not offer particular chapters, added their own distinctive voice to the debates. The mutual respect and sensitivity to alternative positions was apparent throughout the event. My hope is that a flavour of some of this mutual cooperation will emerge in the pages to follow and act as a catalyst for further discussion.

Stephen Clark, commenting on the significance of the new developments in biotechnology with respect to animals, suggested that 'When changes are distant and hardly imaginable it is too soon to take action to prevent them. When they are present realities it is far too late. We live in one of those rare moments when we can just imagine what might develop, and might perhaps avoid it.'[9] It seems to me that a similar critical point has been reached in relation to genetics and the human

---

[9] S.R.L. Clark, 'Thinking about Biotechnology: Towards a Theory of Just Experimentation', in C. Deane-Drummond and B. Szerszynski (eds), *Re-Ordering Nature: Theology, Society and the New Genetics* (Edinburgh: T & T Clark, 2002), p. 177.

genome. There are some changes that we might wish to avoid, others that we might wish to foster. In either event the choices are before us in a way perhaps that they have not been in the past. While there is some fatalism and sense of inevitability in the public response to biotechnology, I suggest that an appropriate response is to resist such fatalism, even though in other respects public attitudes may provide valuable insights in relation to the kinds of development that might be acceptable.[10] Moreover, while this book has necessarily focused on issues in human genetics, this does not thereby imply that genetic issues in relation to non-human species, including plants, are not important. Rather, the modest task set in this book is to promote dialogue between those of different disciplines in the area of human genetics in order to open up discussion for wider debate. It will also be a book that is valuable for students and scholars in the fields of science, genetics, theology, sociology, philosophy and ethics. In addition, it will be of interest to pastors, clergy and health practitioners as well as members of the lay public who are concerned about the way our future is going to be shaped by the new genetics. This generation will bear considerable responsibility for the next in delineating the framework in which new developments in human genetics might take shape. It is the hope of the contributors of this volume that such development will become a shared task in the human communities in which we find ourselves. This book is a small step in this direction.

---

[10] For a discussion of public insights into agricultural biotechnology see C. Deane-Drummond, B. Szerszynski and R. Grove-White, 'Genetically Modified Theology: Implicit Religious Response in Public Attitudes to Agricultural Biotechnology', in Deane-Drummond and Szerszynski, *Re-Ordering Nature*, pp. 17–38.

PART I

What is Genetic Science Doing?

Introduction to Part I

This section looks at what might realistically be possible for genetic science, and outlines some of the basic premises of genetics, especially for those not familiar with the subject. The contributors to this book were clear that without some basic knowledge of genetic science a discussion of the more speculative remarks about the prospects of genetic science by both those inside and outside the field would not be sufficiently grounded in the current state of scientific knowledge.

John Bryant and Peter Turnpenny's chapter draws on their insights from research and clinical experience. It maps some important trends in techniques of genetic manipulation, including the effects of intrachromasomal position on gene expression due to where the genes are inserted into a particular chromosome. The initiative of the Human Genome Project (HGP) is discussed from the perspective of practising scientists, leading on to particular consideration of how genetic knowledge has been used in testing for genetic disease in children and prior to birth through pre-natal diagnostic (PND) methods. The prospects for pre-implantation genetic diagnosis (PGD) through currently available *in-vitro* fertilization (IVF) methods are also evaluated. Their provisional conclusion is that the most fruitful short-term benefit of human genome research is likely to be through improved targeting of drug therapies. Almost inevitably their discussion concludes with a pointer towards some of the ethical issues raised, such as the prospects for germ-line therapy and the difficulties associated with genetic enhancement.

Mary Seller's chapter is a clear guide for the perplexed, yet she does not limit her discussion to the building-blocks of genetic science, but also introduces the reader to some of the prospects as well as the limitations of current research. She scrutinizes common beliefs about genetics, such as the one gene one protein hypothesis. Each cell not only has 'house-keeping' genes in common with all others, but is subject to a cascade of genetic control during development, adding yet more layers to the complexity. Many genetic diseases in humans are related to polygenetic effects. Furthermore, there is a vast amount of non-coding DNA, and differences between individuals are related to small changes taking place at particular sites known as SNPs. While on the one hand Seller is sanguine about the gap between genetic identification and the knowledge required for the treatment of disease, on the other hand she is positive about the prospects of research emerging in the wake of the HGP. The latter is qualified by her suggestion that genetic research needs to be viewed in a realistic way, rather than lead to speculation about designer babies.

1

Genetics and Genetic Modification of Humans: Principles, Practice and Possibilities

John Bryant and Peter Turnpenny

1 Genetic modification

Techniques for the genetic modification of non-human mammals were first developed in the 1980s. There are two basic procedures by which this can be achieved.[1] The more widely used procedure is the introduction of the foreign DNA into an oocyte (unfertilized ovum) prior to *in-vitro* fertilization or into one of the pro-nuclei of the newly fertilized ovum. The genetically modified embryo is then introduced into the uterus in the 'normal' fashion and, provided a pregnancy is established successfully, a *transgenic* (genetically modified) mammal will eventually be born and, further, it will pass on the new gene to subsequent generations. Using mice as the initial experimental animals it was established that not only could foreign genes be introduced in this way[2] but it was possible to control the expression of the genes by the incorporation into the foreign DNA of a gene promoter sequence (essentially a gene's on–off switch).[3] However, the success rate for birth of mice (and

---

[1] Reviewed in N. Maclean (ed.), *Animals with Novel Genes* (Cambridge: Cambridge University Press, 1994), pp. 4–12.

[2] e.g. R.L. Brinster and R.D. Palmiter, 'Transgenic Mice Containing Growth-Hormone Fusion Genes', *Philosophical Transactions of the Royal Society*, Series B 307 (1984), pp. 309–12.

[3] R. Jaenisch, 'Transgenic Animals', *Science* 240 (1988), pp. 1468–74.

indeed other mammals) from embryos that had been genetically manipulated was only about 25 per cent of that achieved
with non-manipulated embryos.[4] Although this figure has been
improved on since then it is still clear that the success rate is
lower with transgenic embryos. Indeed, the overall live birth
rate for transgenic farm animals such as sheep and cattle may
be as low as 2–4 per cent.[5]

An alternative approach, used especially with mice and with
other mammals with a short generation time, is stem cell transformation. Stem cells – cells with the potential to give rise to all
the different cell types within the body – are removed from a pre-
implantation embryo (obtained either by *in-vitro* fertilization or
by embryo rescue) and are transfected with the foreign DNA.
The genetically modified cells are replaced in the embryo which
is then inserted into the uterus and brought to term, and will pass
the foreign gene on to the next generation via the germ-line.

These techniques clearly make possible the genetic modification of human embryos – after all, the second mammalian
species for which successful *in-vitro* fertilization was achieved
was *Homo sapiens*. Further, the feasibility of applying these
techniques to primates was demonstrated in 2001 by the genetic
modification of a rhesus monkey.[6] However, there are some
technical problems that should affect our thinking, at least in a
pragmatic way, about this. First, animal (and indeed, plant)
chromosomes are complex structures and we do not know very
much about the factors that determine where in the
chromosome set (the genome) the new gene is inserted. Thus,
in genetically modified animals, the *level* of expression of the
exogenous gene varies considerably from animal to animal
because of position effects (variation caused by incorporation
of the exogenous gene at different places within the recipient
genome). There has been some limited success in targeting
exogenous genes to specific regions of chromosome in mice[7]

[4] R.B. Church, 'Embryo Manipulation and Gene Transfer in Domestic Animals',
New England Journal of Medicine 341 (1987), pp. 28–37.

[5] H. Griffin, 'Cloning of Animals and Humans', in J.A. Bryant, L.M. Baggott la Velle
and J.F. Searle (eds), *Bioethics for Scientists* (Chichester: John Wiley & Sons, 2002),
p. 286.

[6] G. Vogel, 'Infant Monkey Carries Jellyfish Gene', *Science* 291 (2001), p. 226.

[7] S. Thompson, A.R. Clarke, A.M. Pow, M.L. Hooper and D.W. Melton, 'Germline
transmission and expression of a corrected HRPT gene produced by gene
targeting in embryonic stem cells'. *Cell* 56 (1989), pp. 313–21.

and more recently in sheep.[8] However, this is by no means routine, and thus the researcher must monitor the level of expression of the foreign gene in as many GM animals as possible (which may not be very many given the constraints on numbers imposed by low success rates). Second, the extent to which the gene is expressed in progeny may be variable (possibly because of phenomena such as gene-silencing or genetic imprinting, where a gene or genes in one parental genome remain switched on while the same chromosomal region in the other parental genome is rendered silent). However, these problems have not prevented the use of transgenic animals in research and in biotechnology. For example, mice can be modified with mutant genes which cause monogenic diseases such as cystic fibrosis, Alzheimer's or Huntington's diseases, or with oncogenes that can be activated to induce tumour formation. In the UK alone, tens of thousands of transgenic mice have been used in biomedical research. Farm animals such as sheep can be genetically modified to produce pharmaceutical proteins in their milk. Indeed, one of the motivations for the cloning experiments that led to the birth of Dolly was a wish to be able to maintain a genetic stock in which an economically important gene was expressed at high level.[9]

2   Human genetics and the Human Genome Project

Since the middle of the twentieth century one of the main motivations in the study of human genetics has been to understand the genetic basis of disease. About 4,500 diseases, most of which are rare, are known to be caused by mutations in single genes, whilst approximately 20,000 chromosomal aberrations have been reported to date.[10] Further, as we now know, mutations and polymorphisms within certain genes are involved

---

[8] K.J. McCreath, J. Howcroft, K.H.S. Campbell, A. Colman, A.E. Schnieke and A.J. King, 'Production of gene-targeted sheep by nuclear transfer from cultured somatic cells' *Nature* 405 (2000), pp. 1066–9.

[9] Griffin, 'Cloning of Animals and Humans', pp. 286–7.

[10] T. Strachan and A.P. Read, *Human Molecular Genetics* (Oxford: Bios Scientific, 1996), pp. 367–99; P.D. Turnpenny and J.A. Bryant, 'Human Genetics and Genetic Enhancement', in J.A. Bryant, L.M. Baggott la Velle and J.F. Searle (eds), *Bioethics for Scientists* (Chichester: John Wiley & Sons, 2002), p. 246.

in determining *predisposition* to certain diseases. One of the more common of the monogenic diseases, sickle-cell anaemia, has a very special place in the history of human genetics. It was the first genetic disease for which the specific lesion in the mutant protein[11] was characterized (as long ago as 1957). Elegant work in the 1960s established the genetic code and thus from the lesion in the protein it was possible to predict what change (mutation) had occurred in the gene to produce the malfunctioning protein. However, confirmation of that prediction had to wait until methods became available for determining the sequence of DNA.

Study of genetic diseases in humans is of course limited by our inability to undertake mating experiments. Thus, for example, prior to the advent of DNA analysis, the assessment of genetic risk for a couple wishing to have children depended on the pattern of inheritance of the condition in their family and knowledge of the population frequency of particular gene mutations, which could be calculated by epidemiological studies and statistical methods. There were just a few conditions where the estimates of genetic risk might be informed (not necessarily with great accuracy) by other factors such as biochemical analysis, for example, the detection of elevated levels of particular enzymes in the blood, as with creatine kinase as a possible indicator of Duchenne muscular dystrophy. The development of recombinant DNA technology in the 1970s was therefore very important. The 'growth' of genes (molecular cloning)[12] in microbial cells, combined with a developing ability to characterize particular DNA sequences, meant that it became possible to investigate directly at least some of the genetic changes that lead to the development of a disease. Thus, the genes involved in several heritable diseases, including cystic fibrosis, had been identified, cloned and characterized by the end of the 1980s prior to the establishment of the Human

---

[11] Proteins are the working molecules of cells; the structure of a particular protein is specified by the gene that encodes it. In sickle-cell anaemia the relevant protein is haemoglobin.

[12] Molecular cloning refers to the technique of making many copies of a gene or gene fragment by inserting the gene or gene fragment into a micro-organism. The inserted gene or gene fragment is replicated every time the micro-organism divides, thus generating, in a typical culture of cells, billions of copies of the gene or gene fragment.

Genome Project.[13] This in turn meant that diagnostic and detection techniques based on actual gene sequences were becoming available.

In 1988 a consortium of scientists in the USA persuaded Congress that the time was right for the establishment of a coordinated programme to sequence the entire human genome.[14] The programme was set to run from 1990 to 2005 and, in the USA, $3,000,000,000 was initially allocated to the project. This sum included 5 per cent allocated to study the ethical and social implications of the project. The decision to set up the HGP was not without its critics. In the USA some members of the public (and presumably some members of Congress) believed that the money could have been spent in other ways, raising questions about allocation of limited resources. Even among the science community there were some who, at least at that time, believed the establishment of the project to be a major mistake.[15]

The project also incorporated human gene analysis already in progress outside the USA so that about two-thirds of the work has been undertaken in the USA with most of the rest being split between the UK, Germany, France, Japan and Canada. The results have been spectacular. By the middle of the year 2000, some four and half years before the formal closure of the project, the consensus[16] sequences of the majority of human

[13] Reviewed in Turnpenny and Bryant, 'Human Genetics and Genetic Enhancement', pp. 244–7.

[14] R. Shapiro, *The Human Blueprint: The Race to Unlock the Secrets of our Genetic Script* (New York: St Martin's Press, 1991).

[15] E.g. M.C. Rechsteiner, 'The Human Genome Project: Misguided Science Policy', *Trends in Biochemical Sciences* 16 (1991), p. 455. Critics of the project raised four main points: (a) the amount of money devoted to the HGP would cause other areas of biological and medical research to be starved of funds; (b) such a strong focus on genes gives an unbalanced view of their role in human life; (c) focus on genetic disease would divert attention away from more widespread and pressing causes of disease; and (d) the project would distort the practice of science by training and employing a large cadre of scientists with expertise in a very narrow area of biological science and by spawning and/or supporting a range of narrowly focused journals and other publications.

[16] Consensus sequence: the 'normal' or most common sequence of bases (DNA building-blocks) in any particular tract of DNA. The DNA of any two people when directly compared will reveal that they are 99.9 per cent identical (i.e. the two DNA samples will differ, on average, at one base in a thousand) regardless of population background or ethnicity: see F.S. Collins, 'Human Genetics', in J.F. Kilner, C.C. Hook and D.B. Uustal (eds), *Cutting Edge Bioethics: A Christian Exploration of Technologies and Trends* (Grand Rapids and Cambridge: Eerdmans, 2002), p. 8.

genes were known,[17] as was the identity of many disease-causing
mutations. One interesting and still-puzzling feature to emerge
is that humans, probably in common with other mammals, have
only about 30,000 genes, whereas it had been predicted from
studies of genetics that we would have about 80,000. One
possible explanation for this is that many genes may have
multiple functions (and we certainly already know of some that
do).[18] This in turn implies the existence of complex control
mechanisms that regulate multiple gene functions. It also
implies that genetic modification of mammals may not be as
straightforward as had been previously suggested, notwith-
standing the routine production of genetically modified mice
for use in biomedical research (see also section 1 above).

3   Genetic diagnosis and screening

As described above, the advent of recombinant DNA techniques
led to a previously undreamed-of capability to identify, isolate
and characterize genes, including human genes, and gave a new
impetus to human genetic research, even before the formal
establishment of the HGP. In an astonishingly short period of
time (compared with the rate of progress before the widespread
availability of recombinant DNA techniques) human DNA
analysis will have progressed to rapid, far-ranging and relatively
inexpensive methods of direct sequencing with the potential to
identify very many polymorphisms and mutations.[19] Thus, while
direct genetic diagnosis of a limited number of conditions has
been available for over 20 years, the strong focus on human
genetics since 1990 has seen the addition of many more
conditions to the list for which such diagnosis is possible.
However, this rapid progress is not without problems. First, the
interpretation and health implications of many sequence

---

[17] D. Butler and P. Smaglik, 'Draft data leave geneticists with a mountain still to
climb', *Nature* 405 (2000), pp. 914–15; C. Macilwain, 'World leaders heap praise
on human genome landmark', *Nature* 405 (2000), pp. 983–84; E. Marshall,
'Human genome: rival sequencers celebrate a milestone together', *Science* 288
(2000) pp. 2294–5.

[18] C. J. Jeffery, 'Moonlighting Proteins', *Trends in Biochemical Sciences* 24 (1999),
pp. 8–11.

[19] F. Collins, 'Medical and Societal Consequences of the Human Genome Project',
New England Journal of Medicine 341 (1999), pp. 28–37; Note – a polymorphism is
a genetic variant fixed (i.e. consistently present) within a population.

variations ('mutations') may not be clear for a long time. Many genes may be multi-functional (see above) and further, the penetrance (the extent to which a gene is expressed) of some mutations is variable from person to person. Thus there will be for some conditions an uncertainty in prognosis and for many more, in the short to medium term at least, a paucity of possible beneficial interventions, disappointing the expectations of patients and their families.[20] Second, the applications of the technology will generate a range of socio-ethical dilemmas. These are discussed extensively in subsequent chapters but need to be noted here for future attention.

Despite these problems, it should not be assumed that making genetic diagnoses has no value. For example, negative diagnosis, demonstrating that a person does not carry a particular mutation that is prevalent in their family, can bring great relief.[21] Positive diagnoses may also be beneficial, most obviously when the diagnosis can lead to a specific course of treatment. But even when little change is possible for the affected individual, a diagnosis, a resolution of uncertainty, may empower the patient and/or family because of the specific knowledge of the situation[22] and the senses of both relief and control that may follow.[23] For many parents it is important to be able to explain their child's condition when others ask what is wrong,[24] and in very practical terms having a diagnosis often expedites support through the education and social benefit

---

[20] The discovery of a new 'disease gene' has almost always been hailed as a major breakthrough for the condition in question. It is regarded as a major step in understanding the pathophysiology of the disease, although this is only actually true if the function of the gene product is understood. Hopes are raised because our current thinking is that knowledge of the gene and its product is the first step towards treatment, but we have too often failed to caution that treatment may be years or even decades away. Expectations are further raised by over-enthusiastic reporting in the media which have a strong interest in good news health stories.

[21] See F. Collins, 'The Human Genome Project: Tool of Atheistic Reductionism or Embodiment of Christian Mandate to Heal?', *Science and Christian Belief* 11 (1999b), pp. 99–111.

[22] M. Berkenstadt, S. Shiloh, G. Barkai, M.B-M. Katznelson and B. Goldman, 'Perceived Personal Control (PPC): A New Concept in Measuring Outcome of Genetic Counseling', *American Journal of Medical Genetics* 82 (1999), pp. 53–9.

[23] H. Skirton, 'Genetic Nurses and Counsellors: Preparation for Practice with Families at Risk of Cancer', *Disease Markers* 15 (1999), pp. 145–7; D. M. Webster and A.W. Kruglanski, 'Individual Differences in Need for Cognitive Closure', *Journal of Personality and Social Psychology* 67 (1994), pp. 1049–62.

[24] H. Skirton, 'A longitudinal study of genetic counselling for families – needs, expectations and outcomes', *PhD Thesis*, University of Exeter, UK (2000).

systems and via relevant support groups. Parents may also push for diagnostic 'closure' in relation to resolving the genetic carrier status of their child(ren) with respect to any condition/gene which is present in the family but unlikely to have implications for the child until adult life or leading up to reproductive decisions. The genetic testing of children has been dealt with thoroughly elsewhere[25] and is an important ethical issue in the debate. There can be few objections to testing children if their genetic condition could be managed or treated from a young age. If, however, the condition being tested for is not readily treatable or manageable, whose quality of life is enhanced by the testing? (See above re diagnostic closure.) It could be said that the child has been denied the opportunity to make a fully informed decision about a test that primarily benefits the parents, and in adolescence or adulthood may come to feel that their right to autonomy has been denied. However, the majority of the evidence is that testing in childhood for carrier status is not harmful,[26] although it is noted that some testing is certainly undertaken as a result of parental pressure.[27]

Diagnostic tests for genetic conditions may also be administered pre-natally. The technique of amniocentesis (sampling of foetal cells from the amniotic fluid, generally at about 16 weeks of pregnancy) was first introduced for pre-natal diagnosis in the 1950s for the testing of rhesus blood group status[28] and has been adopted for a range of cyotological, biochemical, chromosomal and, more recently, genetic tests.[29] In the 1970s and 1980s chorionic villus sampling was introduced and developed.[30] This

[25] A. Clarke, *The Genetic Testing of Children* (Oxford: Bios Scientific Publications, 1997).

[26] A. Fryer, 'Inappropriate Genetic Testing of Children', *Archives of Disease in Childhood* 83 (2000), pp. 283–5.

[27] A.M. Proctor, A. Clarke and P.S. Harper, 'Survey of Genetic Testing in Childhood', *Journal of Medical Genetics* 36, Suppl .1 (1999), p. S73.

[28] B.C.A. Bevis, 'Composition of Liquor Amnii in Haemolytic Disease of the Newborn', *Journal of Obstetrics and Gynaecology of the British Commonwealth* 60 (1953), pp. 244–51.

[29] Reviewed in Turnpenny and Bryant, 'Human Genetics and Genetic Enhancement', pp. 250–3.

[30] N. Hahnemann, 'Early Prenatal Diagnosis; A Study of Biopsy Techniques and Cell Culturing from Extra-Embryonic Membranes', *Clinical Genetics* 6 (1974), pp. 294–306; R.H.T. Ward, B. Modell, M. Petrou, F. Karagozlu and E. Douratsos, 'Method of Sampling Chorionic Villi in First Trimester of Pregnancy under Guidance of Real Time Ultrasound', *British Medical Journal* 286 (1983), pp. 1542–4.

essentially involves sampling tissue from the edge of the developing placenta; it can be performed as early as eleven or twelve weeks into a pregnancy and can be used in the same range of tests and diagnoses. The earlier availability of a diagnosis in a pregnancy is regarded as desirable when termination of pregnancy following a diagnosis is a preferred option (see below). However, the vast majority of rare genetic disorders are not tested for in routine pre-natal screening. Instead, tests are administered when the foetus is known to be at risk because of a positive family history where a precise diagnosis has been made, often when a couple have already had an affected child. Pre-natal diagnosis is then a choice based on detailed knowledge of the condition in question, and balanced, if an affected child has already been born, with the effect that a second affected child would have on the family. For many couples the decision is not easy. They may even feel guilty about being parents of one affected child, perhaps now loved and absorbed into family life, but face the prospect of terminating the life of a subsequent affected child *in utero*, and perhaps thereby pronouncing an adverse judgement on their first.

Experience in clinical practice suggests that the decision to undergo pre-natal testing and termination of pregnancy, as a generalization, becomes easier as the severity of the medical condition worsens. Inborn errors of metabolism leading to neuro-degeneration and early death are frequently viewed as being devoid of any real hope because they usually breed true and the outcome is inevitable and predictable. These decisions may be more difficult in the future if realistic treatment options become available.

This is inevitably a recurring issue in the moral and ethical debate. Pre-natal screening, testing and diagnosis in all its forms has greatly extended the element of 'choice' about whether or not to continue an established pregnancy, the principle having been given basic legality in the UK by the Abortion Act of 1967. Nevertheless, concerns have been expressed that pressure may be put on prospective parents to terminate a pregnancy even when the genetic condition detected is manageable within a fulfilled and fruitful life.[31] A further consideration is that

---

[31] T. Shakespeare, 'Choices and Rights: Eugenics, Genetics and Disability Equality', *Disability and Society* 13 (1998), pp. 665–82; H. Kuhse, 'Preventing Genetic

authorities offering testing or screening may be doing so on financial grounds, based on the cost to the community of caring for an affected child. The programme of testing for thalassaemias followed by the ready availability of termination for affected foetuses in Cyprus[32] may be viewed in this light, although less cynically one might ascribe to the programme a desire to reduce human suffering caused by this crippling condition. Further, in countries where healthcare costs are covered by insurance, the insurance companies may well insist on terminations of pregnancy after positive pre-natal diagnosis of a genetic condition.[33] Even more extremely, Edwards, the pioneer of *in-vitro* fertilization, has suggested that 'it will be the sin of the parents to have a child who carries the heavy burden of genetic disease', while an American lawyer, Margery Shaw, has written that it should be a criminal offence to give birth to a child with Huntington's Disease.[34]

Faced with the choice between termination of pregnancy and the birth of a child with a devastating genetic condition, some religious communities have developed other methods for reducing the incidence of such diseases. In New York, Rabbi Joseph Ekstein set up a system for testing all young people for carrier status with respect to Tay-Sachs disease. The results are coded but not revealed to the young people who are tested. However, if two young people begin to think of marrying each other, a call to the office will reveal whether they are carriers of the mutation. If both are, then they are advised not to marry.[35] In Cyprus, within the background of the free testing for carrier status in respect of thalassaemia (initiated in 1978), the Orthodox Church has since 1981 insisted that all couples planning a church wedding should be thus tested, with strong discouragement against marriage should both be carriers.[36]

Impairments: Does It Discriminate against People with Disabilities?', in A.K. Thompson and R.F. Chadwick (eds), *Genetic Information: Acquisition, Access and Control* (New York: Kluwer Academic/Plenum, 1999), pp. 17–30.

[32] R. Hoedemaekers and H. ten Hove, 'Geneticization: The Cyprus Paradigm', *Journal of Medicine and Philosophy* 23 (1998), pp. 279–80.

[33] See J.C. Peterson, *Genetic Turning Points: The Ethics of Human Genetic Intervention* (Grand Rapids: Eerdmans, 2001), pp. 210–11.

[34] Both cited by Peterson, *Genetic Turning Points*, p. 222.

[35] Discussed in S. Jones, *In the Blood: God, Genes and Destiny* (London: HarperCollins, 1996), pp. 74–7.

[36] See Peterson, *Genetic Turning Points*, pp. 221–2.

There are many couples, and not just those with objections on grounds of religious faith, for whom termination of pregnancy is not acceptable as a way of exercising choice in the face of genetic risk but who nevertheless wish to have children. Such couples may opt for pre-implantation genetic diagnosis (PGD): *in vitro* fertilization(IVF) followed by a genetic test on the embryos at the eight-cell stage. Only embryos that are free from the genetic condition will be placed in the uterus of the prospective mother. For individuals and couples who hold the view that full human status begins when a sperm fertilizes an egg, PGD is not an acceptable option. However, PGD is acceptable to many couples who cannot put themselves through the emotional trauma of conventional pre-natal testing and possible termination of an established pregnancy. Nevertheless, IVF itself may cause significant emotional trauma, and thus PGD is not to be undertaken lightly. Further, when the financial burden of such procedures falls on the couple themselves there are ethical issues regarding equality of access to these services, which is part of a wider debate about the rationing of resources and the ethical principle of 'justice' in the delivery of health-care.[37]

Currently, PGD in the UK is only granted a licence when it is undertaken for clear medical reasons, i.e. in situations of known genetic risk. For example, it is not currently permissible in the UK to use PGD for sex selection for purely social or family reasons. However, the ethical debate has been extended recently by the case of the Nash family in the USA. We describe the case more fully elsewhere,[38] but in essence, the couple used IVF and PGD in order to ensure the birth of a child who could be a stem cell donor for an older sister who has Fanconi anaemia.[39] Until recently such selection would have

---

[37] See Turnpenny and Bryant, 'Human Genetics and Genetic Enhancement', pp. 253–4.

[38] Ibid., p. 255.

[39] Fanconi anaemia: although initially described as a blood disorder, Fanconi anaemia is actually a condition of chromosome instability, i.e. increased incidence of chromosome breakage which is inherited as a single recessive mutation. Because of the tendency to chromosome breakage, there is a strong predisposition to malignancies such as leukaemia, although several other types of cancer are possible; there is also a failure to manufacture blood cell lines. The onset of the haematological problems occurs at about the age of eight. Birth defects are frequent, especially upper limb and digit abnormalities.

contravened the guidelines of the UK's Human Fertilisation and
Embryology Authority: selection *against* Fanconi anaemia would
have been permissible but selection *for* a tissue match would not.
However, the HFEA guidelines were altered early in 2002 to
consider, on a case-by-case basis, requests for pre-implantation
genetic diagnosis with tissue typing.[40] The first case in which
permission was granted involved a couple from Leeds who
wished to select an embryo that will be a suitable donor of
umbilical cord stem cells for an older sibling who has thalassaemia. Sadly for the couple, of the fourteen embryos initially
generated by IVF, none were suitable: however, the couple will
continue to attempt this course of action. This of course raises
the issue of 'spare' or unwanted embryos and reinforces the
suggestion that motivation to use the technology in this way
could be regarded as a form of 'commodification', or 'instru-
mentation' – reproductive treatment undertaken to meet very
specific aspirations and needs of the parents. The concept of the
newly created child as a commodity or instrument is an extension
of the normal desire of couples to become parents to a level
where having the child is conditional on certain characteristics or
qualities which the parents require, albeit in these cases with the
very worthy motive of saving the life of an existing child. Indeed,
the UK House of Commons Science and Technology Committee
has very recently published a report criticizing, *inter alia,* the
change in the HFEA guidelines. The report states that such a far-
reaching decision went beyond the Authority's public
consultation on PGD and should have been subject to debate in
Parliament rather than being taken by the HFEA itself.[41]

The development of relatively rapid and less expensive
techniques for analysing hundreds of thousands of DNA
sequences inevitably raises the question of how this might
eventually be applied to pre-natal screening and testing, as well
as to medical examination of adults for employment and

---

[40] Human Fertilisation and Embryology Authority, 'Pre-implantation Diagnosis with
   Tissue Typing', Minutes of Authority meeting, 28 February, 2002:
   <www.hfea.gov.uk/aboutHFEA/archived_minutes/00030.htm>
[41] House of Commons Science and Technology Committee 'Developments in
   Human Genetics and Embryology', Fourth Report of Session 2001–2002
   (London: The Stationery Office, July 2002), pp. 12–15. See also media commen-
   taries by Lorraine Fraser, 'Commons Report to Savage Embryology and Fertility
   Watchdog', *Sunday Telegraph,* 14 July 2002, p. 1, and Sarah Boseley, 'MPs Hit at
   Fertility Watchdog over Designer Baby', *The Guardian,* 18 July 2002, p. 8.

insurance purposes. The latter of course raises extensive possibilities for discrimination on genetic grounds.[42] However, here we focus on pre-natal testing and screening. There is concern that extended pre-natal screening will be perceived as a form of eugenics and the way forward is likely to be very cautious. Indeed, additions to the range of conditions screened will need to be deemed 'serious' in the perception of both the public and relevant medical specialists (although it is admitted that different people will have different views about what is serious). It thus seems likely for the foreseeable future that screening and diagnosis for rare conditions will be restricted to those families directly affected (i.e. there will be no *universal* screening for any genetic condition). However, if extended screening at the embryo stage in PGD, and of the foetus in established pregnancy, becomes feasible for a range of severe mendelian disorders it will also be technically possible to test for mutations and polymorphisms which confer risk, or predisposition, for important medical conditions. Well-known examples of such predispositions are mutations in BRCA1 and BRCA2 for breast and breast-ovarian cancer, and the equivalent mutations in DNA mismatch repair genes for hereditary colorectal cancer. In these familial forms of common cancers the mutations confer a high risk (60–85 per cent) of developing the disease. But other mutations confer much lower risks, and therefore tests have much less predictive value (e.g. the ApoE4 allele in Alzheimer's disease). Many such risk factors are likely to be identified in the next wave of human genome research with so much emphasis on single nucleotide polymorphisms (SNPs),[43] various of which might be found to have different levels of predictive value in, for example, schizophrenia, manic depression, autism, diabetes, and various cancers.

---

[42] See, for example, B.M. Knoppers, 'Genetic Information: Use and Abuse', In J.A. Bryant, L.M. Baggott la Velle and J.F. Searle (eds), *Bioethics for Scientists* (Chichester: John Wiley & Sons, 2002), pp. 233–9, and Peterson, *Genetic Turning Points*, pp. 206–28.

[43] SNP. We have already defined polymorphism as a genetic variant fixed within a population (see note 19). Single nucleotide polymorphisms (SNPs) are variants based on a change at a single position (nucleotide, or colloquially, base) within the DNA. Note that the variation may be 'silent', i.e. has no discernible effects on the carrier of the SNP (although some single base changes have profound effects on the organism).

Will there be requests for tests of this kind if they are technically possible? At present this is difficult to say. Even with a
serious, late-onset degenerative condition demonstrating 100
per cent penetrance, such as Huntington's disease, experience
gathered through the UK Predictive Testing Consortium
indicates that pre-natal tests are relatively uncommon, with
only 208 Huntington's disease tests having been performed
over the complete eight-year period 1994–2001.[44] Indeed,
many couples elect for the time-honoured options of having
children regardless of the risk, or not having any (or more)
children once they know the risk. One of the factors that often
influences their decision, particularly in the late-onset
disorders, is the hope that treatment for the disease will be
found in time to benefit the next generation, and therefore
enhance life for their children.[45]

4   Genetic modification

4.1 Introduction

We have already shown that, despite the difficulties, genetic
manipulation of mammals is possible. Further, the combination
of knowledge and experience in human cell biology, in embryology and in human genetics (including the possibility of
isolating and working with individual genes) sets the scene for
the possible genetic manipulation of humans. There are two
general approaches to this.

4.2 Somatic cell genetic modification and gene therapy

The term *somatic cell genetic modification* means changing the genetic
make-up of cells in the body but not of those cells that will pass the
genetic change to future generations (i.e. the germ-line). It is used
specifically in gene therapy: the treatment of a medical condition
by genetic modification of cells (except germ-line cells) or tissues
in the patient. The concept encompasses many possible strategies
but current approaches generally involve the transfer of genes into

---

[44] S.A. Simpson, personal communication, 2002.
[45] See also N. Stratford, T. Marteau and M. Bobrow, 'Tailoring Genes', in R. Jowell,
   J. Curtice, A. Park and K. Thomson (eds), *British Social Attitudes 16th Report*
   (Aldershot: Ashgate, 1999), pp. 157–78.

the particular cells in which the medical condition is manifest. At present, gene therapy is directed at specifically genetic conditions, attempting to overcome the malfunction of a mutated gene by supplying a fully functional non-mutated gene, but in the future some non-genetic conditions may be treated this way. However, we need to state clearly that at the time of writing, gene therapy is still very much an experimental technique. False hopes have been raised, especially for patients with conditions such as cystic fibrosis, but verifiably successful treatments of genetic conditions have so far been very rare. The recent successful treatment of severe combined immunodeficiency[46] received extensive media attention and once again contributed to the raising of public expectations. However, the development of a leukaemia-like condition in those receiving gene therapy for SCID has brought these trials to a halt. Many clinicians actually consider it more likely that new and effective *drug therapies* will emerge from improved understanding of the molecular pathophysiology of disease rather than the successful development of gene therapy *per se* as a routine treatment. This will involve designing drugs that correct or counteract the cellular lesions that result from genetic mutations rather than correcting the mutated genes themselves. There have already been some encouraging results in clinical trials of a small number of such therapies, including a drug that blocks the cellular lesion in chronic myeloid leukaemia[47] and in laboratory trials with mice of a drug therapy for Huntington's disease.[48]

4.3 Germ-line therapy

Currently in most of Europe and the USA it is illegal to genetically modify germ-line cells, i.e. no *heritable* genetic modification is permitted. The reasons for this legal position are easily

---

[46] S. Hacien-Bey-Abina, F. Le Deist, F. Carlier, C. Bouneaud, C. Hue, J.P. De Villarty, A.J. Thrasher, N. Wulffraat, R. Sorensen, S. Dupuis-Girod, A. Fischer, E.G. Davies, W. Kuis, L. Leiva and M. Cavazzana-Calvo, 'Sustained Correction of X-Linked Severe Combined Immunodeficiency by *Ex Vivo* Gene Therapy', *New England Journal of Medicine* 346 (2002), pp. 1185–93.

[47] M.E. O'Dwyer and B.J. Druker, 'Chronic Myelogenous Leukaemia: New Therapeutic Principles', *Journal of Internal Medicine* 250 (2001), pp. 3–9.

[48] A.Yamamoto, J.J. Lucas and R. Hen, 'Reversal of Neuropathology and Motor Dysfunction in a Conditional Model of Huntington's Disease', *Cell* 101 (2000), pp. 57–66; see also the commentary on this work by Gillian Bates: G. Bates, 'In Reverse Gear', *Nature* 404 (2000), pp. 944–5.

appreciated when there is so much uncertainty about the safety and side-effects of manipulating human genomic DNA at such a fundamental stage. For example, the position effects referred to earlier mean that it is not possible to predict the level at which the inserted gene will be expressed in an individual. This problem will not be overcome until it is routinely possible to insert genes into specified locations within the genome. Safety issues and concerns about the long-term consequences and hazards, possibly persisting over many generations, are additional major concerns about germ-line, as opposed to somatic, gene therapy. We simply do not know enough about the potentially damaging and irreversible perpetuation of genomic changes in succeeding lineages. At present, therefore, there is a consensus that humankind is not yet ready for this. Some take the view that human genetic engineering at the level of the gamete or early embryo will never be acceptable. This is largely because of fears that it represents a new techno-eugenics which will lead ever increasingly to attitudes of genetic determinism in relation to disability and behaviour, and discrimination at all levels in a society driven increasingly by commercial interests. In addition, it may be seen as a step too far in tampering with our own biological nature: the term 'Playing God' is often used, but without necessarily any clear idea of what is meant by the term.[49]

However, let us suppose that gene therapy and genetic manipulation of the germ-line can be developed to become demonstrably safe, effective and workable. There are then likely to be pressures to use these techniques to *prevent* disease in future humans, especially where a family has already been affected. Further, the first case will set the precedent and will thus lead to others. In this context of disease prevention, the Christian ethicist Robin Gill and the lawyer Sheila Dziobon have both argued, using a consequentialist approach, that germ-line therapy does not differ ethically from somatic cell therapy.[50]

[49] See discussion by A.R. Chapman, *Unprecedented Choices: Religious Ethics at the Frontiers of Genetic Science* (Minneapolis, MN: Fortress, 1999), pp. 52–7.

[50] R. Gill, *Moral Communities: The 1992 Bishop John Prideaux Lectures* (Exeter: Exeter University Press, 1992); S. Dziobon, 'Germ-Line Gene Therapy: Is the Existing UK Norm Ethically Valid?' in A.K. Thompson and R.F. Chadwick (eds), *Genetic Information: Acquisition, Access and Control* (New York: Kluwer Academic/Plenum, 1999), pp. 255–65; see also the discussion in Peterson, *Genetic Turning Points*, pp. 275–350.

Indeed, ethically it could be argued that germ-line gene therapy represents a *higher* standard than PGD or termination of pregnancy, in that it does not, in itself, involve the rejection of embryos or abortion of foetuses. However, we note that embryo selection (as in PGD) will almost certainly still be necessary in order to make sure that only embryos carrying the added DNA are implanted. The latter problem would be avoided if genetic manipulation of gametes could be successfully achieved, because most people do not ascribe to sperm and ova the status of 'life' that some ascribe to the early embryo.

But there are also ethical arguments against genetic manipulation of either embryos or gametes. First, there is still concern about the irreversible effects of manipulation for the succeeding lineage even if the process itself has been shown to be safe for the individual who is the subject of the germ-line therapy. Second, as discussed in the context of pre-natal or pre-implantation genetic diagnosis, there is the issue of the acceptance of handicap and disability in society. If we aim assiduously to reduce the incidence of individuals with genetically determined handicaps and disabilities, do we thereby make a statement that the handicapped and disabled have no value, or, if they have value, that it is very much inferior to those who are able in mind and body?[51] Human society may be judged by its level of care for the sick and underprivileged, who will always be there. But the underlying tenets of medicine are to treat and prevent disease, and relieve suffering. It may thus be justified to include genetic manipulation as a form of therapy to prevent handicap and disability while at the same time acknowledging the worth of those judged to be handicapped and disabled.[52]

3.4 Genetic enhancement

Genetic manipulation of embryos and gametes to enhance the resulting person raises images of a brave new world of 'designer babies'. If it becomes possible to modify characteristics such as stature, hair or skin colour, athletic or musical ability, for

[51] Shakespeare, 'Choices and Rights', pp. 665–82; Kuhse, 'Preventing Genetic Impairments', pp. 17–30.
[52] See Turnpenny and Bryant, 'Human Genetics and Genetic Enhancement', pp. 259–60.

example, by genetic engineering, will there be a demand for it? The answer is almost certainly 'yes', especially from those who can afford it, but this does not make it generally acceptable. There is a powerful argument that it represents a form of eugenics, or at the very least, once again, 'commodification' – parents making their children into instruments of their own wishes, meeting their own aspirations rather than fully acknow-ledging them as individuals in their own right. However, it may be difficult to discern between treatment and enhancement. For example, in 'conventional' medicine, is limb-lengthening surgery, undertaken in order to make a young woman tall enough to become an air hostess, treatment or enhancement?[53] The same question may be asked in relation to breast enlargement or reduction surgery, sex change operations for gender identity disorder, and 'pure' cosmetic surgery. The problem here is that one person's enhancement is another person's treatment. Self-image, peer pressure and the cultural norms of a society are all important factors in determining individual perception of enhancement versus treatment. However, in the UK the *Clothier Report*[54] has rejected genetic manipulation for 'cosmetic' reasons.

For many people, genetic enhancement through manipu-lation of embryos or gametes strikes at the very heart of what it means to have one's own identity and dignity. Although this may be ascribing more to genes than is justified,[55] this unease is certainly understandable and is clearly brought out in the 1998 *British Social Attitudes* survey.[56] The survey gave evidence of strong support for genetic research and gene manipulation for the detection, prevention and treatment of *disease* but there was little support for genetic *enhancement.* It will be interesting to see how public opinion will evolve as the technology is developed further. We should not, therefore, assume that human genome research is leading steadily and inexorably towards 'designer babies', for there is no suggestion at present that this is generally acceptable to scientists, clinicians or the public, even if there are individuals in all of those groups who would be comfortable with such developments. Nevertheless, it is

[53] Ibid., pp. 260–1.
[54] Committee on the Ethics of Gene Therapy, 1992.
[55] See Collins, 'The Human Genome Project' pp. 99–111.
[56] Stratford, Marteau and Bobrow, 'Tailoring Genes', pp. 157–78.

important that the ethical debate remains vigorous, keeping pace with scientific progress and seeking broad views through public consultation.

Bibliography

Bates, G., 'In Reverse Gear', *Nature* 404 (2000), pp. 944–5.

Berkenstadt, M., Shiloh, S., Barkai, G., Katznelson, M.B-M. and Goldman, B., 'Perceived Personal Control (PPC): A New Concept in Measuring Outcome of Genetic Counseling', *American Journal of Medical Genetics* 82 (1999), pp. 53–9.

Bevis, B.C.A., 'Composition of Liquor Amnii in Haemolytic Disease of the Newborn', *Journal of Obstetrics and Gynaecology of the British Commonwealth* 60 (1953), pp. 244–51.

Boseley, S., 'MPs Hit at Fertility Watchdog Over Designer Baby'. *Guardian,* 18 July 2002, p. 8.

Brinster, R.L. and Palmiter, R.D., 'Transgenic Mice Containing Growth-Hormone Fusion Genes', *Philosophical Transactions of the Royal Society, London, Series B* 307 (1984), pp. 309–12.

Butler, D. and Smaglik, P., 'Draft Data Leave Geneticists with a Mountain Still To Climb', *Nature* 405 (2000), 914–15.

Chapman, A.R., *Unprecedented Choices* (Minneapolis, MN: Fortress, 1999).

Church, R.B., 'Embryo Manipulation and Gene Transfer in Domestic Animals', *Trends in Biotechnology* 5 (1987), pp. 13–19.

Clarke, A. (ed.), *The Genetic Testing of Children* (Oxford: Bios Scientific Publications, 1997).

Collins, F., 'Medical and Societal Consequences of the Human Genome Project', *The New England Journal of Medicine* 341 (1999), pp. 28–37.

Collins, F., 'The Human Genome Project: Tool of Atheistic Reductionism or Embodiment of Christian Mandate to Heal?', *Science and Christian Belief* 11 (1999), pp. 99–111.

Collins, F.S., 'Human Genetics', in Kilner, J.F., Hook C.C. and Uustal, D.B. (eds), *Cutting Edge Bioethics: A Christian Exploration of Technologies and Trends* (Grand Rapids, MN, and Cambridge: Eerdmans, 2002), pp. 3–17.

Dziobon, S., 'Germ-Line Gene Therapy: Is the Existing UK Norm Ethically Valid?', in Thompson, A.K. and Chadwick, R.F. (eds), *Genetic Information: Acquisition, Access and Control,* (New York: Kluwer Academic/Plenum, 1999), pp. 255–65.

Fraser, L., 'Commons Report to Savage Embryology and Fertility Watchdog', *Sunday Telegraph,* 14 July 2002, p. 1.

Fryer, A., 'Inappropriate Genetic Testing of Children', *Archives of Disease in Childhood* 83 (2000), pp. 283–5.

Gill, R., *Moral Communities: The 1992 Bishop John Prideaux Lectures* (Exeter: Exeter University Press, 1992).

Griffin, H., 'Cloning of Animals and Humans', in Bryant, J.A., Baggott la Velle, L.M. and Searle, J.F. (eds), *Bioethics for Scientists* (Chichester: John Wiley & Sons, 2002), pp. 279–96.

Hacien-Bey-Abina, S., Le Deist, F., Carlier, F., Bouneaud, C., Hue, C., De Villarty, J.P., Thrasher, A.J., Wulffraat, N., Sorensen, R., Dupuis-Girod, S., Fischer, A., Davies, E.G., Kuis, W., Leiva, L. and Cavazzana-Calvo, M., 'Sustained Correction of X-Linked Severe Combined Immunodeficiency by Ex Vivo Gene Therapy', *New England Journal of Medicine* 346 (2002), pp. 1185–93.

Hahnemann, N., 'Early Prenatal Diagnosis; A Study of Biopsy Techniques and Cell Culturing from Extra-Embryonic Membranes', *Clinical Genetics* 6 (1974), pp. 294–306.

Hoedemaekers, R. and ten Hove, H., 'Geneticization: The Cyprus Paradigm', *Journal of Medicine and Philosophy* 23 (1998), pp. 279–80.

House of Commons Science and Technology Committee, 'Developments in Human Genetics and Embryology', Fourth Report of Session 2001–2002 (London: The Stationery Office, July 2002).

Human Fertilisation and Embryology Authority, 'Pre-implantation Diagnosis with Tissue Typing', Minutes of Authority meeting, 28 February 2002: <www.hfea.gov.uk/aboutHFEA/archived_minutes/00030.htm>

Jaenisch, R., 'Transgenic Animals' *Science,* 240 (1988), pp 1468–74.

Jeffery, C.J., 'Moonlighting Proteins', *Trends in Biochemical Sciences,* 24 (1999), pp. 8–11.

Jones, S., *In the Blood: God, Genes and Destiny* (London: HarperCollins, 1996).

Knoppers, B.M., 'Genetic Information: Use and Abuse', in Bryant, J.A., Baggott la Velle, L.M. and Searle, J.F. (eds), *Bioethics for Scientists* (Chichester: John Wiley & Sons, 2002), pp. 233–9.

Kuhse, H., 'Preventing Genetic Impairments: Does It Discriminate Against People With Disabilities?', in Thompson, A.K. and Chadwick, R.F. (eds), *Genetic Information: Acquisition, Access and Control* (New York: Kluwer Academic/Plenum, 1999), pp. 17–30.

Macilwain, C., 'World Leaders Heap Praise on Human Genome Landmark', *Nature* 405 (2000), pp. 983–4.

Maclean, N. (ed.), *Animals with Novel Genes* (Cambridge: Cambridge University Press, 1994).

Marshall, E., 'Human Genome: Rival Sequencers Celebrate a Milestone Together', *Science* 288 (2000), pp. 2294–5.

McCreath, K.J., Howcroft, J., Campbell, K.H.S., Colman, A., Schnieke, A.E. and King, A.J., 'Production of Gene-Targeted Sheep by Nuclear Transfer from Cultured Somatic Cells', *Nature* 405 (2000), pp. 1066–9.

O'Dwyer, M.E. and Druker, B.J., 'Chronic Myelogenous Leukaemia: New Therapeutic Principles', *Journal of Internal Medicine* 250 (2001), pp. 3–9.

Peterson, J.C., *Genetic Turning Points: The Ethics of Human Genetic Intervention* (Grand Rapids: Eerdmans, 2001).

Proctor, A.M., Clarke, A. and Harper, P.S., 'Survey of Genetic Testing in Childhood', *Journal of Medical Genetics* 36, Suppl .1 (1999), p. S73.

Rechsteiner, M.C., 'The Human Genome Project: Misguided Science Policy', *Trends in Biochemical Sciences* 16 (1991), p. 455.

Report of the Committee on the Ethics of Gene Therapy (London: HMSO, 1999).

Report of a Working Party of the Clinical Genetics Society (UK), 'The Genetic Testing of Children', *Journal of Medical Genetics* 31 (1994), pp. 785–7.

Shakespeare, T. 'Choices and Rights: Eugenics, Genetics and

Disability Equality', *Disability and Society* 13 (1998), pp. 665–82.

Shapiro, R., *The Human Blueprint: The Race to Unlock the Secrets of Our Genetic Script* (New York: St Martin's Press, 1991).

Skirton, H., 'Genetic Nurses and Counsellors – Preparation for Practice with Families at Risk of Cancer', *Disease Markers* 15 (1999), pp. 145–7.

Skirton, H., 'A Longitudinal Study of Genetic Counselling for Families: Needs, Expectations and Outcomes', *PhD thesis* (University of Exeter, 2000).

Strachan, T. and Read, A.P., *Human Molecular Genetics* (Oxford: Bios Scientific, 1996).

Stratford, N., Marteau, T. and Bobrow, M., 'Tailoring Genes', in Jowell, R., Curtice, J., Park, A. and Thomson, K. (eds), *British Social Attitudes 16th Report* (Aldershot: Ashgate, 1999), pp. 157–78.

Thompson, S., Clarke, A.R., Pow, A.M., Hooper, M.L. and Melton, D.W., 'Germline Transmission and Expression of a Corrected HRPT Gene Produced by Gene Targeting in Embryonic Stem Cells', *Cell* 56 (1989), pp. 313–21.

Turnpenny, P.D. and Bryant, J.A., 'Human Genetics and Genetic Enhancement', in Bryant, J.A., Baggott la Velle, L.M. and Searle, J.F. (eds), *Bioethics for Scientists* (Chichester: John Wiley & Sons, 2002), pp. 241–64.

Vogel, G., 'Infant Monkey Carries Jellyfish Gene', *Science* 291 (2001), p. 226.

Ward, R.H.T., Modell, B., Petrou, M., Karagozlu, F. and Douratsos, E., 'Method of Sampling Chorionic Villi in First Trimester of Pregnancy Under Guidance of Real Time Ultrasound', *British Medical Journal* 286 (1983), pp. 1542–4.

Webster, D.M. and Kruglanski, A.W., 'Individual Differences in Need For Cognitive Closure', *Journal of Personality and Social Psychology* 67 (1994), pp. 1049–62.

Yamamoto, A., Lucas, J.J. and Hen, R., 'Reversal of Neuropathology and Motor Dysfunction in a Conditional Model of Huntington's Disease', *Cell* 101 (2000), pp. 57–66.

2

Genes, Genetics and the Human Genome: Some Personal Reflections

Mary J. Seller

Genetics and society

'He is the image of his father', people will say. 'She got that from her mother', others may comment about a particular characteristic. The fact that children usually resemble their parents, and that some diseases may be passed on from one generation to the next, has been appreciated from time immemorial. In the mid-nineteenth century Gregor Mendel recognized that there was a verifiable scientific explanation for the inheritance of characters. But it was not until the latter part of the last century that heredity was properly understood and its molecular basis delineated. Now, the beginning of the twenty-first century heralds an exciting era of discovery of the complexity of genetics, and the application of the vast array of our new knowledge to the benefit of humankind, particularly in the field of medicine.

While scientists work unceasingly in their quest to unravel the answers to more and more questions driven by boundless curiosity, the general public expresses some unease. The pace of the scientific enterprise seems unrelenting. Some of the doings of scientists are perceived as overstepping the border of decency and legitimacy, tampering with things that properly should not be tampered with, and challenging certain basic truths such as what it means to be a human being.

Part of the problem is fear of the unknown, because genetics is extremely complex and difficult to understand. Actually, even some geneticists can find it so, so what hope is there of non-scientists understanding all the implications of what is going on? The following account is an attempt to provide some eluci-dation, a simple explanation of some of the genetic terms and processes discussed in the subsequent chapters of this book. It also aims to point to where we are on the genetic road of discovery and to highlight some of what might lie ahead. Moral philosophers, theologians and social scientists contribute their wisdom to the collective guardianship of moral propriety within our society, and discourse between them and scientists should be encouraged to enlighten and enable all members of society to engage in meeting the challenge of contemporary genetic developments.

The genome

The sum total of genetic information for each species is referred to as the genome. In cellular organisms, that is, in all animals and plants, but not bacteria and viruses, the complete genome is carried in every cell of the body, and is contained within a special compartment, the nucleus. So, in humans, all the genetic information necessary to direct and effect our devel-opment from a fertilized egg to our adult form, and to maintain our daily biological existence – metabolism, growth and repair – is present in every one of the billions of cells that comprise the tissues and organs of our bodies.

The genome is made of DNA

The genetic information is carried in the form of a chemical code within a complex macromolecule, deoxyribonucleic acid (DNA). DNA is a chain of nucleotides linked together. Each nucleotide has three components, a sugar – deoxyribose, a phosphate and either a purine or a pyrimidine base. There are two types of purine bases, adenine (A) and guanine (G), and two types of pyrimidine bases, cytosine (C) and thymine (T). Human DNA consists of two polynucleotide chains millions of nucleotides long, running in opposite directions complementary to each other, each with a sugar–phosphate backbone, linked together by their bases, a purine of one chain attached to a pyrimidine of the other, adenine to thymine, and guanine to cytosine – the base pairs. The long, composite chain gently twists like a spiral staircase forming a double helix.

Chromosomes

The DNA of each organism is complexed with special supporting proteins to form chromatin. The total genome of each species is divided into a number of separate units called chromosomes. The number and morphology of the chromosomes is unique to each species. Humans have 23 pairs of chromosomes, one of each pair coming from each parent. Each chromosome consists of a single continuous DNA helix and its associated protein which is tightly coiled and folded to form a relatively compact structure.

Particular segments of the DNA comprise the genes or coding sequences that bear the genetic information (described below). However, in humans, genes comprise only about 3 per cent of the total genome. The remainder consists of DNA that is not apparently used, much of which comprises DNA sequences that are repeated thousands of times throughout the genome. The function of the majority of this DNA is not yet known, although obviously it contributes to the overall structure and integrity of the chromosome. Genes occur linearly along the chromosome, and each individual gene has its own specific position (locus) on a particular chromosome. But genes are not arranged regularly along the DNA like pearls in a necklace. Some chromosomal regions have a large number of genes (hotspots) while others have very few.

The genetic code

The key to the genetic code lies in the arrangement of the nucleotide bases in the DNA. The bases, A, C, G and T, are not necessarily placed in a random order. In the coding sequences, three specific adjacent bases form a 'codon', and this comprises the code for a particular amino acid, a constituent of the polypeptide chain. Polypeptide chains contribute to the protein, the functional end-product of each unit of genetic information. It is proteins that are responsible for the structure, growth, metabolism and all the other workings and life of a cell. As examples, the triplet of bases, T–A–C, codes for the amino acid tyrosine, while C–T–G codes for leucine. Since there are four bases: A, G, T and C, but only three are required for a codon, there are $4 \times 4 \times 4 = 64$ possible codons. However, there are only 20 amino acids in all, so many are coded for by more than one codon. For any polypeptide chain, the order of the amino acids comprising it is the same as the order of codons along the DNA.

Genes

A gene is a unit of genetic information. It is a linear segment of the DNA molecule, and until quite recently a gene was said to be that stretch of DNA that bears the codons for the amino acid sequence of a particular protein molecule, the coding region. However, as our knowledge has advanced, it has transpired that the situation is far more complex. In order for the gene to transmit its information (to be expressed) it has to be transcribed into another nucleic acid, ribonucleic acid (RNA), which, as messenger RNA (mRNA), in turn passes the code to the protein synthesizing machinery of the cell for interpretation (translation). In order for transcription to occur, elements in the DNA immediately preceding the coding region (upstream) need to be activated. This is the promoter region. In addition, transcription is often also controlled by other regions, more distant from the gene, that produce agents called enhancers and transcription factors. These regions may even be located on another chromosome. Further, a segment of DNA after the coding region of the gene is vital for proper stability and transmission of the mRNA through the cell.

Another complication is that although the coding region of the gene is a linear sequence of the DNA, it is split into segments called exons, and separated by intervening sequences of non-coding DNA, called introns. Different genes have different numbers of exons; some may have only a few, while 20 to 30 is common, but larger genes contain more, that for the muscle protein, dystrophin has 79. Both exons and introns are transcribed into the primary RNA, but the introns are immediately excised (spliced out) before formation of the mature mRNA that passes through the cell to provide the template for synthesis of the polypeptide.

Thus, a gene is far more than just the linear coding sequence of DNA. Mutations (changes in the DNA) that cause disease occur not only in the coding regions, but also in the regulatory and other flanking regions, in the regions that produce the enhancers and transcription factors and sometimes in the introns. Furthermore the old genetic adage 'one gene: one enzyme (= protein)' that held for so long has also been proved largely incorrect. For it is now understood that one gene may produce one polypeptide chain or it may produce more than one. Also, one polypeptide chain may constitute one protein, or more than one, or only part of one. For some genes may have alternative promoters that are activated in different cell types, each promoter initiating transcription in a different place in the coding portion of the gene, so resulting in several different end-products. Also, many genes have alternative splice sites so that the same primary transcript can be spliced in a different way. This means that there is more than one way that the exons of a particular gene can be spliced together in mRNA, ultimately giving alternative or different types of proteins. Additionally, there are often post-translational modifications whereby two or more polypeptide chains, the products of the same gene, or of different ones, are combined to form the final complex functional product. Thus, a gene often does not function in isolation.

Genes in action in embryonic development and life

The human genome contains thousands of genes, and until recently the total was estimated to be 80,000 to 100,000 (but see below). A minority of these genes are active in every cell of the body. These are called the housekeeping genes because they encode the genes that are essential for life and survival, that is, those involved in cellular respiration and metabolism. The majority of genes, however, are transcribed only in particular tissues, and often also only for a specific time period. The globin genes are an example: they are only active in the specific erythrocyte precursor cells in the bone marrow when the red blood pigment haemoglobin is being made. Thus, since every cell in the body contains the complete genome, most genes in each cell are inactivated, and only those genes specific to the cell type and the housekeeping genes are switched on, that is, transcribed.

The complex processes of development from a fertilized egg to the mature body form are under strict genetic control, although environmental influences do play some part. Many genes are used only during embryogenesis. Details of the genetics of development are still poorly understood, but a crucial element is a family of genes that produce transcription factors. These regulate gene expression and act by switching genes on and off, that is, initiating transcription or repressing it. They interact with many other genes in a coordinated and sequential cascade, influenced too by signalling molecules and growth factors, themselves gene products. It is thus that the basic body plan is laid down and the body assembled in a precisely ordered fashion. Continuously, from conception right through to our final demise, proper gene function is essential to our development, growth, health, survival and life.

Genes and disease

Changes (mutations) in the DNA can cause serious genetic disease. Mutations can take several different forms: there may be the deletion of a single base, or the substitution of one base for another so altering the codon; or there may be the deletion, rearrangement or addition of larger segments of DNA which disrupt the coding sequences. Mutations in developmental genes are often lethal, but may cause malformations so that a baby is born with malformed body parts. In post-natal life, a mutation in a gene for a specific protein, for example haemoglobin, can cause a severe anaemia, and thus morbidity. Clinically, around 10,000 diseases caused by mutations of single genes of major effect are known. As mentioned, the mutations are most often in the coding sequences, but they may also affect the promoter or other DNA regions. Many of these diseases begin in childhood, but some may not start until adult life. Often these diseases are severe and incurable.

Genetic disease also includes abnormalities of the chromosomes, that is, extra or missing chromosomes, or deletion or addition of parts of chromosomes. Many of these have severe consequences, some less severe, such as an extra chromosome 21, which gives Down syndrome.

The cause of a large proportion of genetic disease is less well understood because it is complex; the underlying cause is not solely genetic, for environmental factors also play a part. These are called multifactorial or complex diseases, and examples are coronary artery disease, schizophrenia and diabetes, and congenital malformations such as spina bifida, and cleft lip and palate. The genetic component is not a single major gene; instead, several, or many genes are involved, originally called polygenes, each of which has a small and additive effect that, rather than causing the condition, creates a susceptibility or a predisposition to it. There need to be other factors, usually environmental, that provide the trigger that causes the condition to be expressed. For instance, there is a polygenic predisposition to peptic ulcers, but the ulcers do not appear until overwork, stress and, perhaps, other environmental factors, come into play. Several normal human characters such as height, intelligence and birth weight are also multifactorially determined.

Finally, that most common disease of modern life, cancer, is basically a genetic disease. An ever increasing number of genes is now known that when mutated result in uncontrolled cellular growth and tumour formation.

Treatment of genetic disease

Some genetic diseases are treatable, for example, insulin therapy in diabetes, but not yet curable; transplantation of pancreatic islet cells would be needed for this. With varying degrees of palliation, surgery can repair a cleft lip, clot-busting drugs can be administered to those with symptoms of coronary artery disease, chemotherapy can be given to cancer patients. But for many, or perhaps most, genetic diseases, sadly nothing can be offered. Tay Sachs disease is typical: parents have to watch their young child from the age of about six months gradually become blind and paralysed, before finally dying around 3–4 years of age. The adult onset, Huntington's disease begins around the fourth decade. There is progressive neurological degeneration lasting with increasing severity for perhaps 20 years or more until death.

Prevention of genetic disease

In some multifactorial conditions such as coronary artery disease, as the precipitating environmental factors are identified, patients can be advised to avoid smoking, high cholesterol diet, obesity, lack of exercise and high blood pressure, to gain some measure of prevention, although hypertension is a multifactorial disease in its own right. Regrettably, most genetic diseases cannot as yet be prevented. But medicine has devised several forms of what may be called 'secondary prevention'. This usually involves the pre-natal diagnosis of the genetic disease and termination of affected pregnancies, or more rarely, *in vitro* fertilization followed by pre-implantation diagnosis with transfer to the maternal uterus of only those embryos free from the genetic disease.

Genetic counselling

Because genetic diseases are hereditary, not only is the affected person involved, but other members of the family may be at risk of either carrying or developing the disease too. Genetic counselling exists to inform and support patients and their families who are confronted by genetic disease. Since individual genetic diseases are usually quite rare; families may not even have heard of the one that suddenly afflicts them. Genetic counsellors provide information on the nature and likely course of the disease, the recurrence risks, probable risks to other relatives, and the options available to modify those risks. Prior to the era of modern genetics, often the only way for a couple not to have another affected child was to avoid having any more children at all. Now with the identity of some of the disease genes known, and also chromosome analysis, and accurate ultrasound scanning that can diagnose many developmental abnormalities *in utero*, pre-natal diagnosis with selective abortion is an option that many couples choose to help them eventually achieve a 'normal' family.

Genetic counsellors are also now becoming involved in the products of newer advances in molecular genetics. In some diseases such as certain inherited forms of breast cancer, it is possible to test for the causative mutation. If a woman is found to be carrying it, there is an 80 per cent chance that she will develop breast, and also possibly ovarian, cancer. That the risk is not 100 per cent emphasizes the complex nature of many genetic diseases: despite a strong genetic element, other factors must be operating. It is the subject of much debate as to whether it is beneficial for someone to know that they have an 80 per cent chance of developing a devastating condition sometime in the future, even though they do have a 20 per cent chance they will not. Some choose to know, and some will go even further and have prophylactic surgical breast and ovary removal. Such complex ramifications lead some to challenge the wisdom of our advances in genetics.

The Human Genome Project

The Human Genome Project (HGP) is an ambitious international collaboration to determine the complete sequence of the entire human genome, that is, the sequence of the nucleotide bases of all 23 chromosomes, and ultimately to find and identify all human genes and their encoded products. Beginning in 1990, it had, by 2001, published a draft sequence, 90 per cent complete.[1] Prior to that, three other organisms had been completely sequenced, the yeast, the fruit fly and a nematode worm (a tiny flatworm as distinct from the more familiar round earthworm). This may appear an odd collection, but they are easy-to-use laboratory organisms spanning a range of body complexity, and since most species have many genes in common, information from them has proved useful in the HGP on several counts, notably in elucidating human gene sequences and the conformation of complex protein molecules.

The results of the Human Genome Project so far

The HGP is ahead of schedule and several remarkable facts have already emerged from the studies; the following points have been selected from the full published account.[2] There are 3.2 billion base pairs in the human genome, and the total number of genes is estimated to be 30,000–40,000. This is far less than the 80,000–100,000 that had been considered likely for several decades previously. Further, this number of genes is only roughly twice that possessed by the fly and the worm. Considering the

[1] International Human Genome Sequencing Consortium, 'Initial Sequencing and Analysis of the Human Genome', *Nature* 409 (2001), pp. 860–921.
[2] International Human Genome Sequencing Consortium, 'Initial Sequencing and Analysis of the Human Genome'.

perceived complexity of the human compared with these other two creatures (although flies can fly while humans cannot), the fact that humans have only twice as many genes as the fly implies that complexity is not related to gene number. Insights into this conundrum have been gained by an analysis of the numbers and types of proteins (the final gene product). Humans have a greater total number of proteins than the fly, and they also have a multitude of specific proteins relating to complex processes: immunity, blood-clotting, cell-signalling and neuronal function, which flies don't have. Since all these are coded for by genes, it may be that it is the nature and quality, rather than the quantity of genes that is crucial for our complexity.

Another finding is that the number of human proteins that exist far exceeds the estimated number of genes. This is partly explained by the fact that alternative splicing appears to be an extremely common phenomenon in humans. It appears that as many as 60 per cent of human genes may be alternatively spliced and, as previously mentioned, this mechanism enables one gene to produce several different protein products. So more proteins are coded for per gene in humans than in flies. Yet a further finding is that in humans the total amount of DNA present in the genome is 30 times that of the worm and the fly. However, since the actual coding sequences are only double, humans, for some reason, have a vast amount of DNA that does not code for protein, the function of which is as yet unknown, while the fly and the worm do not.

Although the approximate number of human genes is now known, their identity and function is not, and that is clearly an important next step in the work. From clinical studies, around 10,000 genetic diseases are known, thought to be caused by mutations of single genes. Prior to the HGP sequence data, a small proportion had been positioned on the human genome by conventional molecular genetic mapping techniques, and, for an even smaller number, the function and molecular mechanism of action had also been elucidated. In the HGP, the genes have been identified solely *in silico*, either by aligning known data on the gene, such as its mRNA or data on the gene from another species, with the genome sequences, or by bio-informatics, using computerized gene prediction programmes. These powerful tools search the DNA sequences for stretches characteristic of genes such as splice sites.

Of enormous relevance to both disease and drug treatment is the finding that every human individual differs from the next by one base pair in roughly every 1,000. These are single nucleotide polymorphisms (SNPs, called snips), and they occur right across the genome both within genes and without. Roughly half of these have already been identified.[3] With the total genome comprising 3.2 billion base pairs, this means that, potentially, we differ from our neighbour, biochemically in our DNA, 3.2 million times! These differences probably account for our varying susceptibilities to complex diseases, our differing response to other diseases in terms of severity or even protection, and our distinct reactions to some drug therapy. It is speculated that such differences may even underpin human variation relating to musicality, creativity and other such characteristics.

Among the other interesting findings reported is that we share a large proportion of our genes with other organisms, including yeast and even bacteria. All the basic biological processes of life such as cellular respiration, metabolism, DNA transcription, are common to all life forms. It seems that the puzzle as to how to do these things has been solved only once, very early in evolution, and then the relevant genes have been passed on unchanged through the evolutionary tree from the lowliest forms, through invertebrates and vertebrates, to humans. Another fascinating discovery that might be salutary for those who are against genetic modification to learn, is that a small number of our genes (possibly around 200) have been obtained directly from bacteria rather than by evolution. Some bacterial DNA has been integrated into, and become a stable part of, our genome. This does not refer to mitochondrial DNA, that was already known to be largely eubacterial in origin (mitochondria are tiny structures within each cell wherein cellular respiration takes place), but it is an observation on human genomic DNA. It is deduced because particular bacterial genes found in humans are not found in invertebrates, contamination in the sequencing process has been ruled out; consequently these genes must have been derived directly from

---

[3] International SNP Map Working Group, 'A Map of Human Genome Sequence Variation containing 1.42 Million Single Nucleotide Polymorphisms', *Nature* 409 (2001), pp. 928–33.

bacteria. Thus, we are genetically modified organisms by natural means!

So what has the Human Genome Project achieved?

The current results of the HGP are of intense interest to the scientific community, as they have given us insights into such disparate realms as evolution, relations between species, human variation, gene action and protein structure and function. But the nature of the results may come as a surprise to lay people who, encouraged by media hype, believe that we now know all that there is to know about human genes, that we will soon be able to cure virtually all diseases, and that we are on the threshold of manufacturing 'designer babies'. This was not the aim of the HGP. Scientists knew that it was to be a long, hard road, and they are delighted with the outcome so far, which has been obtained more rapidly than anticipated. What has been achieved is a draft, but incomplete, human genome sequence. It is already enormously illuminating, and current work under way is concerned with filling in the gaps and producing the complete, definitive sequence.

The estimated total of 30,000 to 40,000 genes was derived *in silico*, and such computer-generated gene prediction is at best a guess. The total comprises genuine genes, but also gene fragments and pseudogenes; furthermore, it undoubtedly omits any number of true genes. We therefore await the precise number – some expect it to be higher, others lower, than the present estimate. But this can only be obtained from painstaking direct experimentation in the laboratory, elucidating individual gene structure and expression, and analysis of its regulatory elements. All this, too, is required before widespread medical applications are feasible. This is not to underestimate the fact that enormous strides in our knowledge have been made by the HGP, the scope of the discoveries summarized above indicates that. But many ask: what does this all mean for us now, and what realistically can be achieved in the immediate future?

Implications for medicine

One of the outstanding features of the HGP has been that as soon as sequences have been reliably determined during the course of the project, they have immediately been published on the HGP website and so have been publicly available to everyone. This has enabled scientists already studying a particular gene to interrogate the HGP sequences *in silico* and quite rapidly determine its position. This circumvents months of painstaking laboratory work in the identification of the gene. The gene can then be sequenced in detail in the laboratory and mutation studies performed in patients with the disease. Quite a number of disease genes have already been identified by this means since the HGP data started appearing in the public domain, and the number will increase rapidly in the near future.

This undoubtedly will lead to more requests to genetic clinics for diagnosis at the molecular level, and for carrier detection, and also for pre-natal diagnosis. This brings mixed blessings to patients; the real benefits will come only when a cure can be offered as well, or at least effective treatment for the condition. Unfortunately, that is not an immediate sequel to gene identification, for that is a far more long-term prospect. If the genetic disease is severe, it is of little help simply to know that one has the mutation, although some people do find a measure of comfort in being able to put a name to the disease that afflicts them. What they really need is to be relieved of the symptoms of the disease. Thus the present application of our new genetic knowledge to patients needs to be undertaken judiciously. It is likely that with more genes identified but no cure, in the short term, there will be an increase in terminations of pregnancy for those diseases.

In order to devise a cure or even treatment, the molecular pathology of the disease has to be determined, and this is a lengthy process. First, the protein product of the normal gene must be found, and how it functions on the body, then how the mutation affects the protein structure and function, and then what the steps are in the disease process. Finally, and perhaps the most difficult, a way has to be found to circumvent all this and effect a cure. It is now over 30 years since the first-ever mutation underlying a genetic disease was identified, that for sickle-cell anaemia, a disease that affects millions of people in the world. But we still do not have a cure. Further, it was always anticipated in medical genetics that knowledge of the causative mutation would perhaps enable completely new forms of treatment to be devised, such as gene therapy. This too has not yet materialized on a wide scale. It has not been without strenuous attempts. However, somatic gene therapy has proved to be much more difficult in practice than in theory. In gene therapy, the idea is to provide the person who bears a gene mutation in all his or her cells with an artificial construct containing the normal counterpart of the defective gene, that will enter at least some of the cells and function normally. Cystic fibrosis has long been a candidate for such therapy, and the gene was identified in 1989. One reason for relative lack of success of gene therapy in cystic fibrosis is that not only are the coding elements of the gene required in the construct, but also the controlling elements, so that there is proper expression of the gene. In cystic fibrosis, the immediate upstream region of the gene, including the promoter, is not sufficient alone to drive gene expression. The gene is also controlled by more distant elements that have yet to be located. Another practical problem relates to tissue-specific expression of many genes. In cystic fibrosis, the lungs, pancreas and sweat glands are the tissues most affected by the disease, so if gene therapy is to be truly effective, the gene needs to be delivered especially to the cells of those tissues, and that problem too remains to be solved. While there has been modest success in a few rare diseases, there are still several technical problems to be surmounted before gene therapy for genetic disease becomes a realistic option. It is entirely possible that before they are solved, other new forms of treatment may supervene, such as stem cell therapy.

Knowledge of the molecular pathology of genetic disease also makes new drug therapies feasible. Drugs can be targeted directly at the molecular mechanism. While this is a possibility, for many genetic diseases it may not happen, for drug research largely takes place in pharmaceutical companies that are driven by profit motives. It is certainly known that they are keen to patent genes and molecular genetic processes that will yield a healthy income for them. But genetic diseases are individually quite rare, and if a new drug is to be targeted specifically to a single gene or its product, there will be only a limited use of each drug. It may not be profitable enough for drug companies to devise drugs for rare genetic diseases, so they will not do so. However, there are other benefits of the HGP work to the pharmaceutical industry. All the present drugs in use depend on a limited number of drug targets.[4] Sequence data on all human genes and proteins offer the opportunity to find new targets. In addition, the discovery that SNPs are so common and so widespread in the human genome, creating individual variation, has implications for personal responses to drugs. From both these sources, pharmaceutical research will find many new targets and new devices with which to refine drug specificity.

SNP research should also help in identifying many of the genes that contribute to the susceptibility to complex diseases. Many research groups are already working in this field as these disorders commonly afflict adult life, causing considerable morbidity. While there is an understandable desire to know what the genetic factors are that are involved in coronary artery disease, hypertension, diabetes and Alzheimer's disease, these are multifactorial diseases, and environmental components also play a distinct part in the aetiology. Thus, application of our knowledge to medicine, once acquired, again demands careful consideration. Having the susceptibility genes for such a condition does not automatically mean that the disease will actually appear. This has already been mentioned with respect to inherited breast cancers, where the genetic element appears to be clearly defined. In complex diseases, the genetic components are multiple and far more diffuse. When our research has led to the discovery of successful treatment or means of prevention, there will be every advantage in applying the genetic knowledge to patient care, but until then, caution seems wise.

One thing definitely not on the horizon in the foreseeable, or even more distant, future, is the so-called 'designer baby'. This commonly seems to feature in the media coverage on advances in genetics, and even in some apparently serious documentary television programmes. The implication is that genetic research will enable parents to select characters such as tallness, high IQ, complexion, sporting prowess, creativity and cultural interests to create their special 'designer children'. While it is not inconceivable that some parents would wish to do

---

[4] J. Drews, 'Drug Discovery: A Historical Perspective', *Science* 287 (2000), pp. 1960–4.

this, scientifically it does not appear feasible. These characters are multifactorial, each determined by numerous genes and also environmental factors. Even if the component genes were eventually identified, and even if, as is mooted, such things as creativity and musicality should turn out to be determined by a particular combination of SNPs and they too are identified, it is difficult to envisage how all these could be selected and transferred to a fertilized egg and then made to function properly. Further, how could the relevant environmental factors be guaranteed? Quite apart from all this, current legislation does not permit such a thing!

The Human Genome Project, its work, and society

Around four decades ago, it was suggested that heart transplants were feasible. Many people were aghast, for they believed that the heart was the seat of the soul, and that if a heart were to be transplanted, irreparable damage would be done to the person (not to their body). Heart transplants were performed. The recipients remained intact as people, most with renewed vigour for enjoying life, delighting in the extra time they had been given. More recently, when human molecular genetics work began, some people were equally aghast, claiming that DNA is sacrosanct, that it is the 'stuff of life', and it should not be tampered with. We have begun to do so. To many of us it has yielded rich bounty, a glittering array of knowledge waiting to be seized upon and investigated further so that it may be used to enhance the lives of people and to enlighten our understanding. Only time will tell whether this opinion is sound, or whether the work is actually to human detriment.

DNA may be the 'stuff of life', but tampering with it has enabled us to discover the, at first sight, astonishing fact that there is a great similarity in DNA between the species of the created order, all species, and both animal and plant species. Perhaps this is an unwelcome challenge to our opinion of ourselves. As humans, we have long regarded ourselves as the pinnacle of creation. Yet the HGP has shown us that we share a large proportion of our genes with, for instance, the lowly, single-celled yeast that makes our daily bread rise.

There is no doubt that the knowledge produced through the HGP will give ever more possibilities for application to the human situation in the future. Of course we do not have to use all of them just because we are able to do so. Society seems to be rather effective at stopping scientists going too far. In the recent past, public outcry in the United Kingdom against human cloning, the therapeutic use of fetal ovaries and germ-line gene therapy, caused legislation rapidly to be introduced that prevented the further development and use of these particular techniques. Society can also set up effective control systems if it feels the need. The UK Human Fertilisation and Embryology Authority was set up in 1990 to allay fears concerning the advances being made in human reproductive technology. But society would still be in the Neolithic Age if it had not accepted at least some innovations arising from human curiosity and creativity through the ages. The HGP and the application of genetics is just another stepping-stone along the way.

Bibliography

Connor, M. and Ferguson-Smith, M., *Essential Medical Genetics*, 5th edn (Oxford: Blackwell Science, 2000).

Drews, J., 'Drug Discovery: A Historical Perspective', *Science* 287 (2000), pp. 1960–4.

International Human Genome Sequencing Consortium, 'Initial Sequencing and Analysis of the Human Genome', *Nature* 409 (2001), pp. 860–921.

International SNP Map Working Group, 'A Map of Human Genome Sequence Variation containing 1.42 Million Single Nucleotide Polymorphisms', *Nature* 409 (2001), pp. 928–33.

Mueller, R.F. and Young, I.D., *Emery's Elements of Medical Genetics*, 11th edn (Edinburgh: Churchill Livingstone, 2001).

Strachan, T. and Read, A.P., *Human Molecular Genetics*, 2nd edn (Oxford: Bios Scientific Publishers, 1999).

PART II

Reinterpreting Life and Death

Introduction to Part II

This part raises important questions about how we perceive ourselves theologically when faced with the possibilities emerging from genetic science. Michael Reiss explores the trajectory of genetic science around the question of longevity, asking us to consider some of the theological and ethical challenges that this might present. What, for example, might happen to traditional Christian notions of eschatology? Our whole concept of death and its meaning starts to take on a radically different interpretation and significance once we believe that it may be possible to extend human life over hundreds of years. Reiss confronts the philosophical and ethical issues associated with such change. Overall he is positive about the use of genetics from a theological perspective, arguing that it could even be seen as reversing some of the damaging effects of the Fall.

Ruth Page, by contrast, is much more sceptical about the possibilities and prospects arising from any scientific judgement, arguing that we always need to take into account unpredictable and diverse effects. Much the same could be said about definitive theological statements, hence ideas such as 'image-bearing' cannot be used to measure a fixed quality of human life against which we assess prospective genetic change. In fact, if anything, genetic science suggests the opposite, so that all our notions of 'image-bearing' could be considered too narrow, so that non-human species are inclusively part of the same circle of life as humans. Overall she is keen to stress the ambiguous nature of human living and knowing, in all its different facets. Such awareness needs to colour and inform the discussion between genetic science and other disciplines such as theology and social science. Her chapter moves into a discussion of ethical and social concerns about the way particular projects are given support.

Together these chapters highlight not just matters of life and death, but the way scientific knowledge can be used and/or scrutinized by those from different theological positions.

3

'And in the World to Come, Life Everlasting'

Michael J. Reiss

I am going to die and I want to live for ever. I can't escape the fact and I can't let go of the desire.

Damien Hirst[1]

We're always thinking of eternity as an idea that cannot be understood, something immense. But why must it be? What if, instead of all this, you suddenly find just a little room there, something like a village bath-house, grimy, and spiders in every corner, and that's all eternity is. Sometimes, you know, I can't help feeling that that's probably what it is.

Svidrigaylov[2]

Introduction

The mapping of the human genome has raised a wider set of questions than most had envisaged when the project began. This chapter concentrates on one specific issue: the possibility of greatly extending human lifespan. Should we settle for three score years and ten? What would be the practical, ethical and religious implications if some people lived for hundreds of years? Can this be seen as a restoration of antediluvian longevity or would it be mere hubris? And what if we could live forever? These questions raise wider issues about the determinacy of

---

[1] C. Hall, *Damien Hirst: Exhibition Catalogue* (London: Institute of Contemporary Arts, 1991), p. 7.

[2] F.M. Dostoyevsky, *Crime and Punishment*, trans. D. Magarshack (Harmondsworth: Penguin, 1866/1951), p. 305.

human genes, the relationship between religion, science and technology, the good life, the nature of personhood and what, if any, should be the limits on scientific research.

The practicalities of greatly extending longevity

In 1900 the UK average life expectancy was about 52 years in women and 49 years in men. By the end of the twentieth century it had grown to about 79 years for women and 74 for men, increases of just over 50 per cent for both sexes. Most of us (i.e. humans) are living longer – though this really depends on when we measure 'us' from. If 'us' is taken not from birth but from conception or some point in the first couple of months of pregnancy, the substantial rises in the abortion rates in many countries over the last few decades considerably decrease these figures. The rise in average longevity is also much more evident in some countries than in others. Indeed, as is widely known, several sub-Saharan countries have seen major falls (around a decade) in average life expectancy as a result of Aids,[3] as have some of the countries in the former Soviet Union subsequent to the collapse of communism.

But my focus is not so much on the impact of socio-political events, or even infectious diseases such as Aids, on average life expectancy; it is rather the age to which someone fortunate enough to be protected from such vicissitudes might expect to live. And here, as is also widely known, things have changed remarkably little over the centuries. When Jeanne Louise Calment died in 1997 she was the first human to have lived to a verified age of 122. But people have been living into their hundreds, albeit in far smaller numbers than nowadays, for centuries or longer. Maximum lifespan has not increased very greatly. One hundred years ago Thomas Emley Young, a former President of the Institute of Actuaries in Britain, verified the age of someone who had lived to 113.[4] So maximum lifespan has perhaps increased by only some 8 per cent in the last hundred years.

---

[3] P.R. Lamptey, 'Reducing Heterosexual Transmission of HIV in Poor Countries', *British Medical Journal* 324 (2002), pp. 207–11.
[4] J. Kingsland, 'Age-Old Story', *New Scientist Inside Science* 117 (23 January 1999), pp. 1–4.

The reason for the difference between the increases in average and maximum lifespans is that while sanitation, better nutrition and medical care have greatly contributed to increases in average life expectancy, little can, as yet, be done to fight off old age for long. But might this situation change? I don't want to spend very long on the practicalities of greatly extending longevity, partly because attempts to predict scientific and technological developments far ahead are almost never successful and partly because I am more interested in what the social and theological consequences of this might be and in whether such greatly extended longevity would be desirable. Nevertheless, it is worth spending some time on the practicalities.

One can envisage two main ways in which human longevity might be greatly extended (say, to several hundred years). One would be in some way to slow the ageing process so that someone aged 200 might look rather like a healthy 50-year-old today. The second way would be for a person to receive various transplants as they aged.

The first possibility can itself be imagined in various ways. For a start, we already know of several ways in which alterations to the environments of non-humans can lead to animals living longer. For example, severely restricting the diet of small mammals can lead to increases in longevity of around 20—40 per cent while feeding certain chemicals that destroy harmful free radicals to nematode worms (much experimented on by today's biologists) increases longevity by around 50 per cent.[5] There is also the evidence that ageing is at least partly accounted for by the gradual loss of telomeres, the ends of our chromosomes, over successive cell divisions. It is not inconceivable that this loss might be prevented or restored in some way.

Then, of course, there are always genes. The Human Genome Project, in particular, has led many to an oversimplified view of the functioning of genes.[6] I was fortunate enough when an undergraduate in the late 1970s to be taught animal behaviour by Pat Bateson, among others. Pat sometimes likened the role of genes to the role of a recipe in making a cake. Genes

[5] D. Concar, 'Forever Young', *New Scientist*, 22 September 2001, pp. 26–33.
[6] E.F. Keller, *The Century of the Gene* (London: Harvard University Press, 2000).

and recipes are essential but it makes little sense to ask what proportion of a good (or a bad) cake is due to the recipe. Nowadays, unfortunately, we live in an age when the role of genes is still widely misunderstood and frequently overemphasized.[7] Genes do, of course, play a major role in almost everything about humans that makes us interesting, including, as I shall consider below, our longevity. But most of the important things about us – such as our personality, appearance, intelligence and longevity – are likely to be determined not by a single gene or even a collection of genes but by a collection of genes operating in interaction with our environment. And part of the especial feature of being human is that our environment consists not just of such physical entities as our diet and the presence and absence of diseases but also of such cultural phenomena as our education, the beliefs in our societies and our own individual aspirations. Further, we have some control over our environments, just as our environments have some consequences for us. Disentangling all this into 'genes' and 'environment' is not merely difficult but of limited meaning and value.

Having said that, the role of genes in human nature often has been and sometimes still is underestimated. A few decades ago psychoanalysts attributed autism only to failures in the environment, typically mother–child relationships.[8] Nowadays we find it easier to accept that there may, at least sometimes, be a genetic basis to autism. Not in the trite sense that there is a single faulty sequence of DNA bases that deterministically and inevitably causes autism, but that certain such sequences make it more likely that a child will develop autism, perhaps as a result of some environmental injury, just as smoking cigarettes (roughly speaking an environmental effect) makes it more likely that a person will develop heart disease or lung cancer, while having one of 'the genes' for breast cancer makes it more likely that someone will develop that disease.

One notable example of an earlier failure to appreciate the possibility of genetic differences between people was the way in

---

[7] M.J. Reiss, 'What Sort of People Do We Want? The Ethics of Changing People Through Genetic Engineering', *Notre Dame Journal of Law, Ethics & Public Policy* 13 (1999), pp. 63–92.

[8] R.D. Hinshelwood, *A Dictionary of Kleinian Thought*, 2nd edn (London: Free Association Books, 1991).

which powdered milk was often sent by Western aid agencies to countries where we now know that almost everyone is lactose-intolerant because they lack the gene that allows people to digest lactose in milk. It is now thought that this lactose intolerance is the ancestral condition. The ability to digest lactose probably evolved only in societies that kept cattle for their milk.

Interestingly, many of the pressure groups that campaign against the new genetics (whether manifested in GM foods or genetic tests for certain conditions such as cystic fibrosis) oscillate somewhat schizoidly between either reifying the gene to the point of demonization – in the process attributing more to genes than do most molecular biologists and sociobiologists – or maintaining that genes have no role in their contribution to such human traits as intelligence and personality.

So how important are genes in contributing to (a better term when discussing gene action than 'determining') longevity? We still don't know for humans. But my prediction would be that within a decade we will find (a) that there are dozens of genes that influence human longevity; (b) that no one of them is overwhelmingly important; but (c) that the combined effects of about four of them make a difference of around plus or minus 10–15 years to both average and maximum longevity (and it may not be the same four genes for both of these). In 1998 a gene was found in the nematode worm *Caenorhabditis elegans* that protects against premature ageing, and later the same year a gene, dubbed *methuselah* – yes, an attenuated memory of religious tales lives even in today's laboratories – was found to enable the fruit fly *Drosophila melanogaster* to live 35 per cent longer. By and large, the message of human genetics over the last few decades is that genes act in a similar way in us but that the results are rarely as dramatic as in other species.

However, it is difficult to imagine that improving our environments or our genes is really going to even double our longevity, let alone enable us to live for many hundreds of years. Which takes us on to the second possibility: transplants.

We are already used to the idea of transplants greatly extending the lifespan of individuals. Indeed, that is pretty much the entire point of them, whether we are talking about blood transfusions or the technically more difficult transplants of whole organs. The early heart transplants provoked both hype and controversy. Success rates were extremely poor; new definitions of death (brain-stem death) were introduced in some countries – an interesting example of the interaction of technology, science and ethics – and some regarded the practice as meddling with the essence of human life. Malcolm Muggeridge referred to it as 'the final degradation of our Christian way of life'.[9] Over the years, though, most people, Christians and others, have come to regard transplants not only as ethically unproblematic but as near-routine.

The most extreme form of transplant that can realistically be envisaged at present is what is sometimes termed a 'whole body transplant'. Most people would call this a head transplant except that our notions of personhood are nowadays tied to the brain, so that head A on body B is presumed to be (pretty much) person A. Actually, the small amount of near-anecdotal data on the feelings of the one or two people who have had hand transplants suggests that some people may not divorce themselves from their bodies quite as absolutely as this. Nevertheless, for my purposes here I take it that one could envisage over time with reference to the same individual, A: (a) head of A receiving a succession of bodies B, C, D, . . .; (b) and head of A receiving new cataracts, lenses, hearing aids and other extra-brain, above-neck restorations; (c) and brain of A itself receiving various treatments (chemical, surgical, psychological) including localized transplants (e.g. using foetal cells) from other individuals. The medical details need not concern us further. Stem cells and so-called therapeutic human cloning may be all the rage today[10] – and may indeed prove the crucial answer – or something else may crop up in a decade. It might – though to some this may sound too much like science fiction – be the case that memories and other aspects of personalities will be able to be stored and transferred to new, younger brains, allowing 'me' (*sensu* my mind) to persist indefinitely through a succession of bodies and brains – cloned or otherwise – or even one day in inorganic form.

[9] R. Hoffenberg, 'Christian Barnard: His First Transplants and their Impact on Concepts of Death', *British Medical Journal* 323 (2001), pp. 1478–80, p. 1480.

[10] M.J. Reiss, 'Ethical Dimensions of Therapeutic Human Cloning', *Journal of Biotechnology* 98 (2002), pp. 61–70..

How long should we live for?

Would greatly extended longevity be a good thing? Given that the overwhelming majority of people have always had a wish to live a long and healthy life, that most people, if physically and mentally at least reasonably well, would like to live longer and that only a small minority of people, whatever their age, truly wish to be dead, the most immediately obvious answer is 'yes'. Actually, the question should be phrased more precisely: 'Would it be a good thing to permit people to live far longer than at present if they wished to?' After all, no-one is proposing or even very likely to propose that it would become a legal requirement for each of us to have a succession of transplants or take the required medication for greatly enhanced longevity. Indeed, the growing practice of 'nursing care only' and 'do not resuscitate' notices, living wills and so on would be likely to proliferate if we really could live for hundreds of years. So what we are talking about is something close to 'Should we forbid people from living very long healthy lives?' and, more immediately, 'Should we forbid researchers from trying to find out ways of enabling us to live for very long periods of time?'

Put like that it seems more difficult to answer 'yes'. I have considered elsewhere the arguments for and against allowing researchers to carry out certain types of research.[11] Suffice it here to say that I consider it (a) extremely unlikely that research intended to extend human longevity will be banned, with the exception, in certain countries, of certain forms of it (e.g. that requiring state funding) which require what are regarded by some as unacceptable procedures whatever the putative desired outcomes (e.g. the use of human foetal tissue for transplantation and the use of human embryos for somatic cell nuclear transfer); (b) difficult to defend a widespread ban on research intended to extend human longevity.

A number of arguments have been advanced as to why greatly extended longevity might not be a good thing. It has been argued that it would be counter to global justice (i.e. that it wouldn't be fair for some people to live very long lives while others are denied the opportunity), that it would lead to too few

---

[11] M.J. Reiss, 'The Ethics of Genetic Research on Intelligence', *Bioethics* 14 (2000), pp. 1–15.

people earning enough to support large numbers of pensioners, and that future people would be denied the possibility of coming into existence (i.e. there wouldn't be either room for them or the wish for them). Such objections, and some others, are carefully considered by John Harris and generally found lacking.[12] For example, Harris argues against the global justice argument by pointing out that this objection holds for any new complex and/or expensive technology, and asserts that this objection 'requires that strenuous and realistic efforts be made to provide the benefits of the technology justly, not that the benefits be denied because of the impossibility of ensuring adequate justice of provision' (p. 6). Although some distributive justice arguments, whether consequentialist or otherwise, would conclude that, at least in certain circumstances, the result of widening inequalities means that forbidding technological developments is the right way forward, Harris makes the interesting point that it may well be more appropriate for the particular issue of greatly extending human longevity to think of it as a side effect of treating various illnesses. It is difficult to imagine arguments that would be convincing (whether ethically or politically) which restrict (let alone prevent) research into cancers, heart disease, mental impairments and so on on the grounds that such research might lead to people living too long.

There have been a number of science fiction writers and others who have explored some of the consequences of extended mortality. In *Gulliver's Travels*, Lemuel Gulliver meets the *Struldbrugs* or *Immortals*. Before he does he waxes lyrical about how he would like to live for ever. However, on meeting a group of *Struldbrugs*, he soon realizes the burden under which they suffer. The reason is that, aside from not dying, all the other consequences of old age attend them:

> At ninety they lose their teeth and hair, they have at that age no distinction of taste, but eat and drink whatever they can get, without relish or appetite. The diseases they were subject to still continue without increasing or diminishing. In talking they forget the

---

[12] J. Harris, 'Intimations of Immortality: The Ethics and Justice of Life Extending Therapies', unpublished lecture (2001). See also J. Harris, 'Intimations of Immortality', *Science* 288 (2000), p. 59 and the various debate responses to it at <www.sciencemag.org/cgi/eletters/288/5463/59hashEL2> (accessed 26 October 2001).

common appellation of things, and the names of persons, even of those who are their nearest friends and relations.[13]

A far fuller fictional assessment of the consequences of greatly extended longevity is provided by Shaw in *Back to Methuselah*,[14] where both positive and negative consequences are presented. John Wyndham's *Trouble With Lichen*[15] features the amusing interview of Miss Diana Brackely, proprietor of Antigerone, an extract of a rare lichen that doubles or trebles longevity, with the hapless Mr Rupert Pigeon of the BBC. (It also includes a worried telegram from the General Council of The Brotherhood of British Morticians to the Home Secretary.) James Blish's four-book series *Cities in Flight*[16] explores further some of the consequences of greatly extended longevity as does Robert Heinlein's *Time Enough for Love*.[17]

Of the science fiction books it is Heinlein's that most fully attempts to deal with the issues of living a very long time (some 2,300 years in this case), though a somewhat cruel, though perhaps accurate, commentary on Heinlein's book is that it is more about the hero having enough time to have a lot of sex (some of it with his grandmother) than about having time enough for love. But the title is an excellent one. For there are surely two main families of arguments in favour of greatly extended human longevity – one to do with the benefits (if benefits there are) for those who live much longer, the other to do with the benefits their extra years might have for others.

Of course, there are those who doubt that benefits would accrue to people able to live for hundreds of years. Perhaps we would get bored. As Kass[18] puts it:

Would professional tennis players really enjoy playing 25 percent more games of tennis? Would the Don Juans of our world feel better for having seduced 1,250 women rather than 1,000? Having

[13] J. Swift, *Gulliver's Travels* (New York: New American Library, 1726/1960), pp. 229–31.

[14] B. Shaw, *Back to Methuselah* (Harmondsworth: Penguin, 1921/1939).

[15] J. Wyndham, *Trouble With Lichen* (Harmondsworth: Penguin, 1960/1963).

[16] J. Blish, *They Shall Have Stars* (London: Arrow, 1956/1974); *A Life for the Stars* (London: Arrow, 1962/1974); *Earthman, Come Home* (London: Arrow, 1956/1974); *A Clash of Cymbals* (London: Arrow, 1959/1974).

[17] R. Heinlein, *Time Enough for Love* (London: New English Library, 1973/1975).

[18] L.R. Kass, 'L'Chaim and Its Limits: Why Not Immortality?', *First Things* 113 (May 2001), pp. 17–24.

experienced the joys and tribulations of raising a family until the last had left for college, how many parents would like to extend the experience by another ten years? Likewise, those whose satisfaction comes from climbing the career ladder might well ask what there would be to do for fifteen years after one had been CEO of Microsoft, a member of Congress, or the President of Harvard for a quarter of a century?

It is difficult to imagine that many will find this argument convincing. After all, watching John McEnroe and Jack Nicklaus along with countless other seniors and veterans makes it evident that there are plenty of professional (let alone amateur) sportspeople who would really enjoy playing 25 per cent more games of tennis or 'just one more round' of golf. Then, as Harris[12] points out, 'if more of the same does not appeal, there is always the opportunity to try something different' (p. 16). Indeed, one optimistic interpretation of boredom is that it is a way of our telling ourselves that there is more to life than what we are currently doing. Even if we accept Kass's argument that being President of Harvard for longer than fifteen years is, quite literally, a fate worse than death (which is what his argument requires), a greatly extended longevity might allow each of us to find more rewarding ways of passing our time.

I doubt that we can learn a great deal about whether or not it would be good to live greatly extended lives from considering those organisms (e.g. many trees, some fungi, giant Galapagos tortoises) that can live for hundreds or even thousands of years. Even less is to be gained from considering those asexually reproducing organisms (e.g. many one-celled creatures, certain plants, even a few species of lizards) that, in a genetic sense, do live forever (well, millions of years). It is virtually certain that none of these various creatures has any more than the most rudimentary degree of self-awareness and reflection and I doubt very much that they have any notion of the passage of time, of their ageing or of their mortality. We are reduced, therefore, to thought experiments and to examining what life is or has been like in societies, past or present, with far higher rates of mortality.

I think it is possible that one disadvantage of greatly extended longevity would be that people would be more fearful of death. People with few possessions don't lie awake at night worrying about burglars. It is difficult to imagine that, as a parent, I would be even more fearful of my child's personal safety if I knew that a fatal accident would rob them of not 70 but 700 years of life, but it is possible that as a 70-year-old I might be more likely to decide never to fly the Atlantic, worried that a crash would rob me not of a few years but of most of my life.

For myself, though, the thought of more time sounds wonderful. On a personal level I could get to know many more people well and know those whom I know well even better; as an academic I could spend far longer thinking and researching before rushing into print; I would have had longer to enjoy the company of my grandparents; perhaps I might become a better person, and so on. Of course, given long enough I might develop the ennui the thought of which evidently so oppresses Kass, but, to emphasize the point made earlier, I could then choose not to postpone death much longer (cf. Isaac Asimov's *The Bicentennial Man*[19] and Doris Lessing's *The Making of the Representative for Planet 8*[20]). I accept, though, that while greatly extended longevity might magnify in someone the virtues of wisdom and love, it might in someone else magnify such vices and shortcomings as selfishness and narcissism, though there would be more time for someone to see, or be persuaded of, the error of their ways – but then there would be more time for others to fall from grace! Old age does seem to bring either the best or the worst out in many people, but then that is true of all of life.

A better country

For a creature with no self-awareness, the difference between living for a very long time and for eternity may only be one of degree. But for creatures such as ourselves, the difference is surely far greater. It was Woody Allen who quipped, 'I don't want to achieve immortality through my work. I want to achieve it by not dying.' No biologists are seriously talking about immortality. Those, such as Michael Rose of the University of California who was reported in a newspaper in 2001 as saying 'I

---

[19] I. Asimov, *The Bicentennial Man and Other Stories* (New York: Fawcett Crest, 1976).
[20] D. Lessing, *Canopus in Argos: Archives. The Making of the Representative for Planet 8* (London: Grafton, 1982/1983).

believe there are already immortal people'[21] probably don't really mean that or haven't thought carefully about the issue. The distinction between not yet dying and living for ever may not be as great as the distinction between being big and being infinite in size, but it is a distinction of kind, of essence. One thinks of the beings in Abbott's *Flatland*[22] who simply couldn't understand the appearance of spheres in their world.

Several reasons why immortality might not be desirable have been proposed, most notably by Leon Kass,[18] though John Harris[12] has again incisively criticized most of Kass's arguments. Harris, though, does use the term very broadly:

> In the remainder of this discussion I shall talk predominantly of 'immortality' and 'immortals' and mean these terms to cover all stages from quite modest life extending therapies to truly indefinite survival. (p. 2)

From a theological perspective I prefer a narrower, more precise understanding of 'immortal', namely living for ever. As a biologist I cannot conceive (in this world) of humans being immortal in this narrow sense. The nearest we might get would be to a situation where only accidents would lead to loss of life. One could then imagine people living to be thousands of years in age, apparently ageless (cf. Ayesha in Rider Haggard's *She*[23]) yet perhaps, in some instances, with the wisdom of ages.

Hiving off theological analysis into a section all to itself could be construed as being implicitly an acknowledgement that theological issues matter only to a minority of people. And there are many for whom a theological treatment of any subject is, at best, meaningless. Yet, unsurprisingly, most of the literature on what it might be like to live for ever is explicitly theological. However, it isn't recent. Although the new genetics in general[24-27]

---

[21] Cited in Concar, 'Forever Young', p. 29.

[22] E.A. Abbott, *Flatland: A Romance of Many Generations* (Oxford: Basil Blackwell, 1884/1974).

[23] H.R. Haggard, *She* (London: Hodder & Stoughton, 1887/1925).

[24] J.R. Nelson, *On the New Frontiers of Genetics and Religion* (Grand Rapids: Eerdmans, 1994).

[25] C. Deane-Drummond, *Theology and Biotechnology* (London: Geoffrey Chapman, 1997).

[26] T. Peters, *Playing God? Genetic Determinism and Human Freedom* (New York: Routledge, 1997).

[27] C. Deane-Drummond, *Biology and Theology Today: Exploring the Boundaries* (London: SCM Press, 2001).

and the Human Genome Project in particular[28-30] have attracted theological analysis, almost nothing has been written about the implications of these for understandings, Christian or otherwise, of the theology of mortality and immortality.

In the Judaeo-Christian tradition, we can start with scripture itself. The early chapters of Genesis[31] portray a world in which the Lord God walked with Adam and Eve, in which humans were naked without being embarrassed, in which agriculture required little toil, in which women could give birth without pain, in which there was no need to eat meat and, perhaps above all, in which there was no death. To the fundamentalists[32] this is read literally; for most of us it is to be understood more figuratively. But to all with a belief in the scriptures it holds up an ideal.

When I turned to Richardson and Bowden's *A New Dictionary of Christian Theology*, I found that the article on 'Life after Death' had very appropriately been written by John Hick,[33] who in his *Death and Eternal Life*[34] provided what is still surely the most intellectually satisfying defence of the doctrine of life after death and one that is not restricted to the Christian tradition but draws deeply on Hindu and Buddhist ideas. To cite from his dictionary entry:

> What is the basis for the Christian belief in life beyond death? ... Today we believe as Christians in 'the life everlasting' for two basic intertwined reasons. One is that Jesus believed this. ... The other reason centres upon the Christian understanding of God as our loving heavenly parent. If God loves each one of us and is seeking to draw us into a perfect relationship both with one another and with the divine Thou, does it not follow that God will hold us in being beyond the end of this short earthly life? Could it be an

[28] J.A.K. Kegley (ed.), *Genetic Knowledge: Human Values and Responsibility* (Lexington, KY: International Conference on the Unity of the Sciences, 1998).

[29] P.R. Sloan (ed.), *Controlling Our Destinies: Historical, Philosophical, Ethical, and Theological Perspectives on the Human Genome Project* (Notre Dame, IN: University of Notre Dame Press, 2000).

[30] A. Mauron, 'Is the Genome the Secular Equivalent of the Soul?', *Science* 291 (2001), pp. 831–2.

[31] Particularly *Genesis 3*.

[32] For example, H.M. Morris, *The Genesis Record: A Scientific and Devotional Commentary on the Book of Beginnings* (Welwyn: Evangelical Press, 1976/1977).

[33] J. Hick, 'Life After Death', in: A. Richardson and J. Bowden (eds.), *A New Dictionary of Christian Theology* (London: SCM Press, 1983), pp. 331–4.

[34] J. Hick, *Death and Eternal Life* (Basingstoke: Macmillan, 1976/1985).

expression of infinite love to create us with immense spiritual potentialities but with so short a career, and often in such inauspicious circumstances, that those potentialities are normally destined never to be fulfilled? (pp. 331–2)

Unsurprisingly, written twenty years ago, Hick needed to take no account of the (logical) possibility that life everlasting might not require life beyond death. And yet the second reason Hick cites for the life everlasting might even be satisfied by a very greatly extended lifespan, let alone immortality in this life. As for his first reason, arguing on the basis of what Jesus believed is often somewhat problematic if only because while much of what we have recorded as being from his lips is clearly intended to be understood literally, some of it is evidently metaphorical or intentional hyperbole. Furthermore, as we hear in the more modern versions of the absolution, we are to be kept in, rather than brought to, eternal life. We may still be far from the kingdom of God, yet it has come upon us.[35] Such an understanding of our positions in time would only serve to underline the appropriateness of an existential worldview in which, using Heidegger's term,[36] our *Dasein* (being) is that into which we grow over time, and for which we have some potential for authenticity, for life in all its fullness, for becoming true to ourselves.

Certainly, were we to achieve immortality through medical advances in this life, there would be major consequences for the exercising of certain of the virtues – such as patience and hope. Clearly, true immortality would also devalue such virtues as physical courage, but then true immortality, in the sense of not being able to die, is not going to be provided by technology. Indeed, it can be argued that there would be more scope to exercise the virtue of physical courage in a world in which one could still expect, if careful, to live for thousands more years. As Christopher Southgate puts it, death 'gives to every breath before we get to work its intensity'.[37]

Immortality may have been lost at the Fall, but scripture records it as taking some considerable time for our present

---

[35] *Matthew* 12.28.
[36] M. Heidegger, *Being and Time* (Oxford: Blackwell, 1927/1962).
[37] C. Southgate, 'Writer's Morning', in *Beyond the Bitter Wind: Poems 1982–2000* (Beeston: Shoestring Press, 2000), pp. 4–5, p. 4.

meagre lifespans to be reached. Adam lived to be 930 years; Seth, Adam's son, 912 years; Enosh, Seth's son, 905 years; and so on. As Jacob said to Pharaoh 'The days of my sojourning are a hundred and thirty years; few and evil have been the days of my life, and they have not attained to the days of the years of the life of my fathers in the days of their sojourning.'[38]

An important distinction between everlasting life (in heaven in God's presence) and interminableness (in hell, where there is said to be 'much time') was made by Augustine and Thomas,[39] while Hannah Arendt discusses the difference between immortality (in these senses of endurance in time and deathless life) and eternity (held by Plato and many Christian writers to be 'unspeakable', and so beyond time).[40] Arendt also develops the classical Greek idea that a person's essence only comes fully into being when they die.[41] In a related vein, early Christian writers discussed what would have happened to Adam as an individual had he not sinned. There would, it was generally held, still have been a need for a transition from this world to the next; from grace to glory.

Contrary to what some notable atheists assert, many of the world's oldest religions, including Judaism, did not, as is widely acknowledged, rely, in any obvious sense, in their earlier formulations on the promise of an afterlife. However one understands Jewish teachings about the resurrection, it was only with the rise of Christianity within its midst that Judaism gave birth, unambiguously, to a sect that fully embraced the notion of eternal life. Among Christians, of course, the mainstream understanding of this, whatever the precise meaning of a new heaven and a new earth and the other complications of Revelation,[42] is of eternal life for all, whether as soon as we die or at the day of judgement. In the incomparable words of Paul:

---

[38] *Genesis* 47.9.

[39] I am particularly grateful to David Jones for discussions about the theology of death. In his DPhil, he valuably analyses the contributions to this field of Paul, Ambrose, Augustine, Thomas Aquinas and Karl Rahner. See D.A. Jones, *Death: A Good or an Evil? A Theological Enquiry*, DPhil thesis (University of Oxford, 2001).

[40] H. Arendt, *The Human Condition* (Chicago: University of Chicago Press, 1958).

[41] I am grateful to Bronislaw Szerszynski for this.

[42] For example, R. Bauckham, *The Theology of the Book of Revelation* (Cambridge: Cambridge University Press, 1993).

Lo! I tell you a mystery. We shall not all sleep, but we shall all be changed, in a moment, in the twinkling of an eye, at the last trumpet. For the trumpet will sound, and the dead will be raised imperishable, and we shall be changed. For this perishable nature must put on the imperishable, and this mortal nature must put on immortality. When the perishable puts on immortality, then shall come to pass the saying that is written:

> 'Death is swallowed up in victory.'
> 'Oh death, where is they victory?
> O death, where is thy sting?'[43]

In the face of such words, we are surely bound to ask what possible connection can the 'promise' of endless transplants or medicines have with such a vision? And perhaps the answer is none – such a promise merely being that of a secularized eschatology.[44] Very probably all the technical advances of medicine may do no more for generations to come than enable a few very wealthy people to live to the age for which Jacob apologized to Pharaoh. More positively, perhaps many of us will be able to live longer, healthier lives than at present and then to have time for amendment of life and a good death.[45]

And yet the interpretation of prophecy is rarely straightforward. As those of us who take seriously the New Testament know, Jewish prophecies can be held to be fulfilled in ways that would have been inconceivable at the time. Consider, for example, how Paul reinterpreted teachings about Israel and circumcision. Today's technological advances could, if interpreted somewhat optimistically, already be seen to have undone some aspects of the original curse. Many women no longer give birth in pain. Many farmers, for all their problems, no longer toil against thorns and thistles. Modern medicines, and to a lesser extent, modern agriculture, have often been seen as God's work. Might it yet be that biotechnological advances

---

[43] 1 Corinthians 15.51–5.

[44] I am grateful to Celia Deane-Drummond for this.

[45] Hauerwas points out that nowadays 'most people when asked how they want to die say in their sleep or suddenly – i.e., in a manner that they do not have to prepare for their dying. In contrast medieval people most feared sudden death since such a death would prevent from preparing for their death both in terms of their social responsibilities and their eternal destiny' (S. Hauerwas, 'Religious Concepts of Brain Death and Associated Problems', in *Suffering Presence: Theological Reflections on Medicine, the Mentally Handicapped and the Church* (Edinburgh: T & T Clark, 1988), pp. 87–99, p. 96).

could help usher in the kingdom of God which, as we are told more than once in the Gospels, is already among us?

Bibliography

Abbott, E.A., *Flatland: A Romance of Many Generations* (Oxford: Basil Blackwell, 1884/1974).

Arendt, H., *The Human Condition* (Chicago: University of Chicago Press, 1958).

Asimov, I., *The Bicentennial Man and Other Stories* (New York: Fawcett Crest, 1976).

Bauckham, R., *The Theology of the Book of Revelation* (Cambridge: Cambridge University Press 1993).

Blish, J., *Earthman, Come Home* (London: Arrow, 1956/74).

Blish, J., *They Shall Have Stars* (London: Arrow, 1956/74).

Blish, J., *A Clash of Cymbals* (London: Arrow, 1959/74).

Blish, J., *A Life for the Stars* (London: Arrow, 1962/74).

Concar, D., 'Forever Young', *New Scientist*, 22 September 2001, pp. 26–33.

Deane-Drummond, C., *Theology and Biotechnology* (London: Geoffrey Chapman, 1997).

Deane-Drummond, C., *Biology and Theology Today: Exploring the Boundaries* (London: SCM Press, 2001).

Dostoyevsky, F.M., *Crime and Punishment*, trans. D. Magarshack (Harmondsworth: Penguin, 1866/1951).

Haggard, H.R., *She* (London: Hodder & Stoughton, 1887/1925).

Hall, C., *Damien Hirst: Exhibition Catalogue* (London: Institute of Contemporary Arts, 1991).

Harris, J., 'Intimations of Immortality', *Science* 288 (2000), p. 59.

Harris, J., 'Intimations of Immortality – The Ethics and Justice of Life Extending Therapies', unpublished lecture, 2001.

Hauerwas, S., 'Religious Concepts of Brain Death and Associated Problems', in *Suffering Presence: Theological Reflections on Medicine, the Mentally Handicapped and the Church* (Edinburgh: T & T Clark, 1988), pp. 87–99.

Heidegger, M., *Being and Time* (Oxford: Blackwell, 1927/62).

Heinlein, R., *Time Enough for Love* (London: New English Library, 1973/75).

Hick, J., *Death and Eternal Life* (Basingstoke: Macmillan, 1976/85).

Hick, J., 'Life After Death', in A. Richardson, and J. Bowden (eds) *A New Dictionary of Christian Theology* (London: SCM Press, 1983), pp. 331–4.

Hinshelwood, R.D., *A Dictionary of Kleinian Thought*, 2nd edn (London: Free Association Books, 1991).

Hoffenberg, R., 'Christian Barnard: His First Transplants and Their Impact on Concepts of Death', *British Medical Journal* 323 (2001), pp. 1478–80.

Jones, D.A., *Death: A Good or an Evil? A Theological Enquiry*, DPhil thesis (University of Oxford, 2001).

Kass, L.R., 'L'Chaim and Its Limits: Why Not Immortality?' *First Things* 113 (May 2001), pp. 17–24.

Kegley, J.A.K. (ed.), *Genetic Knowledge: Human Values and Responsibility* (Lexington, KY: International Conference on the Unity of the Sciences, 1998)

Keller, E.F., *The Century of the Gene* (London: Harvard University Press, 2000).

Kingsland, J., 'Age-Old Story', *New Scientist Inside Science* 117 (23 January 1999), pp. 1–4.

Lamptey, P.R., 'Reducing Heterosexual Transmission of HIV in Poor Countries', *British Medical Journal* 324 (2002), pp. 207–11.

Lessing, D., *Canopus in Argos: Archives. The Making of the Representative for Planet 8* (London: Grafton, 1982/83).

Mauron, A., 'Is the Genome the Secular Equivalent of the Soul?', *Science* 291 (2001), pp. 831–2.

Morris, H.M., *The Genesis Record: A Scientific and Devotional Commentary on the Book of Beginnings* (Welwyn: Evangelical Press, 1976/77).

Nelson, J.R., *On the New Frontiers of Genetics and Religion* (Grand Rapids, MI: Eerdmans, 1994).

Peters, T., *Playing God? Genetic Determinism and Human Freedom* (New York: Routledge, 1997).

Reiss, M.J., 'What Sort of People Do We Want? The Ethics of Changing People Through Genetic Engineering', *Notre Dame Journal of Law, Ethics and Public Policy* 13 (1999), pp. 63–92.

Reiss, M.J., 'The Ethics of Genetic Research on Intelligence', *Bioethics* 14 (2000), pp. 1–15.

Reiss, M.J., 'Ethical Dimensions of Therapeutic Human Cloning', *Journal of Biotechnology* (in press).

Shaw, B., *Back to Methuselah* (Harmondsworth: Penguin, 1921/39).

Sloan, P.R. (ed.), *Controlling Our Destinies: Historical, Philosophical, Ethical, and Theological Perspectives on the Human Genome Project* (Notre Dame, IN: University of Notre Dame Press, 2000).

Southgate, C., 'Writer's Morning', in *Beyond the Bitter Wind: Poems 1982–2000* (Beeston: Shoestring Press, 2000), pp. 4–5.

Swift, J., *Gulliver's Travels* (New York: New American Library, 1726/1960).

Wyndham, J., *Trouble With Lichen* (Harmondsworth: Penguin, 1960/63).

4

The Human Genome and the Image of God

Ruth Page

What is it to be human? And where does the mapping, patenting or therapeutic use of the human genome fit into the definition? Does it assault, or complement, or improve what it is to be human? These are the issues to be discussed here, taking on the one side the Christian affirmation that to be human is to be made in the image of God, an end in itself, and hence not to be violated, even as an embryo, and on the other the pursuit of genetic manipulation with its possibilities for better and worse outcomes.

This is the time for such consideration, for actual, successful examples of cloning or genetic therapy are rare. Steve Jones wrote in 1996: 'The rewards promised so confidently have not materialized and show few signs of doing so.'[1] Little has changed. When a Massachusetts company, Advanced Cell Technology, announced to the media in November 2001 that it had produced the first cloned embryo, it was in the first place bypassing the usual sober process of peer review for the more public route, by which, no doubt, it might encourage more investors. But in the second place it misrepresented its achievements. What the company had succeeded in doing, in Jonathan Cohn's words, 'was to take one person's genes, implant them in an egg donated by another person and get that egg to divide ... twice. Then the egg died.'[2] As the real scientific

---

[1] S. Jones, *In the Blood: God, Genes and Destiny* (London: HarperCollins, 1996), p. xii.
[2] J. Cohn, 'Human Cloning', *Scotland on Sunday,* 2 December 2001, p. 19.

success will be to get the egg to divide dozens of times, this is scarcely a breakthrough. Indeed, as Cohn remarks scathingly: 'Imagine if NASA had announced in 1963 it had won the race to the moon because it had successfully got a rocket to blow up on the launching pad, and you start to grasp the kind of development to which we have been made privy.' Research may be in its early stages, but it seems clear that it will go on, with the safeguards (such as they currently are) of an Act of Parliament. Yet that does not stifle the debate. As Sheila McLean, professor of medical law and ethics at Glasgow University, writes: 'As ever, the hopes of the convinced and the fears of the doubters must be considered seriously: the time for this is now.'[3] Before coming to the specifics of these hopes and fears, however, it is as well to consider the kind of world in which they are expressed, often with great confidence. The basic question here is whether the world is such that unambiguous positions are possible, and if it is not, what that does for the arguments on both sides.

There are three characteristics of the world which challenge all pretension to clear and distinct positions or ideas.[4] The first is change, a matter which has become increasingly clear in such issues as social life, scientific and technological innovation, and even, latterly, climate. Neither things (except the most trivial) nor people remain fixed as what or who they are. Change does not bring chaos, however, but rather a reordering, a movement from one configuration of order to another. Change is often untidy (here but not there) and unpredictable, taking the present settled order by surprise. The new brought about by change must either integrate with what remains of the old order, or overthrow it completely, or occasionally remain as an anomaly in our multiple, and often less than coherent, world. Failure to meet successful changing conditions leads at the least to being sidelined, and at the worst to extinction.

---

[3] S. McLean, 'No Happy Ending Yet to the Gene Debate', *Scotland on Sunday*, 7 April 2002, p. 17.

[4] This view of the world as inherently ambiguous has been developed in much greater detail in R. Page, *Ambiguity and the Presence of God* (London: SCM Press, 1985). Certainly the statement 'everything is ambiguous' is held not to be itself ambiguous, but it is a philosophical phenomenon that the *statement* of what is held to be true does not itself fulfil the *conditions* of truth so stated.

Change is variety down a time-line, but the second characteristic of the world which precludes positivism is diversity, that is, variety at any given moment. That, again, scarcely requires exemplification, for in our shrunken world of global media, and even in ordinary connection with other people, diversity in traditions, faiths, preferences, philosophies, hypotheses and a welter of other instances becomes visible. Out of all the diversity we may make personal or professional judgements on which aspects to adhere to, but there is no human position above and beyond them all from which to judge their merits. Truth, therefore, is a judgement, a conviction (and one worth making), which will be backed up by what seems compelling to the proposer, but not a demonstration obvious to all, or there would not have been so many versions of the conception.

That observation leads to the third characteristic of the world which precludes simple assertions of rightness. That is polyvalence, which is the way in which something is open to multiple interpretations and evaluations on account of the diversity from which it is approached. Words and actions are never simply registered, they are interpreted, and interpreted from a point of view, a set of values, an available vocabulary and so forth. As values and viewpoints differ, so will the interpretations.

These aspects of an ambiguous world do not deny that each person and each affiliation of persons require order for their being and becoming. But that requirement exists in the midst of diverse and fluid orders which may be variously understood. That is never so clear as when two groups disagree. The conclusion is that our world is not so much ordered as orderable, capable of being put into order by whoever or whatever can make a difference. But as 'whoever or whatever can made a difference' can have better or worse effects, sometimes unforeseen effects, there is also moral ambiguity in thought and action. What is better for some person, group or country may simultaneously be worse for others. What seems eminently reasonable from one point of view may appear dangerously inclined from another, a matter exemplified by the debate concerning the uses of the human genome.

Nothing in creation or history is good or bad, better or worse *tout court* (that is, better for all people in all aspects at all times) but better or worse for certain people at certain times and places. Equally, what is good for some people at some point of time may become worse for them as time progresses, or the bad may become better. A relevant instance of such ambiguity over time concerns the future life of 'designer' cloned children, should these become possible. Although they may be just what the parent couple wants at the moment, and hence 'good', one may raise questions about the rights of such children. Will they always have to live out their parents' preferences, in which case the good may become worse for them? From all of this it is evident that there is ambiguity in the very way the world goes, without even mentioning the ambiguity of the human capacity for violence, domination and self-aggrandisement on the one hand, and on the other for care, equality and selflessness. What remains to be seen here is how this ambiguity affects the dispute between some biotechnologists and some Christians (though not every one on each side) and whether the recognition of ambiguity by both groups will make the debate less oppositional.

One of the principal objections raised by those Christians who are against certain uses of genetic manipulation, particularly against the use of embryos for stem cells, is that each human is in the image of God, and as such may not become a means to a medical end. There is a question whether early embryos, whose cells have not yet specialized, may be called life. But for the radical objectors an embryo has all it needs to become a human and may therefore be included in the term. For this argument the value of humans is lodged in their being in the image of God, and they are worthy of respect on that count alone.

But this argument does not escape the incursions of ambiguity. First, the actual meaning of 'image of God' has varied so much during Christian history that no single clear reference emerges and it seems to mean what people want it to mean. Second, the emphasis has made a clear distinction between humans and all the rest of creation. Such anthropocentricity is currently under attack with ontological conceptions of the image (those inhering in the very being of a human) giving way to relational accounts.

A brief survey of the use of image-of-God language will demonstrate the ambiguity of the term. The phrase appears rarely in the Bible (Genesis 1.26, 27; 5.1–3; 9.5, 6), but its importance to theological anthropology has been out of all proportion to its occurrence. The history of its use may be abbreviated into four sections. First comes the possible meaning to the original priestly writer, then its use as the ontological difference between humans and the rest of creation. Third, it has been invoked for the kind of relation held to be desirable between humans and all the rest of creation. Finally, a vague, warm sense of inclusiveness among humans pervades much of its contemporary expression. The diversity of these interpretations, changing as circumstances change, will be seen to diminish the content of the attribution, however emotively it is expressed.

It is possible that the original writer or compiler of Genesis had in mind a physical image, as conquerors left a statue of themselves behind when they departed to remind the conquered people to whom they now owed allegiance. The Old Testament commentator von Rad urges that both the physical and the spiritual make up the whole person and both are involved in the image.[5] In so far as this reference to the physical remained in the tradition as it moved on, it remained as a celebration of humans who are, in Milton's words, 'like God erect'.[6] Only humans stood on their hind legs, and since God was conceived rather literally as personal God was presumed to stand erect also. On the other hand Robert Murray emphasizes a kingly motif behind image-of-God language. God is the supreme being, infinitely wise and powerful, while humans, by virtue of bearing God's image, have vice-regal powers and responsibilities to use their wisdom and power on earth. It was the prophets' complaint that humans failed to live up to these gifts.[7]

These interpretations, whether appealing to the physical or the vice-regal, share the emphasis on superiority, showing how different humanity was from all other creatures on account of its divinely given qualities or endowments. By the Middle Ages, however, only men were considered to show these qualities to the full, for women were held to be inferior types. That gender

---

[5] G. van Rad, *Genesis* (London: SCM Press, 1965), p. 56.
[6] J. Milton, 'Paradise Lost', Book IV.
[7] R. Murray, *The Cosmic Covenant: Biblical Themes of Justice, Peace and the Integrity of Creation* (London: Sheed & Ward, 1992).

distinction was particularly true of rationality as the key human attribute, an interpretation which had earlier come easily to Christian theologians steeped in the categories of Greek philosophy. Women were considered to be not only physically weaker and less able to control their emotions, but also intellectually inferior. Some even questioned whether women were human. Aquinas authoritatively upheld the view that the male was normative, and females defective.[8]

On this account what was mostly held to be important about humanity was not its mere physicality, which other creatures in their own way shared. Rather it was their capacity for theoretical and practical thought, for they wrote books of theology and built civilizations. Further, humans were held to exhibit freedom from the set performance of other creatures as an inherent and unique quality. Both rationality and freedom, therefore, raised humans, especially males, above the rest, cut the connection with non-human creatures, and separated the esteemed qualities from everything to do with the body.

Although God was recognized and praised as the giver of this special connection and likeness, this version undoubtedly encouraged human self-esteem, a recurrent human characteristic not unknown among scientists. That in turn led to problems such as whether those with mental disabilities were or were not in the image of God. But such consideration was never allowed to detract from the glory of attribution. Yet changing circumstances change valuations, and, from a modern perspective, the emphasis on non-human limitations and the superior difference of humanity enabled the mind-set which could exploit non-human nature as so many useful resources which have no independent value to God, while women for centuries could be no more than helpmeets. Further, against the absolute distinction between human and non-human, it is relevant to mention that the coming of genetic information has blurred the clear line. Not only do humans share almost all their genes with other primates, but they have genes in common with such unlikely creatures as butterflies and cress. Neither intelligence, language nor tool-making may now be invoked for that absolute rather than relative difference.

[8] M. O'Neill, 'The Mystery of Being Human Together', in M.C. LaCugna (ed.), *Freeing Theology* (New York: Harper, 1993), p. 43.

To return to the history of the theological use of 'image of God', however, as the nineteenth century advanced the traditional appeal to rationality was already becoming less secure, for now it was science rather than theology which defined how rationality was to be understood. Other human capacities were therefore enlisted as characterizing the image of God. Human moral nature, human creativity, personhood itself were all described in these terms, and concurrently the sense of God changed also. Thus God was described in terms of 'the Archetype of all personality, supremely self-conscious, self-acting, moral', while humans continued to be proclaimed in that image.[9] In this kind of way the specialness of humanity has been consistently maintained in spite of difficulties, although conceptions of what makes for that specialness have quietly altered without advertisement to meet the changing conditions. That humanity at large still considers itself special may be seen from reaction to the cloning of Dolly the sheep. Concern was far less expressed for what that might mean for sheep, but rather for what it might portend for human cloning. It is easy for humans to think themselves special, but the question remains whether image-of-God language should be used in varieties of ways to give an exclusive religious aspect to that sense in every circumstance.

The sense of the term changed again as the changing world brought to light the omnipresence of the ecological crisis in pollution, loss of species, desertification and all the other assorted ills. Christians were charged with culpability for instilling the sense that the world was there for human use: 'The world was made for man and man was made to rule it.'[10] They had to admit there was little in their doctrines which valued the natural world for itself and in the sight of God. At least Christians had done little to stop the exploitation. The crisis provoked a rethinking of the image aimed at reconnecting humans with creation at large, of which Douglas John Hall's *Imaging God: Dominion as Stewardship* is a prime example. First Hall deals a blow to the self-laudatory aspect of the tradition by invoking the New

[9] H.C.G. Moule, *Outline of Christian Doctrine* (London: Hodder & Stoughton, 1905), pp. 57f.
[10] D. Quinn, *Ishmael* (New York: Bantam/Turner, 1992), p. 72.

Testament description of Christ as the image of God (e.g. Colossians 3.9). In that case, 'expecting glory we are shown humiliation; expecting the power of deity we are shown a suffering Son; expecting transcendence we are shown service and compassion'.[11] If that view of the divine were to prevail, instead of the exaltation of the human in the image of God, perhaps therapeutic intervention for the good of others would seem less objectionable.

Hall himself echoes Luther in regarding the image, not as inherent in humans, but as coming about as people respond to God. But he goes further in describing a response and relationship between the human and all creation. He moves from the noun 'image' to the verb 'imaging' and argues that only when humans are actively imaging God in what they do to any part of creation is the term applicable. This is a great remove from the static ontological application of the symbol in which humans had arrived just by virtue of being human. 'Relationship is the essence of the creature's nature and vocation. The relationship to which it is heir is a multiple one; having to do not only with God, whom it is called to image within creation, but also and simultaneously with the other creatures of God, who are served by its peculiar imaging of God.'[12]

Hall's own version of the stewardship of creation does, however, retain some sense of the specialness of humanity, rather like the vice-regal interpretation of Genesis 1, for a steward is different from what is stewarded. The hierarchial view of the superiority of humans remains, since stewards are perceptibly *over* what they steward, rather than with or alongside them. The change therefore in his account is not total. Yet in his descriptions the image of God ceases to be the automatic possession of inherent, divinely given attributes. Rather it is an ascription which has to be earned by what is done. Rationality and freedom give way to relationship, and with that the way is at least open to a renewed sense of male and female equality of possibility, of human bodiliness and creaturely connection.

---

[11] D.J. Hall, *Imaging God: Dominion as Stewardship* (Grand Rapids: Eermans, 1986), p. 80.
[12] Hall, *Imaging God*, p. 107.

There is, finally, another use of image-of-God language at present, which again implicitly stresses the difference between humans and other creatures, for it is aimed at inclusiveness among humanity. What characteristics of humanity make up the image are rarely specified. It seems once more to be enough to be human. The sense of human inclusiveness became important in affirming the humanity of those suffering from HIV/Aids. No human was to be written off as beyond the pale, for all are made in God's image. Again, 'We also affirm that biblical thinking about *Imago Dei* is a powerful appeal for human growth and social transformation. Once each of us can realize that our neighbour too is made in God's image, then we are compelled to treat each other with mutual respect.'[13]

This is, in effect, a denial that only 'normal' or privileged humans are valuable to God, a point worth making, but which does not require the sweeping allusion to image-of-God language to make it. Further, non-human creation is again excluded from this attribution. Since what constitutes the image is not specified, it has become a vague shibboleth rather than a coherent part of doctrine. A relevant recent example of a similar type of use came from the Board of Social Responsibility's Report to the General Assembly of the Church of Scotland in 2001. Although the Board was highly dubious about the use of embryos since that use could be a prelude to human cloning, they nevertheless proposed: 'Should any babies in future be born from human cell nuclear transfer embryos (we) affirm they will be fully human, made in the image of God, answerable to God according to their abilities.'[14]

What sense, then, may finally be made of image-of-God language, especially when that is opposed to what scientists may do with the human genome? As the term has had multiple meanings in its ambiguous history no one authoritative answer may be given. It has changed with changing circumstances and values. The best that can be said of it is that it does connect humans (and other creatures, which would be relevant for some forms of animal treatment and experimentation) with God, so that God is not left out of the argument. But how

---

[13] J. Crawford and M. Kinnamon (eds), *In God's Image: Reflections on Identity, Human Wholeness and the Authority of Scripture* (Geneva: WCC Publications, 1983), p. 56.
[14] Board of Social Responsibility, Report to the General Assembly of the Church of Scotland, May 2001.

humans are connected with God and God with humans remains diverse and often partial in conception. I shall return to make a further critical point on its use after considering what 'playing God' may mean. But already it is clear that this not a sufficiently self-explanatory term to use in a debate as shorthand and without reasoned definition, and therefore its effects are more emotive than rational and may simply alienate scientists.

It remains important that God is not left out of the debate, but not, perhaps, in the way biotechnologists have been accused of 'playing God' in their use of the genome – a phrase much favoured by the tabloid press. As Egbert Schroten comments, 'in this metaphor the view-of-life aspect of some issues in biomedical areas is expressed in a vague way and with a pejorative undertone'.[15] Schroten himself arrives at a positive evaluation of the term: ' "Playing God" is useful as a metaphor for man's stewardship over creation, especially in (bio)-science and (bio)-technology. This duty is a meaningful and responsible task which we are to perform joyfully.' But that eirenic interpretation is rarely the one advanced on the Christian side. Instead it has been argued that 'playing' implies taking on a role which does not belong to the role-players. On this account only God has the wisdom to order creation, and the intervention of scientists arrogates to themselves this prerogative and is thus hubris. Succinctly expressed, 'playing God' implies that, 'In our human pride we are tampering with something which we do not have the knowledge or wisdom to handle.'[16]

Certainly some scientists in reassuring the public seem over-confident about their capacity to bring about a trouble-free future, God-like in that sense, an ambiguity I shall return to. But if the wisdom and knowledge of God in ordering creation is the decisive matter on the Christian side, these have not prevented such anomalies as Siamese twins, or people being born with the gene for Huntington's chorea. There is already the ambiguity of good and bad in the present way the world goes. If God is responsible for present ordering such harmful misordering cannot simply be dismissed as mystery within the good, and

---

[15] E. Schroten, 'Playing God: Some Theological Comments on a Metaphor', in G. van den Brink, L. van den Brom, and M. Sarot (eds), *Christian Faith and Philosophical Theology* (Kampen: Kok Pharos, 1992), p. 195.

[16] D. Bruce and A. Bruce (eds), *Engineering Genesis: The Ethics of Genetic Engineering on Non-Human Species* (London: Earthscan, 1998), p. 85.

should give pause to any version of divine action which implies responsibility for innocent suffering. The optimism of some scientists about their future capabilities may be matched by an equal optimism on the part of some believers about the goodness of the supposedly divinely given state of things when no other intervention has taken place.

Declarations of God's direction of matters in creation, or of human being as in the image of God, always run up against the problem of evil. Were Hitler and Stalin in the image of God? They were, if it is simply enough to be human rather than becoming the image in what is done. It is not surprising that Reformers such as Calvin were sure the image was defaced and had virtually disappeared. For Calvin the image was likened to being a mirror, such that the goodness of God might be reflected in the world.[17] But if that mirror were clouded, or angled towards the self, the image was gone. This is one version of how to ascribe moral evil to human failings and vices, a matter universally agreed among theologians since Augustine.

Moral evil may be attributed to human weakness and sin, but what of natural evil for which humans bear no responsibility? The genetic diseases for which genetic manipulation holds out hope surely come into that category, and are not, as was once believed, the result of sin somewhere in the family. Humans are not responsible for the genes they carry any more than they are responsible for volcanoes. (There is perhaps responsibility over whether to have children and pass on a known faulty gene, but that is a different issue.) If humans are not to blame, is God to blame? At first there appears to be no other candidate.

But there is a way out of attributing to God the mixed better and worse of the natural world, and that is by redescribing God's action in creating. It involves seeing God as both letting go and holding fast. The letting go occurs if, just as God gave humanity freedom of the will to turn to God and do good, or to turn inwards to the self and do evil, so God has given the non-human world freedom to develop as it could right from the beginning. That freedom would account for both volcanoes and faulty genes. At the same time, however, God is holding fast by pervading creation, accompanying and offering it all

---

[17] T.F. Torrance, *Calvin's Doctrine of Man* (Grand Rapids: Eerdmans, 1957), p. 36.

relationship as it has used and continues to use that freedom, but not breaking the relationship by intervening in the world's processes.[18] Yet out of that multiple creaturely freedom some aspects have developed which have hurt humans (and other creatures) in certain contexts at certain times. God is not responsible for volcanoes or Parkinson's disease. Both, like the good which has also appeared, are the results of finite freedoms finding a foothold in the world. Thus moral evil is accounted for humanly and natural evil accounted for naturally. In the end, therefore, the more positive conception of scientists playing God given by Egbert Schroten, such that they become at least stewards of creation, is the more hopeful line to pursue.

As a link between the varieties of theological affirmation and the ambiguities of the biotechnologists' stance, I turn now to the differences among ethical bases. It is clear that what is demonstrated by the appeal to God, on the one hand, however expressed, and the very different approach to benefits in genetic engineering on the other hand, is that the two sides are each proceeding within very different ethical frameworks, which lead to very different stances. These will remain irreconcilable unless in the context of the debate there is at least mutual comprehension of what is ethically valuable on each side, together with an examination of each stance in the light of the other. 'Arguments used both for and against genetic engineering are seen to be related to the different assumptions found among various intellectual traditions in contemporary society, such as the scientist, humanist, Christian and environmentalist.'[19]

On the one hand there are those whose primary value is life as a whole, whether that involves Christian thanks to God, or humanist appreciation of human qualities, or environmentalists' involvement in the natural world. It is the total picture which motivates such groups. On the other hand, scientists, qua scientists, appear to take a more instrumental view of life, such that it may be reduced to its smallest components and altered towards healthier or more socially desirable ends. For some, life as such, life as we have it, is an end which does not justify all

---

[18] These issues are discussed further in R. Page, *God and the Web of Creation* (London: SCM Press, 1996), pp. 11ff.

[19] Bruce and Bruce, *Engineering Genesis*, p. 37.

means, so that those who use it as means have to convince them that a valuable end which does not diminish the whole person is in sight. That in turn is why the possibilities of therapeutic cloning are what is principally made known, while opponents principally fear other developments. Basically for the practice of genetic engineering, life is a collection of programmed systems rather than an interrelationship of whole creatures. Given the notion of such systems, the functions within them may be disembodied, removed and relocated to where they may be useful. Further, there is no essential connection between species and function. Such practical manipulation is new, and Edmund Yoxen, who is fundamentally in favour of the biotechnologists' aims, still suggests that their stance and *modus operandi* require 'dissent, scepticism, appraisal, lobbying for alternatives, political debate and public rumination'.[20]

As part of that public rumination it is reasonable to point out that the divide is not total, since everyone (probably) holds some moral absolutes about life, and has a moral boundary which cannot be crossed. Almost everyone, for instance, believes it is wrong to torture children, even if some information may be gained from the procedure. That is to say, for everyone there are some things which cannot be done to humans. That raises questions concerning the omnicompetence of risk/benefit analysis as all that is ever needed to justify an action, for that would permit the practice of torture if the goods obtained from it were valuable. But if it can be agreed that torturing children is out, the two 'sides' are not totally disparate and one way of describing the ethical differences here is a disagreement on what counts as a moral boundary for what one human can do to another, and the grounds on which that boundary has to be observed or may be infringed if the final goods do not dehumanize but enhance the humanity of the subject.

Yet disagreement over that issue may appear insoluble. Arguments from principle regarding intrinsic worth are sometimes given with a 'take it or leave it' appearance: 'this is just so'; 'here I stand and can do no other', as if the stance alone were enough, in opposition to people who do not share it and cannot understand it. That can stifle debate, as one side is

[20] E. Yoxen, *The Gene Business* (London: Pan Books, 1983), p. 22.

simply excluding the possibilities of the other. When that happens it is easy to see why those with intrinsic beliefs may appear emotive and non-rational to the others, while scientists seem equally impervious to what is important to the objectors. Listening to and understanding those from whom one differs is as important in this case (on both sides) as it is in any other which is to proceed beyond entrenched positions. For it is equally the case that the force of underlying values and attitudes can be seen in those who advocate the use of genetic manipulation. They must all have a basic belief that for certain purposes a human may be reduced to genes, organs or chemicals, which it is all right for them to manipulate. That is at best an assumption, not a scientific 'fact'. Both sides, therefore, are driven by fundamental beliefs.

In so far as the scientific assumptions are ever justified by its proponents, they are justified by results, or sometimes an optimistic, not-yet-proven appeal to health benefits without debilitating side-effects. The ambiguous features of action in the world where multiple components interact are not in view, so the results can be made to seem simple and inescapable. Holding out a possible cure for cystic fibrosis seems powerfully persuasive, so that doubts about the fundamental attitude towards humanity involved may appear, or be represented, as obscurantism. Yet, as Yoxen says: 'I just don't understand how some people can be so certain that the biological future holds no nasty surprises.'[21] Many of the public could echo that and require more than 'Trust me, I'm a scientist' for reassurance.

It is precisely one of the changes of the changing world that society in Britain no longer trusts scientists unquestioningly, as they once did. Science was once a closed book to most, and the results were regarded with awe rather than comprehension. Further, science, and its handmaid technology, have undoubtedly done much good to humanity. But its ambiguous nature as producing both good and evil is now much more perceptible. What is particularly at issue here is the way in which the fascination of research and its success has been separated from its outcomes at large. How is the public to know whether what Oppenheimer wrote of the atomic bomb will not also be true of genetic engineering? 'When you see something which is

---

[21] Yoxen, *The Gene Business*, p. 234.

technically sweet you go ahead and do it, and you argue what to do about it only after you have had your technical success ... that's the way it was with the atomic bomb.'[22]

Pesticides with unwanted knock-on effects and iatrogenic illnesses are two further examples which have diminished society's deference towards scientific 'advance'. As Rosemary Radford Ruether has written: 'The nuclear bomb shattered the naïve faith in science as a tool for inevitable good, and the growing evidence that technology was perhaps doing irreparable damage to the environment eroded faith still more. It seemed more and more likely that the tools created by science might result in the destruction of the earth rather than its decisive establishment on the road to happiness and prosperity for all.'[23] There is thus a fear that although benefits may come from therapeutic cloning, for instance, the door is simultaneously being opened to unknown disasters. At the very least, therefore, caution and advance as slow as it has been in the last twenty years would be more reassuring.

Another cause of public apprehension is the role of pharmaceutical companies in forwarding research or making use of independent research from universities. The prospect of curing disease is positive, but companies which have profits to make may well be interested only in what may be called the 'profitable' diseases, that is, those with a large enough group of sufferers to ensure a return on the costs of research and development. Diseases which are rare but just as distressing do not hold out the same financial incentive. Further, the emphasis is likely to be on curing diseases, not on developing materials or circumstances which would prevent them. It therefore behoves the public to keep asking to what degree biotechnologists are working towards corporate advantage rather than the public good when these do not coincide.

Ethical debates are often decided, not by argument nor by persuasion, but by the power one side has to implement its point of view. In this case it appears that biotechnology and genetic intervention have the government (cautiously)

[22] R. Oppenheimer, cited without reference by T. Shakespeare, in 'Human Cloning', *Scotland on Sunday*, 2 August 2001, p. 13.
[23] R.R. Ruether, *Gaia and God* (London: SCM Press, 1992), p. 36.

and money behind them. That alone could short-cut the whole issue.

> At an institutional level a radical denial of the intrinsic arguments in ethical debate can present real problems to the democratic process. People approach the arguments about genetic engineering in varying relationships of power and influence, both insiders and outsiders, with different and unexposed assumptions and values about the world. In the present context the danger for those who are in positions of power is to assume that intrinsic beliefs are something which only the opponents of technology have, and to be unaware of their own, and of the considerable influence they may already be having.[24]

This quotation implies that the power of scientists to have their own way is finally greater than any objector's. Yet, as has been seen in the outcry over genetically modified crops, objectors may still keep the debate alive, especially if they are well informed, not simply hostile, and do not leave to scientists the rational high ground.

In the case of biotechnology and genetic intervention Edward Yoxen foresees an influential future comparable in its total effects to the immense changes brought about by microelectronics. 'This process of technological change ... is something like a revolution. It is a major economic phenomenon that will have social and political repercussions. It will affect the patterns of trade. It will change the value of some people's assets both positively and negatively. It will force some industries to the wall. It will have profound effects on the global structures of power.'[25] Given this possible outcome, it remains imperative that the early stages are scanned critically, with God's concern over how things are in creation as both the impulse and the criterion for debates. Relevant questions on Yoxen's wider issues include: Who will receive the benefits of work on the human genome? Will the cost be prohibitive for all but the very rich to benefit from it? Will whole countries lose out? As a footnote to this aspect of the debate Yoxen gives an example which shows the worrying possibilities of gene culture, although it is not directly related to the human genome. 'After all, if you can grow opiates in cell culture, what will that do to

[24] Bruce and Bruce, *Engineering Genesis*, p. 83.
[25] Yoxen, *The Gene Business*, p. 239.

the heroin trade in South East Asia or Turkey, or to the cocaine business in Columbia?'

In the end this to and fro of ambiguity on both sides suggests that self-examination should both precede and accompany the debate. Intrinsic beliefs require examination as much as do the consequential attitudes which weigh only costs and benefits. It is not enough to make a vague appeal to God, or God's image, or the good ordering of things as they are. This is not simply a world of beauty, harmony and human flourishing which scientists might destroy. In Christian belief such lack of ambiguity occurs only in the eschaton, the end of time. Among other evils this is a world in which genetic diseases cause untold suffering. If God is concerned that the best possible should take place in creation, and it is the Christian calling to see that all should have the best possible conditions of life, then these conditions may scarcely be withheld from those suffering genetic defects. Genetic biotechnology has the potential for increasing the amount of better over worse in creation and to that extent is to be welcomed. The force of this argument would support a friendly though not uncritical attitude towards therapeutic cloning, but not towards reproductive cloning, which seems much more ethically dubious.

Yet that degree of reconciliation on the one side does not remove the responsibility of all Christians to undertake a very considerable number of tasks. They must watch how scientists use their power, in order to question any over-optimism which might lead to hasty, insufficiently tested results; to ensure that those who cannot be cured by genetic treatment do not suffer disadvantage in terms of employment, insurance or peace of mind; to oversee how accessible cures may be at home and abroad; to investigate the workings of pharmaceutical companies; and to work for the degree of reconciliation with the other side such that unsympathetic scientists may come to perceive and perhaps to question the adequacy of their own intrinsic beliefs about what it is to be human.

Bibliography

van den Brink, G., van den Brom, L. and Sarot, M. (eds), *Christian Faith and Philosophical Theology* (Kampen: Kok Pharos, 1992).

Bruce, D. and A. (eds), *Engineering Genesis: The Ethics of Genetic Engineering on Non-Human Species* (London: Earthscan, 1998).

Crawford, J. and Kinnamon, M. (eds), *Reflection on Identity, Human Wholeness and the Authority of Scripture* (Geneva: WCC Publications, 1983).

Hall, D.J., *Imaging God: Dominion as Stewardship* (Grand Rapids: Eerdmans, 1986).

Jones, S., *In the Blood: God, Genes and Destiny* (London: HarperCollins, 1996).

LaCugna, M.C. (ed.), *Freeing Theology* (New York: Harper, 1993).

Murray, R., *The Cosmic Covenant: Biblical Themes of Justice, Peace and the Integrity of Creation* (London: Sheed and Ward, 1992).

Page, R., *Ambiguity and the Presence of God* (London: SCM Press, 1985).

Page, R., *God and the Web of Creation* (London: SCM Press, 1996).

Quinn, D., *Ishmael* (New York: Bantam/Turner, 1992).

von Rad, G., *Genesis* (London: SCM Press, 1965).

Ruether, R., *Gaia and God* (London: SCM Press, 1992).

Torrance, T. F., *Calvin's Doctrine of Man* (Grand Rapids: Eerdmans, 1957).

Yoxen, E., *The Gene Business* (London: Pan Books, 1983).

PART III

Questioning Implicit Norms

Introduction to Part III

This section takes up and explores some particular issues and scenarios associated with the HGP and subjects these to intensive scrutiny to discern their hidden assumptions. Neil Messer, like Page in the preceding chapter, argues that terms which are commonly used, such as health, normality and disease, are fluid in their meanings. Taking St Paul's thorn in the flesh as a case study for theological reflection on human suffering, he explores the implications it might have for language about health. The medical and WHO definitions could be seen as presenting two opposite poles in the secular debate, so that while the first is narrowly reductionistic, the second tends to weaken a sense of individual responsibility. He draws on a Barthian notion of health as 'God's call', while insisting that even in sickness God's grace can be discovered. He wrestles with the particular problem of how to deal with sickness in terms of genetic manipulation, suggesting that prudential understanding in the context of the Christian community is the way forward in discerning which particular course to take.

Maureen Junker-Kenny's chapter is more explicitly philosophical in orientation. She offers a probing analysis of the assumptions behind genetic science, inviting a deeper exploration of the implicit norms in the HGP, including the claims about human nature buried in the language. Do we go down the path of scientific naturalism, where our concepts of health, normality, illness and suffering are defined by scientific knowledge? She argues specifically for the need for *institutional* ethics in such circumstances, so that ethics cannot simply be confined to individuals, but extends to wider communities and institutions as well. In medical circles ethics seems to have narrowed to a discussion of patient–physician relationships where particular medical risks and benefits are aired. The goal of such methodology is unchallenged. She invites us to consider what might be the social implications of such a narrowing, asking if it creates the social conditions where it is harder to accept disabilities. Provocatively, she suggests that the guardian of human individuality and human dignity is chance. Any ideal of predictability and perfectibility stems from Enlightenment ideals. Her chapter concludes with a discussion of the framework in which ethical judgements might be made, arguing that philosophical anthropology, rather than natural law or virtue ethics, offers the most promising way forward in such debates.

5

The Human Genome Project, Health and the 'Tyranny of Normality'[1]

Neil G. Messer

[T]o keep me from being too elated [on account of visions and revelations of the Lord], a thorn was given me in the flesh, a messenger of Satan to torment me, to keep me from being too elated. Three times I appealed to the Lord about this, that it would leave me, but he said to me, 'My grace is sufficient for you, for power is made perfect in weakness.' So, I will boast all the more gladly of my weaknesses, so that the power of Christ may dwell in me. Therefore I am content with weaknesses, insults, hardships, persecutions, and calamities for the sake of Christ; for whenever I am weak, then I am strong.

(2 Corinthians 12.7–10, NRSV)

Introduction

The human genome project promises to revolutionize our understanding of many human characteristics, including those that have to do with disease and disability. It also offers unprece-dented opportunities for intervening in human heredity in a

[1] I am grateful to my fellow participants in the colloquium for the opportunity to discuss the ideas presented in this chapter, and for the many helpful comments and suggestions they made. I had previously tried out more preliminary reflections on health and disease on my former colleagues and students in the Queen's Foundation, Birmingham, theological educators in the United Reformed Church and other audiences, and am grateful for the helpful discussion, comments and critique from which I benefited on each of these occasions.

variety of ways, for example, through pre-implantation diagnosis and selective implantation of embryos with desired characteristics, pre-natal diagnosis and abortion of foetuses with unwanted characteristics, gene therapy (that is, the treatment of inherited diseases by genetic manipulation) and genetic enhancement (the use of genetic manipulation to 'improve' characteristics that have nothing to do with disease). Some of these applications, such as pre-natal diagnosis, are already well established, but their scope will be greatly extended by the results of the Human Genome Project. Others, such as genetic enhancement, are much more distant prospects (indeed, genetic enhancement is currently illegal in the UK), but are not impossible to contemplate.

These opportunities and prospects raise acute questions about health, disease and human diversity. Most obviously, there are *moral* questions about the right uses of this knowledge and the technology that it makes possible: for example, when if ever is it right to intervene genetically to alter human characteristics, and when should we refrain? Elsewhere I have drawn on Dietrich Bonhoeffer's distinction between the 'ultimate' and the 'penultimate' to argue that *therapeutic* genetic interventions can be considered a legitimate part of the 'penultimate' activity to which humans are called by God; *non-therapeutic* manipulation or genetic 'enhancement', on the other hand, risks becoming part of a grandiose project to perfect the human race by technological means, a project with 'ultimate' or divine pretensions.[2] However, it is often pointed out that this answer is problematic, since the distinction between therapy and enhancement is highly ambiguous and hard to define clearly.

The difficulty of defining a clear boundary between therapy and enhancement arises at least in part because this definition would depend on an understanding of the notoriously elusive and ambiguous concepts of 'health', 'normality' and 'disease'.[3] It becomes clear, then, that behind the practical moral

[2] N.G. Messer, 'Human Cloning and Genetic Manipulation: Some Theological and Ethical Issues', *Studies in Christian Ethics* 12.2 (1999), pp. 1–16; 'Human Genetics and the Image of the Triune God', *Science and Christian Belief* 13.2 (2001), pp. 99–111.

[3] K.M. Boyd, 'Disease, Illness, Sickness, Health, Healing and Wholeness: Exploring some Elusive Concepts', *Journal of Medical Ethics: Medical Humanities* 26 (2000), pp. 9–17.

questions about how to use this knowledge, when to intervene and when to refrain lies a more fundamental question: what do we mean when we speak of health, normality and disease? This question has attracted the interest of scientists, clinicians, artists, philosophers and many others,[4] but a Christian response, while engaging with these different perspectives, must recognize that the question is an inescapably theological one which requires that the distinctive resources of the Christian tradition be brought to bear on it.[5]

Paul's thorn

The theological issue at stake can be drawn out by reference to Paul's famous account of his 'thorn in the flesh', quoted at the head of this chapter. There is very little evidence to suggest what Paul's thorn was: it has been variously interpreted as physical affliction, psychological disorder, persistent temptation and persecution by opponents.[6] But if for the sake of argument we assume that it was some kind of visual impairment,[7] we may re-cast our initial questions along the following lines: how should we understand Paul's thorn – as a disease or dysfunction, something that had gone amiss with the functioning of his body, or as a normal human limitation comparable to the inability to sing in tune or to run a four-minute mile? And (to indulge in a wayward fantasy), supposing that Luke 'the beloved physician' (Colossians 4.14) had been miraculously endowed with the knowledge and the tools of modern scientific medicine (including modern genetics),

---

[4] See Boyd, 'Disease', for a recent survey.

[5] I am aware that this bald assertion begs many questions about theological method; rather than engage in a lengthy discussion of method, it seems best to begin immediately to address the substantive questions that I have raised, in the hope that some of my assumptions about method will become clearer as the discussion unfolds.

[6] See M.E. Thrall, *A Critical and Exegetical Commentary on the Second Epistle to the Corinthians*, vol. II (Edinburgh: T & T Clark, 2000), pp. 809–18, for a comprehensive survey of the theories.

[7] This has been a popular theory, though it does not finally commend itself to Thrall: see *2 Corinthians*, pp. 814–15. John Hull, in his recent book *In the Beginning There was Darkness* (London: SCM Press, 2001), pp. 84–91, considers it possible and comments that though it 'is impossible to say whether Paul was partially sighted or not ... a partially-sighted person reading his letters can certainly feel a sense of communion with Paul' (p. 91).

should he have used these to try and alleviate Paul's condition, or should he have refrained?

Paul's own account, as given in 2 Corinthians, is full of paradox. The thorn was, to say the least, highly unwelcome: it is described as a 'messenger of Satan' sent to 'torment' (*kolaphizē*, lit. 'beat') Paul. He pleaded with the Lord 'three times' to be relieved of it, but his plea was refused, and the Lord told him, '[my] power is made perfect (*teleitai*, which often gives the sense of completion or fulfilment) in weakness'. As a result of this divine answer, Paul has come to see his 'weaknesses' as the things in which he should boast, 'so that the power of Christ may dwell in me'. He is content to experience weakness and suffering, because, as he puts it, 'whenever I am weak, then I am strong'. He appears to be saying at least two related things here: first, that it is his own weakness which forces him to rely most fully on the strength of Christ, and so to experience that strength most fully, and second, that in Barrett's words, 'a display of human weakness is the best possible stage for the display of divine power'.[8] But there are also echoes of the power-in-weakness of the crucified Christ himself, and of Paul's words in 1 Corinthians that 'God's foolishness is wiser than human wisdom, and God's weakness is stronger than human strength' (1 Corinthians 1.25).

The ambiguity and paradox of this passage come in part from its context.[9] Paul's account of boasting in his weaknesses is the climax of his rejoinder to his opponents in Corinth, who have presumably been given to boasting of their superior spiritual credentials and achievements. The Lord's answer, that 'power is made perfect in weakness', reminds us of the necessarily paradoxical nature of any Christian reflection on power and success, since such reflection must take its bearings from the cross of Christ.

Paul's thorn in the flesh is a test case for the theological adequacy of our understandings of health and disease: any Christian account we wish to give must be capable of dealing with the complexity of Paul's story without collapsing his dialectics of power and weakness, suffering and strength. In the

---

[8] C.K. Barrett, *The Second Epistle to the Corinthians* (London: A & C Black, 1973), p. 317.
[9] See Barrett, *2 Corinthians*, pp. 288–318, for a helpful discussion.

following sections I shall use Paul's thorn to evaluate three accounts of health and disease, before making some final comments on the questions about understanding and practice that I raised in the Introduction.

The medical model

One way of answering these questions is to adopt a so-called 'medical model' of health and disease, in which both are defined in purely objective, scientific terms, avoiding the introduction of any value-judgement into the definitions. One prominent exponent of such an approach is the philosopher Christopher Boorse, who defines health and disease in terms of statistical norm and biological function:

> An organism is *healthy* at any moment in proportion as it is not diseased; and a *disease* is a type of internal state of the organism which:
>
> (i) interferes with the performance of some natural function – i.e., some species-typical contribution to survival and reproduction – characteristic of the organism's age; and
>
> (ii) is not simply in the nature of the species, i.e. is either atypical of the species or, if typical, mainly due to environmental causes.[10]

The medical model can give a clear answer to our first question about Paul's thorn in the flesh: to the extent that it interfered with the performance of the natural or species-typical function of (let us say) seeing, of course it was a disease. If that is the case, the answer to the second question may seem obvious: if Paul had a disease and Luke could treat it, then he should. However, Boorse is careful to point out that his definition of disease, being objective and value-free, cannot supply such a conclusion. The practical moral question about Paul's treatment could only be answered by deciding whether Paul's disease also satisfied the further, normative, conditions to be called an *illness*:

> A disease is an *illness* only if it is serious enough to be incapacitating, and therefore is
>
> (i) undesirable for its bearer;

[10] C. Boorse, 'What a Theory of Mental Health Should Be', *Journal for the Theory of Social Behaviour* 6 (1976), pp. 61–84, at pp. 62–3.

(ii) a title to special treatment; and

(iii) a valid excuse for normally criticizable behaviour.[11]

The medical model is an appealing solution, not least because it fits well with the larger project of describing health and disease in terms of biological cause and effect, and so designing biological strategies for overcoming diseases. The sequencing of the human genome is one of the latest and most ambitious expressions of this project: it promises huge advances in our understanding of the causal mechanisms of many diseases, and in our ability to treat these diseases or even eliminate them from the population. Without denying the positive aspects of scientific medicine, however, we can recognize that the medical model is problematic in various ways. First, it is questionable whether we can define health and disease entirely in objective, scientific terms. Richard Hare has noted a number of difficulties with Boorse's definition, most importantly that the concept of 'natural function' is unable to do the work that Boorse wishes it to do:

> [Boorse] is compelled to rely so heavily on the rather wobbly notion of natural function because he wishes to avoid saying that what makes us classify conditions as diseases is that *in general* ... they are *bad* things for the patient to have.[12]

But this, says Hare, is a 'standard constituent' of the concept of disease: the concepts of disease and health involve prescriptive or evaluative terms like 'good' and 'bad', and we cannot avoid value-judgements in talking about health and disease.

Hare raises another difficulty for the medical model. Like Boorse, he is partly concerned with the possibility or otherwise of developing concepts of *mental* health and disease. He wishes to develop concepts which will allow us to describe a relatively uncontroversial condition like depression as a disease, but which are resistant to abuses such as the labelling of political dissidents as mentally ill people who may be forcibly incarcerated and 'treated'. Following his earlier discussion, he argues that to classify a condition as a disease is, by definition, to introduce an evaluative premise into the discussion. Now in

---

[11] Boorse, 'What a Theory of Mental Health Should Be', p. 63.
[12] R.M. Hare, 'Health', *Journal of Medical Ethics* 12 (1986), pp. 174–81, at p. 178.

deciding whether the concept of disease is being rightly used or abused in a particular case, it matters *who* is making the evaluation: in the least problematic cases (like depression), the individual with this condition either makes or readily agrees with the evaluation that it is a bad condition to be in. However, Hare goes on to point out that in some cases, a further difficulty arises. There are two possible reasons why someone in a certain condition judges it a bad one: (i) he or she may dislike the condition as such; (ii) he or she may not mind the condition as such, but may suffer 'social or even legal disabilities' because of it. In the second case, the more appropriate response may be to remove the social penalties associated with the condition rather than seeking to alter the condition itself by medical means.[13] Of course, it is quite possible (though Hare does not spell this out) that in some cases both (i) and (ii) may apply to varying extents.

Although Hare draws attention to this issue in the context of *mental* health and disease, the same question arises and is very vigorously contested with reference to physical disabilities such as blindness and deafness. Medical models of disability would identify the problem as a physical dysfunction which is a proper subject for medical treatment aimed at reversing the condition; 'social' models, by contrast, locate the problem not in the individual's physical condition but in social structures which discriminate against the minority who experience that condition. The proper response is not to try and change the individual's physical condition, but to create social structures which can accommodate diversity and do not discriminate against those who are physically different from the majority. A striking example of this debate is the controversy over the giving of cochlear implants to young children who have been born profoundly deaf. Medical studies suggest that children who are treated in this way can acquire enough speech and hearing to be educated in mainstream schools. The British Deaf Association, however, argues that the Deaf community should be regarded as a linguistic minority whose first language is sign language. It therefore opposes cochlear implantation in young children on the grounds that this may

---

[13] Hare, 'Health', pp. 179–80. The example he uses is homosexuality: a decade and a half after the publication of his paper, the claim that homosexuality is a disease is rarely made, but as the following discussion shows, there are other controversial cases where the question he identifies is very much at issue.

isolate them from the language and culture of the Deaf community without enabling them to be fully integrated into the hearing world.[14]

A similar point is suggested by John Hull with particular reference to blindness in his book *In the Beginning There Was Darkness*. Reflecting on Isaiah 42.16 ('I will lead the blind by a road they do not know, by paths they have not known I will guide them. I will turn the darkness before them into light, the rough places into level ground . . .'), he writes:

> It is all the more remarkable, in view of the popularity of the idea that God would open the eyes of the blind, to find that in [this passage], no such thing takes place. Blind people are not changed, restored or miraculously healed. They are accepted and the behaviour of others around them is modified to give them equal opportunities.[15]

Elsewhere he tells the sad story of a very able man who felt that he had to resign from his responsible job in a government department because he was beginning to lose his sight:

> The intelligence, experience, management skills and creativity of this man were lost to society, and all for nothing, since it would have been possible for him to have continued in his work as a completely blind person.[16]

All this raises the question to what extent visual impairment is a medical problem for which we should seek medical cures, and to what extent the proper response is not to try and reverse the condition but to create structures which do not penalize it. Perhaps (if I may put it like this) it was more important for Paul to have scribes to write his letters and companions to help him travel than for Luke to try and cure him.

---

[14] R. Ramsden and J. Graham, 'Cochlear Implantation', *British Medical Journal* 311 (1995), p. 1588; British Deaf Association, *The British Deaf Association Policy on Cochlear Implants*, <http://www.britishdeafassociation.org.uk/cochlearpolicyfull.html> (accessed 15 February 2002). See, further, N. G. Messer (ed.), *Theological Issues in Bioethics: An Introductory Reader* (London: Darton, Longman & Todd, 2002), ch. 4.

[15] J. M. Hull, *In the Beginning There Was Darkness: A Blind Person's Conversations with the Bible* (London: SCM Press, 2001), pp. 108–9.

[16] Hull, *In the Beginning*, pp. 64–5. Obviously, as Hull acknowledges, some jobs (such as garbage collecting and piloting a jumbo jet) could not be done by a blind person, but in situations such as the one he is describing, 'a highly motivated and organized blind person can be extremely effective. What matters is judgement, efficiency and creativity, not eyes' (p. 65).

There is a further abuse to which medical models may be put (though it is in no way entailed by a philosophical analysis such as Boorse's). This abuse may be described with a phrase borrowed from Stanley Hauerwas: 'the tyranny of normality'.[17] It would be possible to use a medical model of health-as-normality to legitimate our fear of diversity and of those who are different from us. This becomes all the more important in the light of the fact that molecular genetics offers a powerful set of tools with which a society could implement 'quality control' of children and eliminate 'abnormalities' from the population.[18] Hauerwas articulates a very different vision. In the essay from whose title I have borrowed the phrase 'the tyranny of normality', he suggests that one of the gifts that children with severe learning disabilities can give the rest of society is to 'force us to recognize that we are involved in a community life that is richer than our official explanations and theories give us the skill to say'.[19]

In short, a medical model of health and disease gives clear, but ultimately unsatisfactory, answers to the questions that I have raised by means of Paul's thorn in the flesh. The short-comings of the answers are clearly shown by considering some of the issues raised by disability or impairment.

The WHO definition

In sharp contrast to the medical model lies the famous (or notorious) definition adopted by the World Health Organization

---

[17] S. Hauerwas, 'Community and Diversity: The Tyranny of Normality', in *Suffering Presence: Theological Reflections on Medicine, the Mentally Handicapped and the Church* (Edinburgh: T & T Clark, 1988), pp. 211–17.

[18] The established practice of pre-natal diagnosis followed by 'therapeutic' abortion, and the more recent one of pre-implantation diagnosis followed by selective implantation of embryos, could be described as forms of 'quality control' of children. Since the declared intention in current practice is to prevent the birth of children with distressing, painful and frequently fatal genetic diseases, it might be said that 'quality control' is an unduly pejorative description. This observation, however, serves to illustrate the difficulty of saying what we mean by health and disease, and of distinguishing between interventions intended to prevent disease and those intended to eliminate diversity – problems which are major preoccupations of this chapter.

[19] Hauerwas, 'Community and Diversity', p. 231. The language of 'learning disability' is mine, not Hauerwas's: writing in 1977, he used what he described as 'the unhappy word "retarded"' (p. 211).

(WHO) in 1948: 'Health is a state of complete physical, mental, and social well-being and not merely the absence of disease or infirmity.'[20] Those who framed this definition in the aftermath of the Second World War were unashamed to introduce value-judgements into their concept of health, and indeed to promote an all-embracing vision of health as fundamental to peace, security and the well-being of the entire human race.[21]

The WHO definition has commended itself to some Christian writers, such as John Wilkinson, who understand health in terms of biblical concepts like *shalom*.[22] It certainly offers a welcome reminder that there is more to human well-being than the smooth running of a bodily machine, and offers encouragement to those health professionals who wish to take a broad view of their patients' well-being and to collaborate with others in the work of healing.

However, as many critics have pointed out, this definition is by no means without its problems. Indeed, some years ago Daniel Callahan wryly observed that one of the best games in medical ethics was 'that version of king-of-the-hill where the aim of all players is to upset the [WHO] definition of "health" '.[23] The WHO definition equates health with complete human well-being, and as such not only makes a claim about the nature of health, but also implies an understanding of what is meant by well-being. By using Paul's thorn in the flesh as a test case, I shall argue that this definition expresses too *narrow* an understanding of human well-being, but too *wide* a concept of health.

As Paul tells the story of his thorn, he seems to understand it to have had a positive outcome (to use a piece of modern jargon). But this positive outcome cannot be stated primarily in terms of physical, mental or social well-being.[24] In physical terms, he

---

[20] Reproduced on the WHO website, <http://www.who.int/aboutwho/en/definition.html> (accessed 26 April 2002).

[21] D. Callahan, 'The WHO Definition of "Health"', *Hastings Center Studies* 1.3 (1973), pp. 77–87; reproduced in S.E. Lammers and A. Verhey (eds), *On Moral Medicine: Theological Perspectives in Medical Ethics*, 2nd edn (Grand Rapids: Eerdmans, 1998), pp. 253–61.

[22] J. Wilkinson, *The Bible and Healing: A Medical and Theological Commentary* (Edinburgh: Handsel Press; Grand Rapids: Eerdmans, 1998), pp. 11–13, 19.

[23] Callahan, 'The WHO Definition of "Health"', p. 253.

[24] In the following argument, I am assuming as I did earlier that Paul's thorn is a physical condition, perhaps visual impairment; however, the argument would still hold good, *mutatis mutandis*, if the thorn were a non-physical condition such as a mental illness or persistent temptation.

continues to be 'battered' by the thorn, and as for social well-being, he does not seem to find it any easier to get on harmoniously with the Corinthians. While he has achieved a measure of contentment which might be described as mental well-being, this seems to be a by-product of the main 'positive outcome' of the episode: that he has learned to place his hope and trust more firmly in God's grace, and has discovered that even (perhaps especially) when he is at his very weakest, God's strength and unfailing care are more than sufficient to sustain him. In other words, the well-being that Paul has found through this episode is first and foremost that of right relationship to God: a relationship characterized by faith, hope and trust in God's love made known in Christ. This is a kind of well-being of which the WHO definition has difficulty giving an account. To be sure, more recent WHO policy has included some notion of spiritual well-being. For example, the September 2001 *International Classification of Functioning, Disability and Health* includes a reference to 'Religion and Spirituality'. But this is included as one sub-heading under 'Community, Social and Civic Life', and is defined in a somewhat phenomenological tone as

> [e]ngaging in religious or spiritual activities, organizations and practices for self-fulfilment, finding meaning, religious or spiritual value and establishing connection with a divine power, such as is involved in attending a church, temple, mosque or synagogue, praying or chanting for a religious purpose, and spiritual contemplation.[25]

It seems, to put it mildly, rather a weak description of Paul's story to say that he found meaning, religious or spiritual value and established connection with a divine power.

This is by no means to criticize the WHO: it is a welcome development that 'religion and spirituality' is part of the picture of human functioning, and it is hard to imagine how a secular and international organization like the WHO could have done more, or differently. It is simply to say that if we seek to give a Christian account of human flourishing, the WHO definition (*pace* Wilkinson) will not prove to be a summary that does justice to the distinctive sources of Christian faith.

---

[25] World Health Organization, *International Classification of Functioning, Health and Disability* (September 2001), <http://www3.who.int/icf/icftemplate.cfm> (accessed 26 April 2002).

If the WHO definition of health expresses too *narrow* an understanding of human well-being, it has often been said by Christians and others that as a definition of *health,* it is far too wide-ranging – perhaps dangerously so. Callahan points out that by assimilating all human well-being to the concept of health, the WHO definition 'by implication ... makes the medical profession the gatekeeper for happiness and social well-being', and encourages us to seek technological solutions for all kinds of human ills.[26] Taken to its conclusion in relation to the Human Genome Project, this understanding of health would collapse the distinction between genetic therapy and enhancement, and would encourage us to use genetic manipulation, if we could do so effectively and safely, to address any kind of social ill.

Callahan identifies two contrasting but interrelated dangers for the public at large in this development. First, if all suffering and disorder (including social and communal disorder) is classified as a problem of health, it becomes all too easy to describe anyone who contributes to such disorder (which ultimately means all of us) as 'sick'. But as sociologists of health observe, in the 'sick role' one's moral obligations and responsibilities alter so that one may not be held responsible for behaviour which would normally be considered reprehensible.[27] Therefore, if the language of health and sickness is stretched to include social and communal disorder, it may become difficult to speak of our own or others' moral responsibility for the well-being of our community and world. The second danger that Callahan identifies is the other side of the same coin: if health is understood in such a wide-ranging way, it becomes crucial for the survival and well-being of a society that all of its members are 'healthy' in this comprehensive sense. A 'tyranny of health' may then develop in which health becomes a moral and societal obligation, and a society through its health professionals adopts highly coercive policies towards those judged to be 'sick'.[28]

---

[26] Callahan, 'The WHO Definition of "Health"', pp. 256–7.

[27] Cf. at note 11 above.

[28] Callahan, 'The WHO Definition of "Health"', pp. 257–8. Hare's example, alluded to earlier, of the psychiatric 'treatment' of political dissidents in repressive regimes is one extreme instance of this problem, but the questions which are aired from time to time in Britain about the confinement of dangerous offenders

Using Paul's thorn in the flesh as a test case for our understandings of health, a further reason emerges to object to the all-embracing nature of the WHO definition. As Stephen Lammers and Allen Verhey point out, 'if health and human flourishing are rendered equivalent, then we will have lost the capacity to weigh the good of health against other goods'.[29] And if we lose this capacity, Paul's experience – that he is content even in his suffering and weakness because they have been the occasion for him to discover the far greater good of dependence on the strength of Christ – will be unintelligible to us.

Barth on health and disease

Perhaps a more promising approach can be found in Karl Barth's long and subtle discussion of health,[30] which, as Lammers and Verhey observe, 'may be regarded as an extended commentary on these words of Paul'.[31] Barth's account of health forms part of his exposition of 'the command of God the creator' (p. 324): we are called, first, into relationship with God, and, second, into relationship with one another; but there is also a necessary 'third dimension' to this command: 'Obedience to the command of God the creator is also quite simply man's freedom to exist as a living being of this particular, i.e. human, structure' (p. 324). We obey God's command by being the creatures God has made us – by living a human life. This life is a loan from God: in a very important sense, our life is not our own, but God's. Respect for life, according to Barth, should be based on this understanding. Now he is careful to remember that, as he puts it, 'the biblical message is concerned with the *eternal* life of man' (p. 338, emphasis added); but

---

in special hospitals illustrate that these difficult and complex issues are of concern in democratic societies as well as dictatorships. For another trenchant critique of the tendency to hand responsibility for health over to the professionals, see I. Illich, *Limits To Medicine: Medical Nemesis – The Expropriation of Health* (London: Marion Boyars, 1995).

[29] Lammers and Verhey, *On Moral Medicine*, p. 239.

[30] K. Barth, *Church Dogmatics* III/4, §55.1, trans. A.T. Mackay *et al.* (Edinburgh: T & T Clark, 1961). Page numbers in brackets in the following paragraphs refer to this work.

[31] Lammers and Verhey, *On Moral Medicine*, p. 239.

eternal life is still human life, and the hope of eternal life gives a proper value to this temporal life.

It is in this context that we must understand Barth's well-known definition of health: 'Health means capability, vigour and freedom. It is strength for human life. It is the integration of the organs for the exercise of psycho-physical functions' (p. 356). Health is the power to answer God's call to us to live a human life, and this power is itself a gift from God. Therefore, to 'will to be healthy' (p. 357 and *passim*) is both to accept God's gift with gratitude and to obey God's command. According to Barth, all of us, however healthy or sick we are (and as he recognizes, few if any of us are totally one or the other), can and should exercise the will to be healthy within the limits of our condition: 'even those who are seriously ill ... are commanded, and it is not too much to ask, that so long as they are alive they should will this, i.e., exercise the power which remains to them, in spite of every obstacle' (pp. 357–8).

If health has to do with God's call or command, then what are we to make of disease? Barth describes disease or sickness in negative terms, as 'the weakness opposed to this strength' (p. 363).[32] But although it is defined negatively in relation to health, sickness is nevertheless real and serious – it is by no means, as some have claimed, an illusion from which the truly spiritual person can be free (pp. 364–5).[33]

Barth says two things about sickness that may at first seem to contradict one another. First, it is related to sin and death, 'an element of the chaos threatening God's creation'; correspondingly, also, it is a sign of God's judgement on this sin and

---

[32] Barth uses *Krankheit* (rendered 'sickness' in the English translation) to refer in a general way to the opposite of *Gesundheit* or 'health'. He does not make a distinction corresponding to Boorse's between 'disease' and 'illness' ('What a Theory of Mental Health Should Be', pp. 62–3); nor does his use of *Krankheit* correspond to the current use of 'sickness' to denote the sociological phenomenon alluded to at note 26 above, whereby a person is assigned to a particular social role which carries altered expectations and responsibilities. For this differentiation between 'disease', 'illness' and 'sickness', see further S. Pattison, *Alive and Kicking: Towards a Practical Theology of Illness and Healing* (London: SCM Press, 1989), ch. 1. In the following discussion I shall for the most part follow Barth's English translators in using 'sickness' in the general sense of 'the opposite of health', not in the specific sociological sense defined by Pattison. I am grateful to Dr Kathy Ehrensperger for checking the German text of *Kirchliche Dogmatik* III/4 for me.

[33] Here Barth takes issue with Mary Baker Eddy, the nineteenth-century founder of 'Christian Science'.

chaos (pp. 366ff., though as far as I can tell, Barth does *not* mean that diseases are to be understood as God's punishment of individuals for specific sins). Unlikely as it may initially seem, there is good news in this understanding, since God in Christ has already acted to overcome the forces of chaos and evil. This is the significance of Jesus' healing miracles in the synoptic Gospels, which may be understood as signs of God's kingdom breaking into human life and history and overcoming the power of sin and death. If God has shown his faithfulness to us in this way, says Barth, our properly faithful response must be to resist sickness and exercise the will to be healthy with whatever power remains to us.

Before moving on to Barth's second point about sickness, one difficulty must be faced. The call to resist sickness and exercise the will to be healthy seems to be addressed to people who have enough power to exercise some measure of control or will over their own lives. But might there not be people who have been so seriously oppressed or damaged by others, and rendered so powerless, that to exercise the 'will to be healthy' is too much to ask – for example, women or children who have been terribly abused?[34] Barth does not address this question directly, but he does ask whether sickness may not prove so overwhelming a power that any attempt to 'will to be healthy' is simply futile:

> What is man with his health and will for health in face of the invasion of the realm of death to which he himself has deliberately opened the defences? . . . What is there left to will? Strength to be as man? Psycho-physical powers? Is it not almost grotesque from this standpoint to try even to think of a human determination, let alone of human measures, along the lines considered? Are not faith and prayer the only real possibilities in face of this reality of sickness? (p. 367)

His forthright rejection of this view as 'defeatist thinking, and not at all Christian' (p. 367) may not initially seem very

---

[34] I am grateful to the Revd Eve Rose for raising this question with me. It reflects a wider-ranging feminist and womanist critique exemplified by Katie Geneva Cannon, that traditional ethics was written by and for people with power (often socially privileged white men), and is of little use to people with little or no power to determine their own lives and actions (such as, in Cannon's account, African American women during and after the time of slavery). See K. G. Cannon, *Black Womanist Ethics* (Atlanta: Scholars Press, 1988).

promising for those who have been rendered powerless, or nearly so, by the sins of others. But we should recall why he is able to say this: God in Christ has overcome the forces of evil and sickness, and therefore we know that when we will to be healthy, we are willing 'what God has already willed' (p. 368). And for any of us, powerful or powerless, the 'strength for human life' is God's gracious gift, as we noted earlier. When someone has been rendered so powerless that to will to be healthy seems difficult or impossible, part of the work of healing must surely be to enable him or her to find the strength to will what God has already willed – strength that, however mediated through human agency, has its ultimate source in God's love.

Moreover, Barth explicitly recognizes that health and the will to be healthy are not merely individual, but social and structural questions. With relentless logic, he follows through the radical social and political implications of this insight:

> The will for health of the individual must therefore also take the form of the will to improve, raise and perhaps radically transform the general living conditions of all men. If there is no other way, it must assume the form of the will for a new and quite different order of society, guaranteeing better living conditions for all. Where some are necessarily ill, the others cannot in good conscience will to be well. (p. 363)

Mutatis mutandis, the will to be healthy requires all of us to work for individual relationships and social structures in which no-one is rendered so powerless as to be unable to exercise this will for themselves and others.

To recapitulate, the first thing Barth has said about sickness is that it is a result of the world's alienation from God, a sign of God's judgement on the world and a realm of disorder which God has already fought and overcome in Christ; therefore, to will to be healthy is to 'will what God has already willed'. But, second, he says, our present life and health are not eternal, but 'temporal and therefore ... limited possession[s]' (p. 371). Sickness may perhaps be a way in which we can discover our limitation and weakness, and in making this discovery, can also find that 'Christ will be our consolation' (pp. 373f.).[35] Barth

---

[35] In this connection, he quotes Psalm 90.12, 'So teach us to number our days that we may apply our hearts unto wisdom.'

insists that there is no question of setting aside the first view, or capitulating to sickness. But even in suffering and dying, we can discover 'a form of the creative goodness of God beyond death and judgment, of the objectively near promise of His free grace' (p. 374).

By holding in tension these two understandings of sickness, Barth offers an account that can do justice to the complexity, ambiguity and paradox which we have found in Paul's experience of his thorn in the flesh. He helps us to understand that health is a real and precious good, but not the only or the ultimate good; that sickness and physical suffering are real and sometimes terrible torments, signs that the created order is badly astray from God's loving purposes, yet that they can at the same time be occasions for people to discover the goodness and love of God; that the relationship between power and weakness, suffering and success is so complex as to defy easy description.

John Hull expresses something of this mystery and paradox in reflecting on his experience of blindness. In his book *In the Beginning There Was Darkness*, he reproduces a distressingly insensitive letter he received inviting him to seek miraculous healing of his blindness, and to encourage other 'needy and abnormal' (*sic*) people to do likewise. He then gives the letter he wrote in reply, part of which reads:

> you describe me as being needy and afflicted ... However, I do not interpret my blindness as an affliction, but as a strange, dark and mysterious gift from God. Indeed, in many ways it is a gift that I would rather not have been given and one that I would not wish my friends or my children to have. Nevertheless, it is a kind of gift. I have learned that since I have passed beyond light and darkness, the image of God rests upon my blindness ... I am a Christian like yourself. My Christian life has deepened since I lost my sight. This loss has helped me to think through many of my values in living, and in a way I have learned a greater degree of intimacy with God.[36]

Conclusion

By using Paul's thorn in the flesh as a test case, I have argued that both the medical model, with its precise, narrow and purportedly objective definitions of health and disease, and the

---

[36] Hull, *In the Beginning*, pp. 46–8.

WHO definition of health, as complete human well-being, are theologically inadequate for the task of giving an account of health and disease that will enable us to address the questions raised by the Human Genome Project. I have argued that Karl Barth's account does greater justice to the mystery and paradox with which Paul's story of the thorn is shot through – mystery and paradox echoed in John Hull's reflections on his experience of blindness. If I am right that the most theologically adequate account of health and disease is one that is irreducibly paradoxical and ambiguous, then there will be no clear procedure for distinguishing between disease and 'normal' human diversity: the conditions of all our lives are a curious mixture of suffering and strength, and a particular experience may be at one and the same time both an occasion of suffering and a 'dark and mysterious gift', in Hull's words.

Nor is there likely to be any clear and unambiguous procedure for deciding when and how to intervene medically and when to refrain. This is borne out by the experience of pre-natal testing for Down's syndrome, a well-established procedure in clinical genetics.[37] It is standard clinical practice that the parents-to-be rather than clinical staff make the decision whether to have a pre-natal test, and if it proves positive, whether the pregnancy should be terminated. Yet what appears to be an individual, autonomous decision of parents takes place in a wider medical and social context. Parents only have these decisions to make because researchers and clinicians have developed techniques for pre-natal diagnosis and because the law allows the termination of pregnancies on medical grounds.[38] Some parents report that they are strongly advised to

---

[37] I am grateful to my fellow participants in the colloquium, particularly Mary Sellar, Ruth Page, Celia Deane-Drummond, Bron Szerszynski and Robert Song, for much of the information, experience and argumentation in this paragraph.

[38] In many areas of medicine, decisions about when to treat and when to refrain are made *de facto* by governments, regulatory authorities or funding agencies. For example, in May 1999, Frank Dobson, then UK Secretary of State for Health, announced that the anti-impotence drug Viagra would only be available through the National Health Service to men whose impotence was caused by one of twelve specified medical conditions which between them account for only 20 per cent of cases of impotence: A. Ferriman, 'UK Government Finalises Restrictions on Viagra Prescribing', *British Medical Journal* 318 (15 May 1999), p. 1305. Obviously, economic as well as philosophical, scientific and clinical criteria influence such decisions. This is particularly clear in systems where much healthcare provision is by commercial organizations: see H.O.J. Brown, 'A Patient's Experience', in

have a pre-natal test: if they refuse, their decision is respected, but considered odd, by clinical staff. Furthermore, the attitudes of both parents and clinical staff are inevitably shaped, whether they realize it or not, by the wider community or culture to which they belong: it is sometimes observed that some cultures and ethnic communities are more accepting than others of disabilities, and that this may be a factor in the lower take-up of genetic services in those communities.[39] And it is questionable whether such decisions can be regarded as wholly private, individual decisions, since they have both future implications and wider social effects.[40]

In other words, even what appears at first to be a simple decision-making process – for example, that decisions about pre-natal testing and termination of pregnancy should be made by the parents with appropriate information and support from clinical staff – turns out to be a much more complex process which necessarily involves explicit or implicit assumptions about health, disease, diversity and suffering. These assumptions are shaped by the overlapping contexts (such as the familial, clinical and wider social contexts) in which the individual decision is made; but the decision that is made also changes those contexts and makes its own contribution to the shaping of future decisions.

All this is to reinforce what I have already argued: that it is almost certainly impossible to spell out a simple procedure for

---

J.F. Kilner, R.D. Orr and J.A. Shelly (eds), *The Changing Face of Health Care: A Christian Appraisal of Managed Care, Resource Allocation and Patient–Caregiver Relationships* (Grand Rapids: Eerdmans; Cambridge: Paternoster, 1998), pp. 10–16.

[39] This suggestion is made with reference to the African-American community by M.B. Mahowald, *Genes, Women, Equality* (New York and Oxford: Oxford University Press, 2000), pp. 108–12. Note, however, that many other factors may play a part, such as socioeconomic disadvantage with corresponding lack of access to health services, and mistrust of the medical system engendered by past experiences of discrimination and prejudice: see Mahowald, ibid., and J. Telfair and K.B. Nash, 'African American Culture', in N.L. Fisher (ed.), *Cultural and Ethnic Diversity: A Guide for Genetics Professionals* (Baltimore and London: Johns Hopkins University Press, 1996), pp. 36–59. My thanks to Robert Song for these references.

[40] I owe this point to Bron Szerszynski, who suggests that the shape of the clinical encounter may 'construct' parents-to-be in this situation as individuals making private choices, by analogy with Michel Foucault's claim that the practice of the confessional played a key role in constructing an interior life or discourse of 'sexuality': M. Foucault, *The History of Sexuality*: vol. I: *An Introduction*, trans. R. Hurley (London: Allen Lane, 1979).

understanding the meaning and significance of an individual's condition. Nor is it likely to be possible to write an adequate algorithm or step-by-step process for deciding when and how it is right to intervene medically in that individual's condition and when to refrain. Such understanding and decision-making calls for a complex and subtle kind of discernment that requires the exercise of the virtue known as 'prudence' or 'practical wisdom' (Gk. *phronēsis*). This virtue is famously expounded by Thomas Aquinas in the *Summa Theologia*:[41] for Thomas, in Jean Porter's words, 'prudence determines which courses of activity and specific actions would instantiate the virtues in the specific situations that make up our lives'.[42] Porter goes on to argue that prudence is needed to give substance to the first principle of practical reason (that good is to be done and evil to be avoided). While this principle, according to Thomas, is self-evidently true, its substantive content is not self-evident, because a concrete and specific account of the human good would be required in order to specify the outworking of the first principle in a particular situation. Prudence supplies this account in a particular context, 'determin[ing] what amounts to a substantive theory of the human good, at least as it applies to this individual in his particular setting'.[43] Furthermore, in his account of 'political prudence' Thomas emphasizes that prudence is not only concerned with the good of the individual, but also with the common good; thus there is a communal dimension to the determination of what the human good means in particular concrete situations.[44]

Stanley Hauerwas has frequently emphasized that the right discernment and practice of the virtues requires a 'community of character' whose identity and common life are shaped by a particular narrative.[45] Thus both the understanding and the practice of Christian virtue depend crucially on the Church,

---

[41] See especially Thomas Aquinas, *Summa Theologiae* II–II, Q47.
[42] J. Porter, *The Recovery of Virtue: The Relevance of Aquinas for Christian Ethics* (London: SPCK, 1994), p. 159.
[43] Porter, *The Recovery of Virtue*, p. 162.
[44] Thomas Aquinas, *Summa Theologiae* II–II, Q47, arts. 10–12. See Porter, *The Recovery of Virtue*, pp. 162–5, and C. Deane-Drummond, *Creation Through Wisdom: Theology and the New Biology* (Edinburgh: T & T Clark, 2000), pp. 99–107.
[45] See e.g. S. Hauerwas, *A Community of Character: Towards a Constructive Christian Social Ethic* (Notre Dame: University of Notre Dame Press, 1981). For a critique, see Porter, *The Recovery of Virtue*, pp. 28–31.

called to be a 'community of character' which trains its members in the discernment and practice of virtue by repeatedly retelling and participating in its distinctive narrative, by enabling the development of virtuous habits and by providing saints (both famous and obscure) as 'significant examples' of Christian living.[46]

If Hauerwas is right, then Christians who wish to discern the significance of someone's condition and the appropriate response to it in a theologically adequate way cannot do without the Church. This claim is beautifully illustrated by Hauerwas and William Willimon's story of Dorothy:

> In the church where one of us was raised, Dorothy was a perpetual member of the third grade church school class . . . She had even been in the class when some of our parents were in the third grade. Dorothy was in charge of handing out pencils, checking names in the roll book, and taking up the pencils. It was much later, when we were nearly all grown up and adult, that the world told us that Dorothy was someone with Down syndrome. At the church, we were under the impression that Dorothy was the teacher's assistant. When Dorothy died, in her early fifties – a spectacularly long life for someone with Down syndrome – the whole church turned out for her funeral. No one mentioned that Dorothy was retarded or afflicted. Many testified to how fortunate they had been to know her.[47]

Hauerwas and Willimon connect Dorothy's story with the episode in Matthew's Gospel in which the disciples ask Jesus who is the greatest in the kingdom of heaven; Jesus replies by placing a child among them and saying, 'Whoever becomes humble like this child is the greatest in the kingdom of heaven' (Matthew 18.1–4). They continue:

> In placing Dorothy, someone quite insignificant and problematic for the world, in the middle of the third grade Sunday school class, Buncome Street Church was reenacting Matthew 18:1–4 and practicing ethics in the ordinary, unspectacular yet profound and revolutionary way the church practices ethics.[48]

My purpose in reproducing this story is not primarily to argue that the world regards Down's syndrome as an illness but that

---

[46] For 'saints as significant examples', see S. Hauerwas and W.H. Willimon, *Resident Aliens: Life in the Christian Colony* (Nashville: Abingdon Press, 1989), pp. 98–103.
[47] Ibid., p. 93.
[48] Ibid., p. 97.

the Church should not – though something like that may well
be true. It is rather to illustrate Hauerwas and Willimon's point
that

> ethics is first a way of *seeing* before it is a matter of *doing*. The ethical
> task is not to tell you what is right or wrong but rather to train you
> to see. That explains why, in the church, a great deal of time and
> energy are spent in the act of worship: In worship, we are busy
> looking in the right direction.[49]

Allowing for some possible hyperbole, this statement and the
story which illustrates it seem to me to express something very
important about a Christian response to health, disease and
diversity. If we are to respond to these phenomena in a way that
does justice both to them and to the distinctive sources of
Christian faith, we will need to be trained, by participation in
the life and worship of the Church, to 'see' Down's syndrome,
visual impairment and so on truly – or more accurately, to 'see'
truly the concrete instances of Down's syndrome, visual
impairment and so on in the individual and unique lives which
they play a part in shaping. If we learn to 'see' them truly, we
will have some hope of responding to them well, as Buncome
Street Church did to Dorothy.[50]

In short, I have argued that an adequately Christian account
of health, disease and diversity is so laden with paradox and
ambiguity as to make it impossible to set out, in general and in
advance of particular cases, procedures for distinguishing
between disease and diversity and for determining the appropriate response to each. To understand a person's condition
truly and to respond rightly require a kind of discernment
which cannot be fully described in the abstract, but must be
learned through the training in 'seeing' and living which the
Church is called to supply. In other words, my argument tends

---

[49] Ibid., p. 95 (italics original).

[50] This kind of claim has laid Hauerwas open to accusations of naivety, since his
account of the Church can seem somewhat unreal and detached from real
churches, which often seem to make a poorer job of 'seeing' truly and responding
well than the secular society around them. But he is more aware of this difficulty
than his critics sometimes give him credit for: for example, he comments that 'I
find I must think and write not only for the church that does exist but for the
church that should exist if we were more courageous and faithful' (*A Community
of Character*, p. 6). For a sympathetic but critical insight into the ongoing difficulties with Hauerwas's presentation of the Church, see R.B. Hays, *The Moral
Vision of the New Testament* (Edinburgh: T & T Clark, 1997), pp. 264–6.

to support Hauerwas's oft-repeated claim that, both to support its practice and to render it intelligible, medicine needs a community very like the Church.[51] This needs to be said of our attempts to discern how to use well our knowledge of the human genome, no less than it does of any other area of medical understanding and practice.

Bibliography

Barrett, C.K., *The Second Epistle to the Corinthians* (London: A & C Black, 1973).

Barth, K., *Church Dogmatics* III/4, tr. A.T. Mackay *et al.* (Edinburgh: T & T Clark, 1961).

Boorse, C., 'What a Theory of Mental Health Should Be', *Journal for the Theory of Social Behaviour* 6 (1976), pp. 61–84.

Boyd, K.M., 'Disease, Illness, Sickness, Health, Healing and Wholeness: Exploring Some Elusive Concepts', *Journal of Medical Ethics: Medical Humanities* 26 (2000), pp. 9–17.

British Deaf Association, *The British Deaf Association Policy on Cochlear Implants*, <http://www.britishdeafassociation.org.uk/cochlearpolicyfull.html> (accessed 15 February 2002).

Brown, H.O.J. 'A Patient's Experience', in J.F. Kilner, R.D. Orr and J.A. Shelly (eds), *The Changing Face of Health Care: A Christian Appraisal of Managed Care, Resource Allocation and Patient–Caregiver Relationships* (Grand Rapids: Eerdmans; Cambridge: Paternoster, 1998), pp. 10–16.

Callahan, D., 'The WHO Definition of "Health"', *Hastings Center Studies* 1.3 (1973), pp. 77–87; reproduced in S.E. Lammers and A. Verhey (eds), *On Moral Medicine: Theological Perspectives in Medical Ethics*, 2nd edn (Grand Rapids: Eerdmans, 1998), pp. 253–61.

Cannon, K.G., *Black Womanist Ethics* (Atlanta: Scholars Press, 1988).

Deane-Drummond, C., *Creation Through Wisdom: Theology and the New Biology* (Edinburgh: T & T Clark, 2000).

Ferriman, A., 'UK Government Finalises Restrictions on Viagra

---

[51] See Hauerwas, 'Salvation and Health: Why Medicine Needs the Church', in *Suffering Presence*, pp. 63–83.

Prescribing', *British Medical Journal* 318 (15 May 1999), p. 1305.

Foucault, M., *The History of Sexuality*, vol. I: *An Introduction*, trans. R. Hurley (London: Allen Lane, 1979).

Hare, R.M., 'Health', *Journal of Medical Ethics* 12 (1986), pp. 174–81.

Hauerwas, S., *A Community of Character: Towards a Constructive Christian Social Ethic* (Notre Dame: University of Notre Dame Press, 1981).

Hauerwas, S. *Suffering Presence: Theological Reflections on Medicine, the Mentally Handicapped and the Church* (Edinburgh: T & T Clark, 1988).

Hauerwas S. and Willimon, W.H., *Resident Aliens: Life in the Christian Colony* (Nashville: Abingdon Press, 1989).

Hays, R.B., *The Moral Vision of the New Testament* (Edinburgh: T & T Clark, 1997).

Hull, J.M., *In the Beginning There was Darkness: A Blind Person's Conversations with the Bible* (London: SCM Press, 2001).

Illich, I., *Limits To Medicine: Medical Nemesis – The Expropriation of Health* (London: Marion Boyars, 1995).

Lammers, S.E. and Verhey, A. (eds), *On Moral Medicine: Theological Perspectives in Medical Ethics*, 2nd edn (Grand Rapids: Eerdmans, 1998).

Mahowald, M.B., *Genes, Women, Equality* (New York and Oxford: Oxford University Press, 2000).

Messer, N.G., 'Human Cloning and Genetic Manipulation: Some Theological and Ethical Issues', *Studies in Christian Ethics* 12.2 (1999), pp. 1–16.

Messer, N.G., 'Human Genetics and the Image of the Triune God', *Science and Christian Belief* 13.2 (2001), pp. 99–111.

Messer N.G. (ed.), *Theological Issues in Bioethics: An Introductory Reader* (London: Darton, Longman & Todd, 2002).

Pattison, S., *Alive and Kicking: Towards a Practical Theology of Illness and Healing* (London: SCM Press, 1989).

Porter, J., *The Recovery of Virtue: The Relevance of Aquinas for Christian Ethics* (London: SPCK, 1994).

Ramsden, R. and Graham, J., 'Cochlear Implantation', *British Medical Journal* 311 (1995), p. 1588.

Telfair, J. and Nash, K.B., 'African American Culture', in N.L. Fisher (ed.), *Cultural and Ethnic Diversity: A Guide for Genetics Professionals* (Baltimore and London: Johns Hopkins University Press, 1996), pp. 36–59.

Thomas Aquinas, *Summa Theologiae* II–II, Q47.

Thrall, M.E., *A Critical and Exegetical Commentary on the Second Epistle to the Corinthians*, vol. ii (Edinburgh: T & T Clark, 2000).

Wilkinson, J., *The Bible and Healing: A Medical and Theological Commentary* (Edinburgh: Handsel Press; Grand Rapids: Eerdmans, 1998).

World Health Organization website, <http://www.who.int/aboutwho/en/definition.html> (accessed 26 April 2002).

World Health Organization, *International Classification of Functioning, Health and Disability* (September 2001), <http://www3.who.int/icf/icftemplate.cfm> (accessed 26 April 2002).

6

Genes and the Self: Anthropological Questions to the Human Genome Project

Maureen Junker-Kenny

Questioning implicit norms in the Human Genome Project (HGP) presupposes a vantage point from which certain assumptions can be recognized as hidden norms and evaluated. The critical backdrop against which the HGP has to be assessed is, in my proposal, the understanding of self, intersubjectivity and society based on the concepts of freedom and justice as it has been worked out in philosophical anthropology. Besides its antique Greek and Christian heritage it shows the traces of historical struggles for the equal dignity of every human being, regardless of natural endowment or social position, sex or age. As a philosophical discipline, it is based on self-reflection and life experience, not on detached empirical observation. It investigates how the basic human condition marked by invariant features, such as language, sociability, agency, embodiment, and finitude, finds expression in different historical life-forms and constructions of the place of the human in nature and society.[1] While the very nature of its theme, the struggle between interpretations of the mystery of being human, means that it can never be concluded in one unified theory, its reality is not limited to seminar discussions. Insofar as the normative concept of human dignity has become institutionalized in the UN Declaration of Human Rights, in EU conventions as well as

[1] Cf. R. Wimmer, 'Anfragen an die Integrative Ethik Hans Krämers aus philosophisch-anthropologischer Perspektive', in M. Endreß (ed.), *Zur Grundlegung einer integrativen Ethik* (Frankfurt: Suhrkamp, 1997), pp. 56–72, pp. 67–8.

116

in many national Constitutions, the philosophical anthropology in which it is rooted exists and offers resources for the interpretation of 'dignity' in new situations.

What are the implications of the HGP, both in its basic assumptions and its possible applications, for human dignity? Any assessment of this question will have to include considerations on the kind of knowledge that the HGP provides (section 1) and the ways in which the HGP, or more generally, the 'genetic paradigm', affect our image of the human person. I want to explore especially the danger of scientific naturalism, the standards for defining normality, health, illness, and suffering, as well as the implicit assumption that our individual lives will flourish once we are able to mend and enhance our genes to suit our life projects (section 2). I will, third, try to identify which aspects of the HGP have a specifically theological significance. What is called for is a distinctively Christian response that can nonetheless be mediated in the public forum (section 3). In this way, Christian ethics will contribute to identifying and renewing resources for a public morality in civil society. Yet resources need structures, ideas institutions; relevant links need to be established between civil society and its agents, including the churches and affected groups and individuals, the various expert cultures (scientific, legal, ethical), and politics. The need for such an institutionalization of ethics is obvious in a situation where science is a major factor for economic growth, but its consequences on our life-world are seen to be ambivalent and contradictory.[2] Do the assumptions that carry our everyday self-understanding – a concept of human nature, accountability, the human dignity of every human being, mutual and anticipatory recognition, solidarity with the weaker, spontaneity and an open future as elements of a flourishing life and community – have to be reassessed and

---

[2] Examples of this ambivalence are hopes for prevention and cure over against the fear of losing the sense of an open future by being diagnosed with genetic predispositions to diseases that still remain untreatable; gains in rational life-planning from knowing one's personal genetic status, yet being saddled with the burden of proof of risk-free insurability and employability; the individualization of healthcare and prevention based on one's personal gene profile, over against a new social ideal of genetic perfection coupled with the risk of the rise of a two-class society of the 'genetically endowed' versus the 'genetically flawed'; the justification of the $3 billion research funds spent by the high aim of hoped-for therapies, over against monopolies for biotechnological companies on possible cures secured by patenting legislation.

modified in the light of new genetic possibilities? Or do they have to be defended against new forms and qualities of domination and exclusion, control and social engineering, streamlining and reduction that arise in the attempt to harness the molecular basis of our physical lives?

It is becoming increasingly clear that the 'application of biotechnology concerns basic moral questions of our future and the power to shape them ... Bioethics should be part of a political ethics of institutions.'[3] Christian ethics can contribute its specific insights to this discourse and help restore ethics as the discipline of argumentation on matters of conflict against the political temptation to mere 'consensus management'.[4]

1   Scientific insights and ethical conclusions

Two scientific insights that have received great attention because of their relevance for our self-understanding as persons are the number of genes (a), and their diversity (b).

(a) It was a surprise to find that the number of human genes turned out to be not 80–100,000, as expected, but just 30–40,000.[5] Thus, the distinction of humans from other living entities could not lie in the number of genes. We 'share many gene sequences with other living beings. We discover ourselves as genetic relatives of baker's yeast and the fruitfly. 99% of our gene sequences are identical with those of the chimpanzee.'[6] So what is the reason for our difference?

---

[3] D. Mieth, *Die Diktatur der Gene* (Freiburg: Herder, 2001), p. 7. All translations from books and articles in German are my own.

[4] 'Pragmaticians like to sacrifice debate and search with statistical means for the "overlapping consensus" or the mere minimal consensus. But one does not need ethics for that. Consensus management ultimately gives social scientific descriptions of moralities the privilege of regulating their relations' (Mieth, *Diktatur der Gene*, p. 37).

[5] I am leaving aside the question whether 'genes' constitute separate and stable entities of any kind, or whether they are a scientific hypothesis or substantializing projection that posits a basis for certain effects. L. Honnefelder quotes the molecular biologist W. Gelbart's statement that 'contrary to chromosomes genes are not material objects but merely concepts that have acquired a lot of historical baggage (*Ballast*) in the last few decades' (p. 15). C. Deane-Drummond speaks of 'regions of nuclear acids that may be activated at different times'. The terms used to describe their function are metaphors from human interaction, such as 'information', 'command', and 'code'. The uncertain epistemological status of the concept of 'gene' in the following summary of results has to be kept in mind.

[6] L. Honnefelder, 'Einführung', in L. Honnefelder and P. Propping (eds), *Was wissen wir, wenn wir das menschliche Genom kennen?* (Köln: Dumont, 2001), pp. 9–25, p. 11.

Decisive is not the (finite) number of genes but the complexity of their multiple interactions. Researchers do not get one gene with a predictable effect; there are networks of interacting genes which have a cumulative effect. D. Mieth concludes that the wealth of data gained on the one hand only indicates the poverty of our knowledge on the other: 'Genetics as knowledge is ... both a place of triumph and a place of modesty.'[7]

> The *genome* is matched by a *proteome* that is 10–100 times bigger, which itself is only a partial factor in the *physiome* the size of which cannot even be estimated. Which sequences have to be related to which functions, can only be found through the complete analysis of the interconnection of genome, proteome, and physiome.[8]

How the organism reacts with the outside world is a further question. And the decisive philosophical enquiry only begins here: whether it is justified in the face of all these predetermining interactions still to assume the freedom to act and to take a stand towards, for example, one's various genetic and other predispositions. But independent from this principal debate, the scientific insight that there is no 1:1, 1 gene = 1 trait, relationship, but that one gene carries several informations is ethically relevant: if all one may be able to do is to 'disturb the complexity of reciprocal effects', instead of being able to modify features directly, the first ethical conclusion is to advise the scientific community to decide not to interfere with these networks. Researchers cannot oversee what effect their interventions would have on these complex connections and what unintended damage could be caused.[9]

So the very feasibility of an 'anthropotechnique', of the purposive elective breeding of a superman, which the philosopher Peter Sloterdijk demanded in 1999, is disputed. This has not stopped philosophers, cultural critics, and journalists debating the proposal as if it was a real possibility. Indeed, the question, 'Should we want such genetic self-designing?' needs to be discussed. What is at stake is the relationship between the two opposite poles of the human constitution: givenness and openness, nature and freedom: 'How can the

---

[7] Mieth, *Diktatur der Gene*, p. 12.
[8] Honnefelder, 'Einführung', p. 11.
[9] Ibid., p. 18.

balance be formulated between self-transcendence and embodiment, project-openness and predetermination, change
and maintaining identity?'[10]

(b) The second unexpected insight concerns the diversity
and lack of normality in the human genome. 'Genetic polymorphism is what is normal; every one deviates from the genetic
norm. Normality is really only statistical frequency. It is a
genetic variant in the frame of genetic variability in humans.'[11]
This finding, polymorphism, provides an argument from
science against genetic determinism.[12] It also leads to a second
ethical conclusion, namely the call to recognize instead of
pathologize diversity.

Results such as these should be welcomed not least for their
potential to chasten scientific objectivism and positivism already
on scientific grounds, not to mention philosophical ones. Yet
the scientists' public announcements of the significance of their
findings do not always reflect their awareness of the internal
limits posed by these insights for analysis and intervention,
medical diagnosis and therapy. John Sulston of the Sanger
Center in Cambridge, where a third of the human genome was
unravelled, declared: The point in human history has been
reached 'where for the first time we hold in our hands the set
of instructions to make a human being'.[13] Quite apart from the
initial exaggeration, as if the analysis could ever be concluded,
and the added hyperbole, as if the ability to analyse something
was the ability to construct it, this is a telling formulation:
'Making' indicates a relationship of domination, not of recognizing equally original freedom.To be made to someone else's
specifications violates the original equality of children with
their parents which is everybody's birth-right.[14]

Two further ethical insights from the debate concern
the inappropriateness of risk/benefit comparisons (c), and the

---

[10] Ibid., pp. 18–19.
[11] D. Lanzerath and L. Honnefelder, 'Krankheitsbegriff und ärztliche Anwendung',
in M. Düwell and D. Mieth (eds), *Ethik in der Humangenetik* (Tübingen: Francke,
1998), pp. 51–77, p. 66.
[12] Cf. Honnefelder, 'Einführung', p. 21.
[13] *Irish Times*, 1 July 2000.
[14] The formulation in the Creed, 'begotten, not made' that expresses Christ's being
of the same essence as the Father, has been aptly used by O. O'Donovan as the
title for his reflections on ethical issues in assisted reproduction: *Begotten or Made?*
(Oxford: Oxford University Press, 1984).

need for a sober analysis of the likelihood of designing therapies (d).

(c) A consequentialist risk analysis is not sufficient, even if already the pragmatic reason of inadmissible risk arising from the insight into the multiple interactions between genome, proteome and physiome counsels against any type of intervention. Since the reconstruction of these complex effects is an interminable task, the benefits envisioned are more a matter of luck than of predictably steady, straightforward progress in 'unravelling' the genome in its interaction with the physiome.

The ethical shortcomings of a risk/benefit balance are:

> It reduces the assessment of harms and gains to the narrow sphere of the patient–physician relationship and leaves the question of whether societal values, goods and rights could be endangered out of the picture. Being interest- , not dignity-oriented, it may harmonize conflicts of interest, e.g. between parents and children, or between currently suffering and future patients.

> It takes the goal for granted and only questions the intermediate steps for their safety. At most, it will reject the technology for the lack of controllability of these steps.

> As an empirical argumentation, it does not reach the level of an ethical analysis which needs the concept of human dignity as a marker of the non-instrumentalizability of one person by another. Thus, no reason can be given other than self-interest why risks should be excluded.

Thus, the evaluation of risks against benefits normally concentrates on the technology itself and does not include a genuinely ethical reflection on the values and historical achievements in human self-understanding and normative social relations that would have to be sacrificed for such technological advances. For a full assessment of the biomedical

---

[15] Julie Clague provides such a framework in her contribution to this volume (Chapter 9). It would be interesting to specify the concept of 'common good' by applying it to the idea of a life-world that embodies historically achieved standards of social interaction and cooperation, such as a concept of justice oriented towards including the most disadvantaged members of society, the equality and relationality between spouses, and parents' recognition of their perfect and imperfect duties to their children. On the way in which these duties may be rendered conditional by the move from a 'given' to a 'chosen' relationship through genetic selection, see O. O'Neill, 'The "Good Enough" Parent in the Age of the New Reproductive Technologies', in H. Haker and D. Beyleveld (eds), *The Ethics of Genetics in Human Procreation* (Aldershot: Ashgate, 2000), pp. 33–48.

principles of beneficence/maleficence, a social framework is needed.[15] D. Mieth calls for 'consensus formation to orient itself by the maximum of basic rights that is needed to have all human beings participate'. Against the seemingly 'unhaltable progress of knowledge to application not only a technology assessment, but a society assessment is needed, ... an evaluation that is directed in advance by basic values and basic rights. It establishes first of all what cannot be put into question by technological developments.' Thus, the 'effects of newly generated life worlds, e.g., in the information society, on private lives and structural questions' are taken into the balance before the projects are allowed to go ahead.[16] An evaluation can only be called ethical if it goes beyond an empirical risk/benefit calculation and is able to conceive of limits that can be drawn categorically.[17]

(d) The final point to check in argumentations is whether the promises held out are realistic, or whether hopes for cures continue to be treated as virtual realities, 'virtual' being understood not as merely fictitious, but as not yet realized, yet sure to come. D. Mieth speaks of the 'normative power of fiction',[18] observing that in the name of hoped-for cures for future patients, existing bearers of rights, such as embryos, or persons incapable of consent, are in danger of being sacrificed or subjected to research which is anything but therapeutic for them.

It is true that most human geneticists are not endorsing large-scale unspecific genetic enhancement; they are working hard to relieve future and present patients of the fate of horrifying illnesses. There is no need to doubt their good intentions. It is positive to be able to access conditions of illness also through genetic information. Nothing can be said against, but everything for, painstaking, patient research which keeps within the limits that can be ethically justified. The demand for strict justification of genetic intervention is all the more urgent in

---

[16] Cf. Mieth, *Diktatur der Gene*, p. 43.

[17] Honnefelder, 'Einführung', p. 23: 'Should germ-line interventions only be prohibited because up to now they carry incalculable risks, or are there limits to be drawn categorically in view of the experimentation on humans necessary for them and of the claims of future bearers of the modified genome?' Cf. M. Junker-Kenny, 'Categorical Arguments: Pro-Life Versus Pro-Choice?', in E. Hildt and S. Graumann (eds) *Genetics in Human Reproduction* (Aldershot: Ashgate, 1999), pp. 147–55.

[18] Mieth, *Diktatur der Gene*, p. 21.

view of the uncontrollable complexity of interacting factors which exacerbates the always existing conflict of interests between a clinician's role as physician and as researcher. Responsible care for an existing patient excludes human medical experimentation on which the hoped-for research insights for future patients may be based.

Yet, it needs to be kept in mind that 'unravelling' the genome, 'comparing health sequences to, e.g., cancerous ones, is not yet a cure'. Against the 'euphoric misunderstandings' of procedures called 'therapeutic' where 'the way is named after the goal', it should be admitted that 'in reality, help for the incurably ill ... is still in the stars, since not even the first beginnings of a causal gene therapy have been mastered. A responsibility argument would have to start out from the real technical possibilities and realistic prospects.' Instead, there are grounds for suspicion that legitimate hopes for cures are being instrumentalized to push through applications of genetic knowledge out of fear that this knowledge 'will turn old before it has returned the costs invested in it'.[19]

2 The 'geneticist paradigm' and the concept of the human person in philosophical and theological anthropology

We have seen that the HGP's major findings – first, that there is no direct causal relationship from gene to trait, but rather an infinite number of interactions between genome, proteome, physiome, and then between the organism and the environment to produce a trait, and, second, that diversity, not uniformity, is 'normal' – show the questionability of determinist interpretations; yet, the HGP implicitly, by its very research focus, tends to reduce the human person to the sum of her genes. It thus reinforces the existing division between two concepts of being human: one objectifying scientific, the other reflecting our everyday self-experience as 'self-interpreting animals'.[20] I want to treat three kinds of implicit norms associated with the HGP, even if they cannot be sustained by its very findings: the 'geneticist' paradigm, definitions of sickness,

---

[19] Ibid. pp. 56, 52.
[20] C. Taylor, 'Interpretation and the Sciences of Man', *Review of Metaphysics* 25 (1971), pp. 3–51. Reprinted in *Philosophy and the Human Sciences, Philosophical Papers 2* (Cambridge: Cambridge University Press, 1985).

and the idea behind enhancement, of matching one's genes to one's vision of an ideal life.

The 'geneticist' and the philosophical/theological images of the human person

'geneticist'	*philosophical/theological*
Scientistic objectifying	'self-interpreting animal'
predetermination	freedom
person = qualities of consciousness	person = self-reflective + relational
autonomy = ability to choose	autonomy = self-legislation – unconditional recognition of the other
agency	facticity, receptivity and agency
empirical concept of dignity	transcendental concept of dignity
progress + frontier mentality	human finitude
control	spontaneity
perfectibility	temptability, fallibility
eliminate suffering/potential sufferers	accept human fragility and inevitable suffering

In order to understand the above juxtaposition of catchwords that summarize two different perspectives on human personhood, it is important to keep in mind that the two organizing labels, 'geneticist' versus 'philosophical/theological', are to denote tendencies but not unified or coherent 'schools'. The first, 'geneticist', column includes both a neo-naturalist scientism,[21] and a non-deterministic but still reductionist philosophical account of personhood. The move in the interpretation of human personhood to 'qualities of consciousness' with its implicit segregation of mere 'human beings' from 'persons' (with its effect on rights to protection at the beginning and end of life and for people with mental impairments) begins with the

---

[21] In Chapter 13, Peter Scott speaks of 'scientific naturalism'; in Chapter 7, Bronislaw Szerszynski observes the reduction of 'essence', i.e. the 'opacity and open-endedness of the human', to 'behaviour' or a 'spatialized genetic code'.

philosopher John Locke. The emphasis on 'agency' in the first paradigm is typical of particular brands of Neo-Kantianism, e.g. of Alan Gewirth and even of the theory of communicative action of Jürgen Habermas (which itself has to be understood in its critique of both Karl Marx's and Max Weber's concentration on purposive, object-oriented, or 'instrumental' rationality). In the second, philosophical/theological, paradigm, the theories of action that restore the abiding element of 'receptivity' to a full understanding of human agency tend to come from a hermeneutical background, such as Paul Ricoeur's. Kant's own definition of autonomy belongs to this second view, being based not on an empirical, but on a transcendental concept of dignity for which the 'capability' (not the actuality) for morality is central. His position allows for an anticipative acknowledgement of nascent autonomy. It can neither be used to exclude mere 'human beings' from the ranks of personhood, as if this was a knighthood specially reserved and awarded for deserving services; nor can autonomy be identified with the faculty to choose which is a basic cultural tool in consumer societies but reduces autonomy to 'optionalism' (D. Mieth). As self-legislation by reason, it has an inherent connection to the categorical imperative never to use anyone only as a means but always also as an end in himself. The recognition of the equal dignity of the other that was subsequently conceptualized as 'unconditional recognition' by Johann Gottlieb Fichte manifests an understanding of the human person as both self-reflective and relational, two aspects that cannot be reduced to each other.

Yet, even if the positions summarized in the first column stem from different backgrounds which are in tension with each other, they are made 'scientistic' by their practical stance. The ideals of controlling nature, the 'frontier' and 'breakthrough' mentality[22] do not allow for doubts about the identification of scientific and human progress. The simple distinction of pleasure from pain as the goal of human existence makes the elimination of suffering the highest aim. This appreciation stays below the level of the insight expressed

---

[22] In *Diktatur der Gene*, p. 13, Mieth speaks of the 'fundamentalism of a horizontal breakthrough mentality which only knows an orientation forward, a "futurum", i.e. a progressive prognosis from the present, and no longer knows what is coming towards us'.

in John Stuart Mill's distinction between higher and lower pleasures, that a certain kind of suffering or lack of fulfilment may be due to the human constitution. It is exemplified in the insight that the deepest need of human freedom, namely to be recognized by another, cannot be realized by oneself. Instead of being requisitioned, it has to be offered freely, or else it is not the fulfilling response sought. Suffering from unrequited recognition is a pain specific for human freedom, and it could only be abolished together with the orientation towards the other's freedom. One other form in which suffering is inevitable is in the consciousness of human finitude. To insist on the validity of these insights does not imply that the many forms of suffering which can be abolished should not be tackled. But an awareness of the *internal* limits to human happiness guards against utopian concepts of a pain-free existence. It is an insight missing in the frequent identification of a state free of suffering with (an empirically understood) 'dignity'. This is contrary to Kant's understanding of dignity, which includes the realization that dignity is not at our disposal and that the specific difference between 'having dignity' and 'having a price' means that we cannot take stock of our or anybody else's lives.[23] The transition from the wish to eliminate suffering towards eliminating sufferers, e.g. by preventing potential sufferers from being born, cannot claim Kant's concept of dignity for justification.

It is in the context of the understanding of suffering and finitude that the significance of the Christian heritage comes out strongest. Yet it also appears in the appreciation of the need for a hermeneutics of healthy self-suspicion, i.e. in those insights that stress the temptability and fallibility of the human person. Philosophical anthropologies in the twentieth century have taken on board the insight that the human capability to make mistakes includes the fact that we cannot retrieve the consequences of our actions.[24] It marks the idea of 'perfectibility' as a dangerous illusion which was already discredited within the Enlightenment by Kant's acknowledgement of the existence of a 'radically evil' element in

---

[23] I. Kant, *Groundwork of the Metaphysic of Morals*, trans. H.J. Patton (New York: Harper, 1964), pp. 102–3. Cf. D. Mieth, *Was wollen wir können? Ethik im Zeitalter der Biotechnik* (Freiburg: Herder, 2002), p. 484.
[24] Cf. Mieth, *Diktatur der Gene*, p. 82.

human nature. It is also a profound misunderstanding of the human condition to think we can optimize ourselves in such a way that all illness and suffering is abolished. What is at stake in the conflict between the two paradigms is what concept of the human person will reign in the future: Will the insight into human finitude, fallibility and fragility be suppressed and replaced by a quest for perfect humans (by whose standards?), e.g. the ideal of totally healthy and perfectly adjusted, happy, high achievers?

Norms for health and illness

If the above empirical assumption of what constitutes a fulfilled human life is not an implicit norm, it is difficult to say what is. It would, however, be too easy a target if it was not true that 'the more society is fixated on the conception of a happy life free of suffering, the more are conditions created which add further difficulties to the aim of disabled people of fulfilling their social roles and realizing the goals and projects of their lives'.[25]

As a consequence of the HGP, concepts of normality, health and illness are coming under renewed debate.[26] The promises and problems of predictive genetic testing were already under discussion long before its conclusion.[27] Different visions of enhancement were being assessed before the practical difficulties of targeted intervention had become obvious. To have the breathing space for a debate on normality, diversity and illness is rare enough at the accelerated rate of change that marks biomedical ethics. What is again decisive, also with regard to definitions of illness, is that the understanding of the human person as a 'self-interpreting animal' is taken seriously. This understanding excludes an objectifying concept based solely on 'biological disfunctionality' that does not take the subjective evaluation of the patient into account. From the various concepts on offer ('biological' and 'system theoretical

[25] Lanzerath and Honnefelder, 'Krankheitsbegriff', p. 64.

[26] In Chapter 5 of this volume, Neil. Messer questions definitions of illness and calls for medicine to be set in the tradition of a community, which would help define its horizon of meaning. The role I see for philosophical anthropology is similar to this service of a tradition.

[27] H. Müller, 'Predictive Genetic Testing: Possibilities, Implications, Limits', in H. Haker *et al.* (eds), *Ethics of Human Genome Analysis* (Tübingen: Attempto, 1993), pp. 136–46.

disfunctionality', the consensus of several practitioners, and a 'practical' definition of illness arising in the interaction between patient and doctor),[28] the latter dialogical definition takes both the self-experience of the patient and the expertise of the physician seriously. Since quality of life expectations, cultural definitions of normality, and so on go into conceptions of illness, nobody should be declared a patient based on unexamined 'objective' findings. Implicit norms should be made explicit and discussed.

Genetic make-up and life project

What anthropological assumptions are behind the view that knowing, and possibly enhancing, our personal gene profile will increase our freedom? Do they continue and reinforce the misunderstanding mentioned above of the conditions that need to be met in order to lead a happy life? Is the fate of being genetically disposed towards unchosen directions a feature that should, if possible, be changed, or is it more in keeping with the human constitution that this should remain so for the very possibility of our dignity and happiness?

In the analysis of the philosopher Ludwig Siep, the guiding conception behind the purpose of making our genes fit our life project is that a flourishing life is believed to be possible only under unlimited natural conditions. What is overlooked here is that such fulfilment only arises from the relationship that a person is able to develop not just towards her potentials for development, but also towards her limits.[29]

For him, it is the way a person copes with her genetic as well as her other unchosen heritages that offers the possibility for fulfilment, rather than the genetically enhanced realization of preconceived ideals. Instead of seeking salvation in the 'progressive liberation from the natural limits of our life planning', Siep suggests a different route: the satisfaction of solving problems.

> From a philosophical perspective, it is questionable whether the guiding idea of instrumentalizing everything given as means of individual wish-fulfilment is realistic and meaningful ... Human

[28] Cf. Lanzerath and Honnefelder, 'Krankheitsbegriff', pp. 53–62.
[29] Ibid., p. 64.

beings as natural and as cultural beings are to a much greater degree than we want to recognize at present reacting, problem-solving and task-resolving beings. They still can do that only through a large degree of taking over traditions (learning) and adaptation to given conditions.

Self-discovery as well as contentment comes from being able to master existing tasks:

> A considerable part of the experience of what is valuable, satisfying and fulfilling results from the mastering of problems and the fulfillment of tasks recognized as necessary and meaningful ... It is less in the realization of projects than in the discovery of what we are good at, and in the often surprising insights into what we really care about that we encounter meaning in life. And these discoveries are by no means always along the line of our dispositions.

If these anthropological insights are true, help is not to be found in genetic enhancement (which will always remain incremental and finite, and is based on an artificial and empty idea of self-design), but in knowing oneself and one's limits:

> It is neither realistic nor advisable to regard our body and our environment as mere material for self-projections. If this thesis is true, then the long-term goal to give as much information and possibilities for 'optimizing' one's genetic heritage must be viewed sceptically ... How many have produced major achievements without the support of specific dispositions, or even against them? How much fulfillment grows from activities for which we were not particularly endowed as long as we were able to know our limits?[30]

His conclusion resembles the point Lanzeroth and Honnefelder made regarding the guiding idea that only optimal biological conditions allow for a life to be happy. Judging from an anthropological perspective, of all the norms implicit in the HGP this is the one that seems the most misguided:

> With regard to goals for the future, it should be the subject of public discussion how good it is for the human person to measure her natural 'start conditions' solely by the scope of possible self-projects, and maybe try to optimize them. Genetic and cultural fate,

---

[30] L. Siep 'Genomanalyse, menschliches Selbstverständnis und Ethik', in L. Honnefelder and P. Propping (eds), *Was wissen wir* (Köln: Dumont, 2001), pp. 196–205. All the following quotes are taken from pp. 199–200.

unless it predisposes to misery or severe illnesses, does not have to be a barrier (*Fessel*) for wishes and plans. This fate can also lead to meaningful tasks and experiences of value, which we could not have invented or dreamt of better ourselves. (p. 203)

What needs to be developed, instead, is an anthropology of finite freedom[31] that does not see the naturally given specificity of a person's existence as an enemy to be combated or material to be processed but as the basis of our ineffable individuality. It is on this question that two eminent schools of social philosophy come to radically opposing answers. Is this givenness something that needs to be respected, or is it something individuals are free and called to improve on? Alan Buchanan and Norman Daniels see the use of the dawning possibilities of genetic intervention for preventing disease and enhancing capabilities as mandated by Rawls's principle of justice. Jürgen Habermas fears the principle of fundamental equality between present and future generations endangered if parents are given the unilateral power of altering the genetic make-up of their offspring. For him, there is a principal difference between the genetic and the environmental, i.e. educational, shaping of one's children. Children are free to react to and negate the socialization they received; yet they are condemned to live with the specificity *(Sosein)* their parents chose for them in an act of domination which can neither be reciprocated nor got rid of. The imminence of this new situation of irreversible basic inequality forces Habermas to call for a 'species ethic', thus enlarging the task of ethics which he had restricted to clarifying procedures for deciding on the 'right' and shunning all 'evaluative' questions of the good. To renounce to such a 'moralization of human nature' could result in not allowing our descendants to voice their views, and to put an end to the reciprocity of cultural traditions and processes of formation.[32] The polar opposition in normative judgement on genetic intervention between these two deontological theories can be traced back to the difference in their key concepts: there is a direct connection between Habermas's guiding concept of mutual

---

[31] Cf. Mieth, *Diktatur der Gene*, pp. 82–7.

[32] J. Habermas, *Zur Zukunft der menschlichen Natur. Auf dem Weg zu einer liberalen Eugenik?* (Frankfurt: Suhrkamp, 2001). English translation, *The Future of Human Nature* (Cambridge: Polity Press, 2003).

recognition, and the idea of human dignity. By comparison, the Rawls school arrives at only a qualified 'right of children to an open future' indirectly by way of indirect argumentation in which the recognition of one's children as free is just an intermediate step. In order to educate their children towards reasonable respect for reasonable world views or 'comprehensive doctrines', parents have to acknowledge their descendants' freedom and consequently their right to an open future.[33] The dilemma posed is not between human dignity and instrumentalization, but between justice and parents' rights to reproductive freedom. Consequently, the focus is more on parents being restricted in their rights, not on children being dominated by their parents' designs. Habermas observes that the authors only sense danger from 'communitarian' (*sive* extremist political and religious groups) or state-led measures, not from parental initiatives of liberal eugenics. The lack of prominence of the concept of human dignity may not be surprising in a theory that proposes a 'wide reflective equilibrium' as the method of finding moral norms. Its fear of 'foundationalism' goes so far as to ignore human dignity as foundational for discourse, tolerance, and justice and not at the disposition of society. It cannot be up for a bargaining process of a minimal 'overlapping consensus'.[34] These minimalist norms are then claimed as a position that is respectful of the existing pluralism of values. As becomes clear in the debate on the future role of genetics, it is a model of political philosophy which does not have the resources to resist, but only to adapt to, and by its acceptance promote, technological changes to our life-world and historical self-understanding.[35] It is only consequent that it even envisages 'dispensing with' the concept of human nature in the distant future.[36] The alternative model is

[33] A. Buchanan, D.W. Brock, N. Daniels and D. Wikler, *From Chance to Choice: Genetics and Justice* (Cambridge: Cambridge University Press, 2000), pp. 175–6.
[34] Cf. D. Mieth, 'Reply to Ludwig Siep's Commentary' (on D. Mieth's 'Common Values in Europe'), *Biomedical Ethics* 5 (2000), p. 88.
[35] Cf. H. Peukert, 'Beyond the Present State of Affairs. *Bildung* and the Search for Orientation in Rapidly Transforming Societies', *Journal of Philosophy of Education* 36 (2002), pp. 421–35, p. 427. Instead of insisting on the unconditional elements within a truly human life-form and measuring technological progress by them, the current new naturalism delivers the future to a comprehensive process to which one continually is to adapt *post factum*: 'Adaptation would be the new catchword for "*Bildung*".'
[36] Buchanan *et al.*, *From Chance to Choice*, pp. 18, 25.

to 'embed' normative ethics in an anthropology or species ethics, as Siep and now also Habermas demand.

To summarize the problems that arise from the norms implicit in the HGP: even if the scientific evidence discloses diversity, not normality as standard, the interest in turning the new-found knowledge into profitable applications promotes a social norm of 'iron health' as one major determinant of a person's market value. This norm is sought at the expense of values and standards that have been won in arduous historical battles. They are already under pressure now but very likely to be more so with the diagnostic tools of the HGP:

Solidarity used to be the willingness to support the weaker members of society. It is now being redefined as the obligation of these weaker members not to burden society with their (genetic) imperfections.[37] With regard to procreation, this implies the voluntary submission to the norm of 'flawless babies', which ignores their right to life independent of 'quality control'; it turns the first half of pregnancy into a trial period for the foetus to qualify for birth, puts attachment on hold, and reduces choice for parents.

Equality: To be destined by one's genes towards unchosen directions is an insight that can be assimilated by human freedom, just as everyone's other concrete 'givens' of culture, historic period, language, family and gender can. To be predestined at the wish of another human being towards specific directions, however, introduces an element of domination that did not exist with the 'lottery' of natural chance which up to now has been the inevitable fate of every human born. Habermas envisions the psychological effects on the receivers, their resentment of such induced endowments. The fact that the natural equality and 'equal birth' (*Ebenbürtigkeit*) of parents and children is compromised by parents specifying the offspring they want, leads him to demand the 'embedding' of discourse ethics in a species ethic. We now have to choose for or against the conditions that make a true, unrestrained consensus possible. If those conditions of equality are violated from the start, the next and future generations will not have equal access to establishing their consensus but will have been predetermined, i.e. dominated by their parents' ideas of what is desirable and

[37] E. Hildt ends her review of R. Chadwick *et al.* (eds), *The Right to Know and the Right Not to Know* (Aldershot: Avebury, 1997), with the prognosis, 'bad times for a right not to know ...', *Biomedical Ethics* 2 (1997) pp. 92–3.

acceptable. And in contrast to the process of education, they cannot escape, resist or deny their heritage since it has been decided as part of their bodily make-up. Thus, Habermas views positive eugenics' interference with the genome as a fundamental breach of the congenital equality between parents and children. In addition to the central criterion of the equality that comes with being 'begotten, not made', another aspect that has to be evaluated is that parents are destining their children to compensate for the genes they are unhappy with themselves. The lack of self-acceptance revealed by this urge to modify and enhance the personal genetic inheritance one has passed on to one's descendants in itself forebodes trouble. Genetic engineering has to help to bring out 'the best' in parents, as suggested in the film *Gattica*.

To equate *autonomy* with rational life-plans and a self-control extended to one's genes falls short both of Kant and of his critics. For Kant, autonomy meant self-legislation over against one's natural inclinations and dispositions, genetic and other. His critics point out the lack of relevance of the affective, emotional sides of subjectivity. The assumption that once people know their genetic risks, they will choose a lifestyle that minimizes them is rationalistic to a worse degree than Kant's ethics. Such caution, measure, and prudence is rendered even more unlikely by a culture which builds its economic success on consumerism and permissiveness, not on restriction and present sacrifices for future gains. Autonomy may also be endangered by another aspect of the HGP: as long as predictive genetic diagnosis is not matched by existing therapies, the advance knowledge of genetic risks may put an end to freedom as spontaneity. Yet without the sense of an open future, the most immediate experience of freedom will be lost.

The contemporary ideal of authenticity presupposes confidence in one's *individuality*. If 'elective breeding' were technically possible and were to be allowed legally, it would mean the end of Western civilization's idea of individuality from Boethius through Schleiermacher to postmodernity. It is only now, with the possible thought of fixing features in advance, that we discover that the guardian of individuality (as well as of human dignity) is natural chance.[38]

---

[38] Instead of being regarded as a threat to be minimized, natural chance needs to be acknowledged as the guardian of freedom. The philosopher Michael Baumgartner states: 'The idea of human dignity is to be realized for the individual subject only if his beginning is not marked by the will *(Willkür)* of other human beings. Thus it can be said: only if a facticity untouched by humans and, in this sense, "fate", stands at the beginning of their own lives, can human beings

One does not have to negate the role which health plays for human flourishing to be critical of the following traits that come with the practical coalition between proponents of autonomy as the ability to express one's interests and promoters of genetic health:

> the restriction of personhood to an exclusive ('aristocratic') feature of fully-fledged autonomous adults, segregating a gentlemen's club of conscious persons from the hoi polloi of mere humans;

> a determinism in the shape of a double reduction that reduces person to body and body to genes;[39]

> unbroken allegiance to the idea of 'perfectibility' typical of eighteenth-century Rationalism, unchallenged by later ninteenth-century insights into negativity and twentieth-century evidence of human commitment to evil, fallibility, temptability, and tendency to rationalize rather than admit guilt;

> a belief in the ability to fix human nature technically, espécially evident in media headlines on 'genes predisposing to aggressiveness' and 'criminality'.[40]

Philosophical answers critical of this new situation include the

---

determine themselves freely and, that is, independently of the will of other human beings. This signifies: The dignity of the human being as a being who determines himself presupposes fate. He can only be an end in himself according to the Kantian formula if what he is from his natural basis is not calculated into a context of purposes in which the human being affected can only be a means for the ends of other human beings. It may sound provocative to name this "fate"; the point is to see that this undisposability at the beginning of human life is the condition of the truly free self-determination of a being who ... unites *animalitas* and *rationalitas* in himself. ... The beginning of the human being is not marked by the will of another of his kind, but by a facticity free of will. The human being is creature, he is given to himself (*factum*) as a task (freedom), but he is not the creature of the human being. It is not the human being who stands at the beginning of human life.' (M. Baumgartner, 'Am Anfang des menschlichen Lebens steht nicht der Mensch', in O. Marquardt and H.-J. Staudinger (eds), *Anfang und Ende des menschlichen Lebens. Medizinethische Probleme*, vol. iv (Paderborn, 1987), pp. 40–3, pp. 42–3.)

[39] H. Haker, 'The Perfect Body: Biomedical Utopias', in R. Ammicht-Quinn and E. Tamez (eds), *The Body and Religion, Concilium* 38 (2002), pp. 9–18, p. 10.

[40] In his introduction to *From Chance to Choice*, p. 24, A. Buchanan describes this as one of the 'genetic determinist fallacies' which 'promotes a worshipful attitude toward genes and genetic science'. If one believes with J. Watson that 'our fate is in our genes', our admiration for the achievements of genetic science leads us to look to our genes for the source of all our problems and to molecular biology for their solution. We thereby conveniently blind ourselves to the uncomfortable possibility that many of our most serious problems result from our social practices and institutions.

call for a 'species ethic' (Habermas) and for an anthropology in which the abilities to learn, adapt and solve problems even against the odds are seen to have special importance for human flourishing (Siep). The idea that human fulfilment would be increased if people were given the best headstart genetically reveals itself as a misguided and illusionary approach.

3 Theologically significant aspects of the HGP

Two features of the HGP stand out that have special relevance for a theological understanding of the human person: the idea of human perfectibility, and the belief that humanity can be improved in a technical way. I will conclude this evaluation by indicating which type of theological ethics I consider best able to contribute to modern ethics in its interdisciplinary constitution.

Some of the promises held out by proponents of positive eugenics seem to revive the idea of the 'perfectibility' of the human person, typical of early Enlightenment rationalism and optimism. It was already resisted by Kant in his acceptance of a 'radically evil' propensity in humans, and by Friedrich Joseph Wilhelm Schelling in his 1809 analysis of human freedom as the double capacity for either good or evil. Both philosophers were reformulating in anthropological terms the Christian analysis of the human duality of being made in the image of God, and of sin. In his 'Christian Faith', the dogmatics that were to meet the challenge posed by Kant's critique of the traditional proofs of God's existence, Friedrich Schleiermacher made special reference in his Christology to the shallow concept of the human person on which such reform-happy rationalism was based. It is typical of their successors, too, to locate the alienating element outside the will of the human person, in civilization, nature, class structures, the reactive forces of life, patriarchy, systemic imperatives, or anti-social genes. It is a denial of human agency and responsibility to claim all the successful outcomes for the human subject and blame the history of suffering committed by the same subject on other factors, as J.B. Metz has shown in his classical contrast of 'emancipation and redemption'.[41] The least that can be asked

---

[41] J.B. Metz, *Faith in History and Society* (New York: Crossroad, 1980), ch. 7.

from genetic utopias of perfection is to take on board the insight into our voluntary 'complicity' with the forces of domination, as feminism has done, and engage in more in-depth analyses of the sources of evil and ways of fighting and transforming them.

It is through the combination of 'fantasies of perfection' (*Vollkommenheitsphantasien*, R. Spaemann) with a mentality of technological fixes that the application of the HGP receives its totalitarian potential. Misconceptions of human nature, such as down-playing human finitude and advocating at the same time the possibility of a life free of suffering, are not harmless even as theoretical proposals; when they become guiding ideas behind research programmes, however, they acquire the power of social engineering.[42]

I have argued that genetic technology as a product and as an expression of contemporary culture points to the need for redeveloping a philosophical anthropology, compatible, however, with the modern loss of teleology and essentialism. The norms implicit in the hopes put forward by genetic technology, some of them secular equivalents to the promise of salvation, should be spelt out and put up for discussion against the backdrop of a shared concept of human nature. From life experience and self-reflection, people could agree that the meaning of life cannot be made dependent on specific events or specific endowments such as genes, and that the meaning of life is not at our disposal. One primary function of a philo-sophical anthropology would be to correct such false self-understandings.[43] The insights into human finitude and fallibility are results of self-reflection which are ignored to our detriment.

Which type of theological ethics is best suited to contribute to the joint enterprise of interdisciplinary ethics and to the necessary public debate on which life-world, concept of

---

[42] The declaration of the human genome as the 'common heritage' and property of humanity is an alarming sign in this context. It may be meant to save the genome from private interests in patenting, but in fact it may result in relativizing and sacrificing inalienable individual rights, e.g. to life, bodily integrity and privacy. A 'symbolic' understanding of the human genome, as the 'common heritage' of humanity in the context of individual human rights that are not at the disposal of a majority, may be better capable of protecting human dignity which, after all, was attributed to the 'humanity in each person' by Kant.

[43] Wimmer, 'Anfragen', p. 63.

humanity, and vision of society we should strive for in the future? The revival of virtue ethics in the past twenty-five years against overly act-centred, proceduralist and rationalist ethics already makes the step to basing ethics in anthropology. A theory of human nature is presupposed and implicit in its idea of human flourishing.[44] Equally, the revisionist natural law approach starts out from a concept of human nature that is based on shared human experience and acknowledges the role of interpretation in its findings and ensuing moral demands; yet, its very strength, the move from a 'physicalist' and 'biologist' to an interpretive understanding of human nature also makes it more prone to endorsing the spirit of the times. Its lack of critique of the goal of enhancement is an example of this vulnerability. Even if the physicalist approach lacked any hermeneutical awareness of changing interpretations, e.g. of female over against male nature, it did contain the idea of a limit based on the givenness of natural structures. A third concept of Christian ethics, 'autonomous ethics in a Christian context', sees the guiding idea of human dignity as setting the limit against instrumentalization. Since this approach combines rational communicability and Christian specificity (contained in the heuristic context, horizon of meaning, motivational and integrative potential, and its subordinating of morality to the need for redemption),[45] I see it as the most encompassing type of Christian ethics.

While all of these approaches share some commitment to philosophical reflection and interdisciplinary dialogue, the exception seems to be Stanley Hauerwas's ecclesial communitarianism. However, its extrinsicism and separatism prompts the question of its relevance to the Christian communities it addresses, whose members are residents of other worlds besides the Church. Full-time professionals in matters of faith and theology may overestimate the Church as the 'only true foundation in a world without foundations', and underestimate their fellow-Christians' sense of shared human fellowship in being partners, parents, colleagues at work, and co-citizens.

---

[44] Cf. ibid., p. 56.
[45] See the summary of this approach in Mieth, *Was wollen wir können?*, p. 464.

Open questions that need to be addressed in collaborative investigations by the integrating disciplines of philosophy and theology and the individual empirical human sciences include the role of health in human life.

(1) Some questions at the deontological level are: What presuppositions are made when one distinguishes negative from positive eugenics, thus allowing for germ-line interventions and pre-implantation selection against severe genetic disorders, but not for measures of 'enhancement'? Would positive genetic interference violate only equality, or also autonomy?[46] If one restricts eugenics to preventative measures, is one endorsing the premise of the right to have a child, and a healthy child?

(2) Examples of questions at the teleological level of striving for a fulfilled life are: What significance does the sense of an open future have for personal identity? What role should the ideas of a rational life-plan and of self-control that are inherent in the medical hopes associated with the diagnostic potential of the HGP have in a person's life project? How does suffering affect biographical, moral and religious identity?

(3) Questions for philosophical and theological ethics include the status of the relevant principles, e.g. equality and autonomy: Are they universally valid principles of reason which can stand and be sustained on their own, or are they marked by their contingent origin in the history of Western thought? Can they survive without the resources of meaning that accompanied their conception, i.e. the context of hope in ultimate meaning engendered by faith in God's power of creation and God's deeds of redemption? Are the specific conclusions drawn from these principles merely their application, or are certain demands, e.g. for justice, marked by a concrete history of values[47] which cannot deny its theological roots? Then Christian specificity would not only be present in ecclesial communities. It needs to be discovered and recognized in the humanistic assumptions of our culture. The challenge to 'sustain humanity

---

[46] Cf. L. Siep, 'Moral und Gattungsethik', *Deutsche Zeitschrift für Philosophie* 50 (2002), pp. 111–20, pp. 112–13.

[47] Cf. Siep, 'Moral und Gattungsethik', p. 113, n. 5. This question arises *a fortiori* with regard to the consensus proposed by the authors of *From Chance to Choice* that remedial genetic intervention is a demand of justice. In the case of compensating for undeserved disadvantage through genetic engineering, however, a particular understanding of justice is pursued at the expense of other values.

beyond humanism',[48] however, may need the resources of renewal and hope that believing communities can offer after their runaway secular offspring has spent its fortune and is running short of means and meaning. Will an ethics of Christian inspiration have more to offer to contemporary struggles than verdicts of a 'culture of death' and superior disengagement?

Bibliography

Baumgartner, Michael, 'Am Anfang des menschlichen Lebens steht nicht der Mensch', in O. Marquardt and H.-J. Staudinger (eds), *Anfang und Ende des menschlichen Lebens. Medizinethische Probleme,* vol. iv (Paderborn, 1987), pp. 40–3.

Buchanan, Alan, Brock, Daniel W., Daniels, Norman and Wikler, Dan, *From Chance to Choice: Genetics and Justice* (Cambridge: Cambridge University Press, 2000).

Habermas, Jürgen, *Zur Zukunft der menschlichen Natur. Auf dem Weg zu einer liberalen Eugenik?* (Frankfurt: Suhrkamp, 2001).

Haker, Hille, 'The Perfect Body: Biomedical Utopias', in R. Ammicht-Quinn and E. Tamez (eds), *The Body and Religion, Concilium* 38 (2002), pp. 9–18.

Honnefelder, Ludwig and Propping, Peter (eds), *Was wissen wir, wenn wir das menschliche Genom kennen?* (Köln: Dumont, 2001).

Junker-Kenny, Maureen, 'Categorical Arguments: Pro-Life Versus Pro-Choice?', in E. Hildt and S. Graumann (eds), *Genetics in Human Reproduction* (Aldershot: Ashgate, 1999), pp. 147–55.

Kant, Immanuel, *Groundwork of the Metaphysic of Morals,* trans. H.J. Patton (New York: Harper, 1964).

Lanzerath, Detlev and Honnefelder, Ludwig, 'Krankheitsbegriff und ärztliche Anwendung', in M. Düwell and D. Mieth

---

[48] The cultural diagnosis that we are living in an age of 'posthumanism' is reflected in recent conference titles, such as this one organized by the European Ethics Network at the European Parliament in Brussels, August 2002, which contains a section on 'Bio-ethics and the *Humanum* in Question'.

(eds), *Ethik in der Humangenetik* (Tübingen: Francke, 1998), pp. 51–77.

Metz, Johann Baptist, *Faith in History and Society* (New York: Crossroad, 1980).

Mieth, Dietmar, 'Reply to Ludwig Siep's Commentary' (on D. Mieth's 'Common Values in Europe'), *Biomedical Ethics* 5 (2000), p. 88.

Mieth, Dietmar, *Die Diktatur der Gene* (Freiburg: Herder, 2001).

Mieth, Dietmar, *Was wollen wir können? Ethik im Zeitalter der Biotechnik* (Freiburg: Herder, 2002).

Müller, Hansjakob, 'Predictive Genetic Testing: Possibilities, Implications, Limits', in H. Haker *et al.* (eds), *Ethics of Human Genome Analysis* (Tübingen: Attempto, 1993), pp. 136–46.

O'Neill, Onora, 'The "Good Enough" Parent in the Age of the New Reproductive Technologies', in H. Haker and D. Beyleveld (eds), *The Ethics of Genetics in Human Procreation* (Aldershot: Ashgate, 2000), pp. 33–48.

Peukert, Helmut, 'Beyond the Present State of Affairs. *Bildung* and the Search for Orientation in Rapidly Transforming Societies', *Journal of Philosophy of Education* 36 (2002), pp. 421–35.

Siep, Ludwig, 'Genomanalyse, menschliches Selbstverständnis und Ethik', in L. Honnefelder and P. Propping (eds), *Was wissen wir* (Köln: Dumont, 2001), pp. 196–205.

Siep, Ludwig, 'Moral und Gattungsethik', *Deutsche Zeitschrift für Philosophie* 50 (2002), pp. 111–20.

Taylor, Charles, 'Interpretation and the Sciences of Man', *Review of Metaphysics* 25 (1971), pp. 3–51; reprinted in *Philosophy and the Human Sciences, Philosophical Papers 2* (Cambridge: Cambridge University Press, 1985).

Wimmer, Reiner, 'Anfragen an die Integrative Ethik Hans Krämers aus philosophisch-anthropologischer Perspektive', in M. Endreß (ed.), *Zur Grundlegung einer integrativen Ethik* (Frankfurt: Suhrkamp, 1997), pp. 56–72.

PART IV

Discerning Historical Trajectories

Introduction to Part IV

A number of authors thus far have hinted at the importance of historical analysis for consideration of shifting ideas about human identity (Page) or human perfectibility (Junker-Kenny). This section explores some of the historical issues in more detail, while pointing to particular implications and social recommendations in our present context. Bronislaw Szerszynski's chapter is particularly concerned with the way we use language. The emerging sciences of the seventeenth century developed a universalized reference language of inter-dependent propositions. In the emerging scientific world view of the seventeenth century, God became the object of language, which facilitated the eventual removal of God-language altogether. Controversially, he suggests that the Human Genome Project and associated disciplines are likely to contribute to a similar loss in language about the human. While the idea of human beings as knowing, representing subjects was incorporated into scientific knowledge later in the nineteenth century, he considers that the reordering of sciences is threatened by the dominance of molecular biology. In this scenario, DNA becomes the deep surface to which all else about the human person relates, so that ambiguities about human action appear more superficial. If humanity can be 'plotted' and 'mapped' through the Human Genome Project, might it also in some sense be 'destroyed'?

Robert Song's chapter explores the potency of genetics as an emerging cultural symbol. He asks how it was that such a reductionist understanding could ever take hold? With the demise of eugenics, he suggests that the social acceptance of genetics has been predicated on its claim for medical and health benefits. The ideal of freedom from disease has roots in the early project of Francis Bacon, who considered science to be used in the service of humankind's estate, challenging the fateful and inevitable course of mortal existence. In Francis Bacon we find ideals are subject to the limits of religious concern, while contemporary movements are detached from such explicit religious concerns and instead become a secularized and surrogate form of soteriology. The HGP is a particularly symbolic representation of this soteriological trajectory. He is sharply critical of the obsession with the elimination of suffering and fetishization of health that seems implicit in the new genetic technologies and which ignores wider issues such as global poverty.

Both chapters are concerned to view the wider social issues implicit in the HGP in the light of changes that were set in place during the emergence of experimental science in the seventeenth century. Both see the outcomes of such a trajectory as problematic, or at least ambiguous in their outcomes. While Szerszynski is concerned about the damaging effects, as he sees it, on our understanding of the human person as a social and complex self, Song is concerned about the incursion of science into areas more properly considered to be theological. Both authors find implicit religious norms in the HGP and challenge the scientism arising out of it.

7

That Deep Surface: The Human Genome Project and the Death of the Human[1]

Bronislaw Szerszynski

Introduction

In the development and application of new technologies such as agricultural and human biotechnology it is becoming increasingly common for policy-makers to turn to philosophers, theologians and religious leaders to make ethical judgements on specific developments. There seem to be two assumptions underlying this kind of approach. The first assumption is that science and religion can be regarded as complementary activities, whose truth claims cannot directly conflict with each other. According to this widely held view, science is the arbiter over questions of ontology and causality – over what *is*, and how it came to *be* what it is – whereas religion can answer questions of meaning and purpose about the reality that is determined by science. Similarly, whereas technology determines what it is possible to do, and how it might be achieved, religious values and ethical reasoning can determine whether it is permissible or desirable. Put crudely, once science and technology have determined what we *could* do, religion can serve as an ethical resource that can help us determine whether we *should* do it or

[1] I am extremely grateful to John Brooke, Ruth Chadwick, Celia Deane-Drummond, Robin Grove-White, Alan Holland, Margaret Lock, Maureen McNeil, Stephen Pumfrey, Jackie Stacey, Nikolas Rose, Pete Rogers, Claire Waterton, Brian Wynne, and the participants of the *Brave New World?* colloquium, for invaluable suggestions and responses to earlier drafts of this chapter, and to Nina Moeller for fruitful discussions on the philosophy of technology.

not. The second, related assumption in this approach is that the key questions that should be asked are ones about specific technological advances, about specific applications of such new technologies, or about specific consequences of their application.

In this chapter I want to suggest that at least *some* of the questions we might want to ask about the Human Genome Project (HGP) are ones that require us to set aside both of these assumptions. I do not want to deny that at certain times it is entirely appropriate for policy-makers to turn to religious and other experts for their judgements about specific proposals. Nevertheless, there is a danger that some more fundamental issues raised by technological development are thereby neglected. I will spend most of the chapter developing an argument against the first assumption mentioned above, suggesting that modern science, conceived as the theoretical and practical mastery of nature, is itself a partly theological project, one with a specific religious construal of the world and of the human place in it. If I am right, approaching human genetics as posing a series of discrete challenges, to be judged one at a time against ethical and religious criteria, risks obscuring a deeper challenge posed by genetic science to the language we use to describe the human – and thus to the human itself.

In questioning both of these assumptions I am seeking to develop a more specific argument – that the HGP[2] can be seen as a new and significant phase in a theologico-scientific project, originating in the early modern period, to render existence according to a *mathesis universalis,* a universal formalized reference language. In particular, I suggest that the HGP is an attempt to complete this rendering, through the extension to *humanity* of certain theological moves made in that earlier period in relation to *God.* And just as this rendering of God in embodied and univocal terms rendered him[3] ultimately expendable – as famously captured by Laplace's purported comment to Napoleon that he had no need of that particular

---

[2] At least as it is interpreted by some of its key commentators and advocates.

[3] I have chosen to use the masculine pronoun for God in this chapter not for theological reasons, but in order to be consistent with the usage in the period about which I am writing.

hypothesis – so too does the HGP threaten the future of the human person as we understand it.

This might be seen as a rather paradoxical claim: at most, the HGP might be seen as a project to *map* the human being. How could mapping something thereby threaten it? Of course, in relation to many episodes of world history, mapping places and things has indeed been a prelude to their destruction – wilderness areas, for example. Reassuringly, I do not think that the human being is the kind of thing whose mapping lends it to being threatened in *this* way.[4] However, the very features of the human being that make it *less* vulnerable to destruction by mapping in this sense make it *more* vulnerable in another, because of the way that our subjectivity is constitutively shaped by the languages we use to understand it.[5] As Hannah Arendt wrote of theories of behaviourism, which stand in the same tradition of attempts to theoretically reduce the human, the trouble 'is not that they are wrong but that they could become true'.[6] The worry I am focusing on in this chapter, then, is less about the material effects of human genetics, and more about the effects such technologies might have on our language about human beings – and thus on ourselves.[7]

But as well as being counterintuitive, my claim is also a rather apocalyptic one. While it is also possible that the ideas and practices of human genetics may simply provide additional conceptual and explanatory resources to add to the rich panoply of ways that modern humans have of talking about themselves and others,[8] this more positive outcome cannot be

[4] Though of course there are many issues of ownership and patenting in human genetics that at least threaten people's possession over themselves and their powers, in the sense that Macpherson described as 'possessive individualism'– see C.B. Macpherson, *The Political Theory of Possessive Individualism: Hobbes to Locke* (Oxford: Clarendon Press, 1962).

[5] P. Heelas and A. Lock (eds), *Indigenous Psychologies: The Anthropology of the Self* (London: Academic Press, 1981).

[6] H. Arendt, *The Human Condition* (Chicago: University of Chicago Press, 1998), p. 322.

[7] In this way I am drawing on the *substantive* approach to the philosophy of science and technology, as contrasted with the *instrumental* approach. Rather than understanding technologies as neutral instruments or means that can be used for the pursuit of different (and morally assessable) ends, the substantive approach sees a specific technology or technology itself as having an essential framing quality that tends to gather the world around it in a particular way. It is in this way that I am approaching the Human Genome Project.

[8] C. Taylor, *Sources of the Self: The Making of the Modern Identity* (Cambridge: Cambridge University Press, 1989).

assumed. There are real signs of a kind of genetic reductionism starting to invade the way that we talk about human persons, a change that might start to alter fundamentally our conception of the human, to the point at which the connection becomes attenuated to breaking point. It is not necessary to posit an essential 'human nature' in the way that Francis Fukuyama does in his own apocalyptic account of genomics in order to be deeply concerned about what might be happening to our language of human persons.[9]

I will develop my argument by way of a three-part narrative: the death of nature; the death of God; the death of the human. First, in the development of modern science nature was 'killed' in the sense of being known in a new kind of way, one which stripped it of active power and meaning. Second, in the reordering of the concept of knowledge and truth which this involved, divine attributes were de-metaphorized and mapped on to specific aspects of reality as it was coming to be understood by natural philosophers, thus laying the ground for God's eventual dismissal as unnecessary. Third, by situating the HGP in this larger historical narrative I hope to illuminate ways in which genomic science might similarly threaten the existence of the human person, through its reordering of the language of 'depth' in relation to the human, and the reduction of the opacity and open-endedness of human identity to a spatialized genetic coding.[10]

---

[9] F. Fukuyama, *Our Posthuman Future: Consequences of the Biotechnology Revolution* (London: Profile Books, 2002). By being apocalyptic, of course, I am assuming that it is worth being so at this stage in the hope of being proved wrong later.

[10] I am focusing here on the fate of the human as an *object* of knowledge in genetic science. There are other theological questions raised by the new role of (some) human beings as *subjects* and wielders of genetic knowledge and technology. Robert Song (Chapter 8 in this volume) traces the roots of the activist and ameliorative construal of science and technology that he sees as animating the Human Genome Project back to a set of beliefs and attitudes initially assembled in the seventeenth century. Others, notably T. Peters, *Playing God* (London: Routledge, 1997), take this line of thought further in their construal of the genetic scientist as co-creator with God. An exploration of these and other rather different and non-reductive conceptions of the human in genetic science is outside the scope of this paper. Nevertheless, as John Brooke points out in a personal communication, there is an irony if we become more like God and erase ourselves with the same gesture – or, to use Song's more cautious language, if in the name of humanitarianism we erase the human.

The death of nature[11]

According to many accounts of the scientific revolution of the sixteenth and seventeenth centuries, this period was a crucial stage in the separation of science from religion. In terms of institutions and practices, this is indeed the case, with the birth-pangs of this separation perhaps most graphically dramatized in the persecution by the Church of Galileo for his public support of the Copernican, heliocentric model of the cosmos.[12] However, as the historian Amos Funkenstein has convincingly argued, the work of Galileo and Descartes, Newton and Leibniz, Hobbes and Vico may in other ways be seen as a high point of *convergence* between science, philosophy and theology.[13] Funkenstein describes the activity of many natural philosophers of the time as a 'secular theology', and this in two senses. First, theirs was a theology practised by the laity rather than by clergymen, and by those without advanced degrees in divinity. Secularization of theology in this sense, its appropriation by laymen, had of course been encouraged by the Reformation. But, second, this was a theology oriented to the 'world' in a way that had not been the case before, a world increasingly seen not as a transient stage for the development of human souls, but as having its own religious value, both as a dwelling place and as a creation whose study can reveal the mind of its creator. As Funkenstein puts it, '[t]he world turned into God's temple, and the layman into its priests'. Theology was increasingly expected to import ideas and forms of reasoning from other disciplines, such as mathematics, and in turn 'God ceased to be the monopoly of theologians'.[14] In a related development, from

---

[11] My argument in this section is broadly compatible with that made by Carolyn Merchant in her book of the same name. However, while her account prioritizes the shift from organic to mechanical metaphors for nature, as the key move in the death of nature, I follow Foucault and Funkenstein in seeing this as merely part of a more general epistemic shift. See C. Merchant, *The Death of Nature: Women, Ecology, and the Scientific Revolution* (San Francisco: Harper and Row, 1980).

[12] W.R. Shea, 'Galileo and the Church', in D.C. Lindberg and R.L. Numbers (eds), *God and Nature: Historical Essays on the Encounter between Christianity and Science* (Berkeley: University of California Press, 1986), pp. 114–35.

[13] For a less controversialist account of the scientific revolution than Funkenstein's, but one that nevertheless also argues for a far more complex relationship between science and religion than that of separation and conflict, see J.H. Brooke, *Science and Religion: Some Historical Perspectives* (Cambridge: Cambridge University Press, 1991).

[14] A. Funkenstein, *Theology and the Scientific Imagination from the Middle Ages to the Seventeenth Century* (Princeton, NJ: Princeton University Press, 1986), p. 6.

the fourteenth century onwards, barriers between disciplines
had been progressively eroded, not least with the rise of the
peripatetic programme transmission as a model competing with
the medieval university. Even as new disciplines emerged
through this erosion of boundaries, the idea of a unified
'system' of thought and knowledge, conceived as 'a set of inter-
dependent propositions' and based on one method, gained
increasing currency, especially from the seventeenth century.

These changes were accompanied by another, related
change in the understanding of nature which rendered it
available for reinterpretation by modern science. According to
the earlier, symbolist mentality of the Middle Ages, objects,
plants and animals have been understood as *signs*, implicated in
endless chains of resemblance.[15] As codified by Origen and
Augustine, the medieval *Quadriga* gave rules for the interpretation of both scripture and nature, in terms of literal,
allegorical, moral and supernatural levels of meaning. Through
this method of interpretation, which formalized and to some
extent attempted to 'tame' a broader symbolic approach to the
natural world,[16] natural objects and not just words were seen as
referring, either to other objects and events in nature and
history, or to moral and spiritual truths as laid out in scripture.[17]

However, the Protestant Reformation saw a profound
transition in Europe, one which included a shift of emphasis
from image to word,[18] and from allegorical to literal meaning.
As Peter Harrison argues, the search by Protestant reformers for
a stable, unambiguous religious authority in the Bible led to an
insistence that it should be interpreted literally, withdrawing
intelligibility and meaning away from objects themselves and
reserving such properties for words alone:

> The sacred rite which had lain at the heart of medieval culture was
> replaced by a text, symbolic objects gave way to words, ritual
> practices were eclipsed by propositional beliefs and dogmas. In the

[15] M. Foucault, *The Order of Things: An Archaeology of the Human Sciences* (London:
Tavistock, 1970).
[16] K. Thomas, *Man and the Natural World: Changing Attitudes in England 1500–1800*
(Harmondsworth: Penguin, 1984).
[17] P. Harrison, *The Bible, Protestantism, and the Rise of Natural Science* (Cambridge:
Cambridge University Press, 1998), p. 15.
[18] E. Duffy, *The Stripping of the Altars: Traditional Religion in England, c.1400–c. 1580*
(New Haven: Yale University Press, 1992), p. 591.

course of this process, that unified interpretive endeavour which had given meanings to both natural world and sacred text began to disintegrate. Meaning and intelligibility were ascribed to words and texts, but denied to living things and inanimate objects. The natural world, once the indispensable medium between words and eternal truths, lost its meanings, and became opaque to those hermeneutical procedures which had once elucidated it.[19]

Harrison can be accused of making this shift appear too stark – as if there were no proponents of literal truth in the Middle Ages, and there were no symbolic interpreters of nature in the seventeenth century. Nevertheless, the move away from symbolic interpretation – sometimes hesitant, sometimes robustly asserted – laid nature increasingly open to the radically new modes of ordering offered by the emergent natural sciences. These orderings were based not on similitude and analogy but on the precise comparison of sameness and difference – either through mathematics, an approach that reached its epitome in Galileo, or through taxonomy, for example, in the work of John Ray.

It is important to try to grasp the distinctiveness of this emergent theologico-scientific project of the theoretical mastery of nature. It was the quest for a *mathesis universalis* – an unequivocal, universal, coherent, yet artificial language in which could be formulated the clear and distinct ideas of science.[20] The search for this purified, formalized language played a crucial role in the idea of truth which science assumed, whereby '[w]ord and thing are brought to coincide in the sense that the former is a completely adequate and transparent representation of the latter'.[21] According to Michel Foucault, the Classical *episteme* of the scientific revolution was characterized by the use of this artificial, precise but arbitrary reference language to analyse the world into elementary elements, and at the same time to specify how they combine to form more complex phenomena:

> In the Classical age, to make use of signs is not, as it was in preceding centuries, to attempt to rediscover beneath them the

---

[19] Harrison, *The Bible, Protestantism, and the Rise of Natural Science*, p. 120.
[20] Funkenstein, *Theology and the Scientific Imagination*, pp. 28–9.
[21] T.J. Reiss, *The Discourse of Modernism* (Ithaca, NY: Cornell University Press, 1982), p. 36.

primitive text of a discourse sustained, and retained, forever; it is an
attempt to discover the arbitrary language that will authorize the
deployment of nature within its space, the final terms of its analysis
and the laws of its composition. It is no longer the task of
knowledge to dig out the ancient Word from the unknown places
where it may be hidden; its job now is to fabricate a language ... as
an instrument of analysis and combination.[22]

The whole Classical *episteme*, for Foucault, ultimately
conceives of knowledge in the form of a unified table – a
spatialized grid of interdependent but unequivocal propositions. In a complementary account Funkenstein describes
modern science as the convergence of four ideals –
homogeneity, univocity, mechanization and mathematization.[23]
Each of these ideals has an often long history prior to the seventeenth century, but in the *episteme* of modern science they come
together in a distinctive and powerful way. The ideal of
homogeneity assumes simplicity in *things*, that the universe is
the same everywhere – the same matter, the same kinds of
motion, ultimately the same laws. Univocity requires simplicity
in *language* – that terms unambiguously denote their referent in
terms of relations of identity and non-identity, rather than
through similitude, analogy and metaphor. Mathematization
involves not as it had for Plato and Pythagoras that *things* were
mathematical, in the sense that nature takes simple, geometric
forms, but that scientific *language* should be mathematical in
order to perform its analytic and combinatory functions.
Finally, mechanization required the expulsion of teleology,
final causes and intentions from nature; matter was conceived
as passive, its behaviour determined by causal relations and
natural laws.[24] Nature in this *episteme* is no longer alive with
agency, *telos*, meaning and mystery. Its death in this sense was
necessitated by the very project of analysing and mapping it.

---

[22] Foucault, *The Order of Things*, pp. 62–3.
[23] Funkenstein, *Theology and the Scientific Imagination*, pp. 28–42.
[24] G.B. Deason, 'Reformation Theology and the Mechanistic Conception of Nature',
in D.C. Lindberg and R.L. Numbers (eds), *God and Nature: Historical Essays on the
Encounter between Christianity and Science* (Berkeley: University of California Press,
1986), pp. 167–91. For Foucault, mechanization and mathematization were not
constant features in the origin of all sciences; what the latter did have in common,
nevertheless, was the ideal of generating an ordered system of knowledge based
on an artificial reference language, analysis and recombination – see Foucault,
The Order of Things, p. 57.

The death of God

However, in this secular theology God was still alive and needed, but needed in new ways – ways which would easily render him just as unnecessary as at this point he was necessary. What was different about the secular theologians' discourse of God? In medieval thought God had characteristically been seen as the ground of language and meaning itself, rather than as an object of language.[25] Similarly, in liturgical understandings of language, God is more than an object of speech; he is an addressee or a speaker, an I or a Thou.[26] But in the secular theology of Descartes, Galileo and Newton, God was made necessary in a different way, by making him perform specific functions within the emergent scientific understanding of the world. While many natural philosophers were concerned to emphasize the transcendence of God from his creation, they did so in ways that actually made him vulnerable to being cut adrift altogether.

This was partly to do with the way that these thinkers brought theology within the systematization of thought mentioned above, and thus subject to the drive towards unambiguous speech that was occurring in science and elsewhere. For, whatever their differences, the progenitors of modern science agreed that what was crucial for the securing of truth about the world was the purification and formalization of language. The advocates of this perspective argued like Hobbes that knowledge depends on 'Perspicuous words ... purged from ambiguity', rather than 'Metaphors, and sense-lesse and ambiguous words', relying upon which 'is wandering amongst innumerable absurdities'.[27] Some, such as Francis Bacon and John Wilkins, broadly following the classical distinction of logic and rhetoric, distinguished the precise, artificial, universal language required for scientific work from the rhetoric of common speech, ethics, and poetry. But others such as John Locke wanted all speech to be purified of ambiguity, part of a trend which at this time saw history and

---

[25] N. Frye, *The Great Code: The Bible and Literature* (London: Ark, 1983).
[26] C. Pickstock, *After Writing: On the Liturgical Consummation of Philosophy* (Oxford: Blackwell, 1998).
[27] T. Hobbes, *Leviathan* (London: Dent, 1914), p. 22.

law, and even religion and morality, experiencing new fashions for 'plain speech'.[28]

For our secular theologians this desire for univocity involved the refiguring of theological discourse along the same lines, stripped of the analogical and symbolic relations between signs, ideas and things that had been central to the main currents of theological reasoning for centuries. Whereas for Thomas Aquinas all talk of God's attributes – even concerning his very existence – could only be analogical, Descartes, Newton, More and Leibniz aspired for a clarity and distinctness in their ideas about God which paralleled that which they sought in relation to nature. Language about God's attributes – about his very being – had to be stripped of its analogical character and rendered univocal; similarly, talk of the relation between God and his creation had to be clarified and purged of mystery. 'The medieval sense of God's symbolic presence in his creation, and the sense of a universe replete with transcendent meanings and hints, had to recede if not to give way totally to the postulates of univocation and homogeneity in the seventeenth century. God's relation to the world had to be given a concrete physical meaning.'[29]

Thus, rather than God holding meaning in place, meaning came to hold God in place. God's being was made the prisoner of a language that was understood as immanent, transparent, given and univocal. For example, it was necessary for the secular theologians to reject medieval ideas of God cooperating with vital principles immanent within nature. One of the preconditions of their project of the mechanical description of the world according to mathematical laws was that matter had to be seen as wholly passive, containing no vital force or *nisus*. Mechanical philosophers such as Boyle and Newton thus stressed the absolute sovereignty of God and the dependency of matter on him for its continued existence and movement. For Newton, for example, lifeless nature was only animated by God's continuing intimate, active but predictable involvement in the world, as manifest in the operation of forces such as gravity.[30]

[28] B.J. Shapiro, *Probability and Certainty in Seventeenth-Century England: A Study of the Relationships between Natural Science, Religion, History, Law, and Literature* (Princeton, NJ: Princeton University Press, 1983), pp. 242–3.

[29] Funkenstein, *Theology and the Scientific Imagination*, p. 116.

[30] Deason, 'Reformation Theology and the Mechanistic Conception of Nature'.

In different ways, then, God's attributes were stripped of metaphor and allegory and allotted specific functions in the emerging scientific understanding of the world. Ironically, this disambiguation of theological talk was associated sometimes with an emphasis on Divine transcendence, sometimes with a radical immanence; but either way the end result was similar. The de-metaphorization of God's attributes and being directly laid the grounds for his disappearance from Western science. As Funkenstein graphically puts it, '[i]t is clear why a God described in unequivocal terms, or even given physical features and functions, eventually became all the easier to discard . . . all the easier to identify and kill'.[31]

The fusion of science and theology thus ultimately led to a science that refuses to speak of God. Yet if this science is atheological, it is so not in the sense of not having a theology, but in the sense of having a theology without God. Futhermore, the period of 'secular theology' that Funkenstein describes was more than simply a transitional period, a not-yet-complete separation of science from religion. The theological elements in the thought of Descartes and Newton played an important role in the formulation of their scientific concepts. And, more importantly, rather than their talk of God representing merely a temporary resistance to the arrival of an atheological science, it was their very disambiguating of theological language in order to fit it for their project that laid the grounds for the later disappearance of God. This irony will become particularly relevant later when I turn to the possible irony that the Human Genome Project might destroy the human by mapping it. One might say that God was killed on the scientists' table – by his incorporation into the *mathetic* project of separating signs into words and things, rendering language arbitrary and unequivocal, banishing allegory and symbol, and construing knowledge as a spatialized grid of statements.[32]

Other accounts of Newton's work put greater stress on the diversity in his treatment of gravity – see, for example, E. McMullin, *Newton on Matter and Activity* (Notre Dame: University of Notre Dame Press, 1978), and B.J.T. Dobbs, *The Janus Face of Genius: The Role of Alchemy in Newton's Thought* (Cambridge: Cambridge University Press, 1992). Nevertheless, the particular version I am stressing here is the one which is closest to the *mathetic* project.

[31] Funkenstein, *Theology and the Scientific Imagination*, p. 116.
[32] Dobbs poignantly describes the irony of this outcome in respect of Isaac Newton,

The death of the human

Could the human ever suffer its own obsolescence in a similar way? The final stage of my narrative is indeed to ask this question, to wonder whether the human might suffer a parallel fate to that suffered by God. But what might it *mean* for the human to die as God has in mainstream Western culture? In my use of the term 'human' here I am not referring to the biological human species,[33] but to a specific, contingent, historically situated phenomenon, one that came into being at a particular historical moment and could perhaps as accidentally depart. Foucault uses 'man' in this kind of way when, inspired by Nietzsche, he suggests that man, who has killed God, might himself be in the process of being erased – 'that man is in the process of perishing as the being of language continues to shine ever brighter upon our horizon'.[34] However, although Foucault is here using 'man' in a formally similar sense, as a historically specific formation rather than a biological species, there are also significant differences in our prophecies – and not just in terms of Foucault's apparent lack of alarm at the prospect he describes.

Foucault is using 'man' to refer to the object studied in and constituted by the human sciences, such as sociology, psychology and linguistics. 'Man' in this sense is that being which lives through representations – of itself, of the world, and of its actions – and was only constituted as a potential object of knowledge with the rise of the human sciences in the nineteenth century. In fact, Foucault's 'man' only appears when the *mathetic* project stumbles. In the Classical *episteme* of the seventeenth and eighteenth centuries that we were exploring above, in which knowledge was understood as transparent and

---

whom she presents as attempting to prove divine activity in nature, in order to stem the tides of mechanism and atheism. Far from the rise of atheological science representing Newton's triumph, Dobbs makes us see it as Newton's failure – see B.J.T. Dobbs, 'Newton as Final Cause and First Mover', in M.J. Osler (ed.) *Rethinking the Scientific Revolution* (Cambridge: Cambridge University Press, 2000), pp. 25–39. The deeper irony, of course, lies not in the dominant misrepresentation of Newton as a scientist who was only accidentally a theologian, but in the fact that Newton's secular theology in the long run had the opposite effect to that which he had hoped.

[33] Although the future of the human in this sense too might be in question – see Fukuyama, *Our Posthuman Future*.

[34] Foucault, *The Order of Things*, p. 386.

objective, 'man' as a subject which represents and posits knowledge had to remain invisible, outside the table of knowledge which he drew. 'The personage for whom the representation exists ... is never to be found in the table himself.'[35] Within this *episteme*, the human could only appear as a material object but not as a knowing, representing subject.

In the nineteenth century this human-as-subject *was* incorporated into scientific knowledge. However, this incorporation, rather than reducing and destroying the human, in many ways has added to and enhanced the vocabularies of the 'self' available to modern subjects.[36] What had happened to science – to the theologico-scientific project of the theoretical mastery of nature – that allowed the human-as-subject to survive its incorporation in a way that God-as-subject had not? I want to suggest that a precondition for this safe incorporation was not just the rise of the specifically human sciences, but also a transformation of the natural sciences, and of the relationship between the sciences – a precondition which might be threatened by the development of genomics.

As Foucault recounts, many sciences underwent a transformation in the nineteenth century, departing from the methods of analysis and recombination that had characterized the *mathetic* project of the seventeenth and eighteenth centuries. Rather than areas of knowledge being organized in terms of a horizontal table of similarities and differences, many of them thus started to be reorganized according to a new spatial metaphor – one of hidden unities lying underneath a surface of differences.[37] Take, for example, the shift from Linnaeus's natural history to Cuvier's biology. Linnaeus approached the study of living beings by analysing and measuring their visible similarities and differences – in an explicit rejection of the medieval search for analogies and similitudes, he wrote that the natural historian 'distinguishes the parts of natural bodies with his eyes, describes them appropriately according to their number, form, position, and proportion'.[38] Cuvier, by contrast, looked at the organs of the body in a very different way, prioritizing function over physical arrangement in what amounts to a

---

[35] Ibid., p. 308.
[36] Taylor, *Sources of the Self*.
[37] Foucault, *The Order of Things*, p. 251.
[38] Ibid., p. 161.

return to Aristotelian ways of thinking about organisms. As Foucault puts it, 'from Cuvier onward, function ... is to serve as a constant middle term and to make it possible to relate together totalities of elements without the slightest visible identity'.[39] Thus beneath the surface of the differences between species and species, and between organisms and their environment, lie the great unities of function – respiration, digestion, sensation and so on – not reducible to constituent material elements or visible to the senses, but nevertheless in many ways more ontologically fundamental.

In biology as elsewhere thus arose a language of surfaces and depths in a shift which amounted to the abandonment of the narrowly referential understanding of language that had dominated the last two centuries. Instead, there was a growing recognition of the enigmatic profusion of language as an evolving and complex human creation, and a return of exegesis and interpretation – the analogies binding objects together, the forces operating under the surface were not visible to the eye, but had to be discerned. Similarly, as the human sciences emerged they adopted similar metaphors of surfaces and depths. This was true of economics and sociology, but also psychology and wider culture, which saw the articulation of the psyche, 'a psychological space ... between the body and its organs and the person and his or her conduct' that added a new language of 'depth' to our understanding of the human person.[40] This articulation was noticeable in the rise of 'literature', a use of language oriented to its own sheer power of disclosure and expression in relation to this psychological space, but also in that of the human sciences, which sought to know in a more systematic way the human being as a representing and knowing subject. It was these depths that at once reformulated the concept of the human, and gave it a safe place in which to dwell within the realm of positive knowledge. The non-reductive spatial metaphor of surface and depth, and the giving way of the idea of a unified system of thought to a more decentred system of ordering within and across disciplines, made space

[39] Ibid., p. 265.
[40] C. Novas and N. Rose, 'Genetic Risk and the Birth of the Somatic Individual', *Economy and Society* 29.4 (2000), pp. 485–513, p. 508.

for the human as subject in a way that was not possible before.

Unlike Foucault I am less interested in 'man' as an object of various forms of knowledge that emerged in the nineteenth century than I am in the way that these new knowledges became extra 'sources of the self' – new resources for the way that human persons can talk about themselves and each other.[41] The surface–depth metaphor and the lack of unified tabular ordering across disciplines meant that social scientific and psychological knowledge did not successfully locate and pin down the human in the way that had happened to God. But now we have genomic science, which seeks to unravel the code that makes us human, and that makes us who we uniquely are, and to do so in a way that signals a robust return to *mathesis* – to the visible and measurable, to the method of analysis and recombination – and to the aspiration to unify the sciences. The dominance of molecular biology, with its strongly reductionistic aspirations, threatens a reordering of the sciences, as human behaviour is seen as reducible to biology, and biology to physics and chemistry.[42]

In a genetic science dominated by molecular biology, the surface of the DNA molecule and its sequences now becomes the real, a 'deep surface' which can be mapped and measured. The ambiguities of human action and identity become by contrast a 'superficial depth', a vague and disordered space of forces and conations which can only be given determinate meaning by being mapped and flattened on to that deep surface. DNA has become the 'Book of Man'[43] in terms of which human behaviour, predispositions and competences should be interpreted. Rather as natural objects were interpreted in the Middle Ages as signs that allegorically or symbolically refer to spiritual truths laid out in the Bible, human behaviour is now increasingly interpreted in terms of the meanings inscribed in

[41] Taylor, *Sources of the Self*; A. Giddens, *The Consequences of Modernity* (Cambridge: Polity Press, 1990).

[42] P.R. Sloan, 'Introductory Essay: Completing the Tree of Descartes', in P.R. Sloan (ed.), *Controlling our Destinies: Historical, Philosophical, Ethical and Theological Perspectives on the Human Genome Project* (Notre Dame: University of Notre Dame Press, 2000), pp. 1–28.

[43] D. Nelkin and M.S. Lindee, *The DNA Mystique: The Gene as a Cultural Icon* (New York: W.H. Freeman, 1995), pp. 52–3; W. Bodmer and R. McKie, *The Book of Man: The Quest to Discover Our Genetic Heritage* (London: Abacus, 1994).

the sacred text of the human genome. Forms of human action such as criminal behaviour, promiscuousness or alcoholism, for example, are interpreted as the working out of various genetic predispositions,[44] as 'natural signs' of deeper, molecular-biological arrangements.[45]

For two centuries the human person has had a place to dwell in knowledge. The human has inhabited the depths – spaces ordered not by a horizontal grid of similarities and differences but by a contrast between surface differences and deep unities, not by the visible but by the invisible, not by identity and non-identity but by analogy and function. The human has also been able to slip through the gaps *between* disciplines, to avoid capture and redundancy by virtue of the impossibility of a unified *mathetic* method and language for the sciences. In the new genomic future, with a colonization of these depths by the *mathetic* grid and a new spatial metaphor of deep surface, and a renewed attempt to reductionistically unify the sciences, the human's ability to escape the fate of God in Western knowledge – our ability to retain a fully humanistic language of the human person – seems less certain.

I have suggested above that the HGP should be engaged with as a species of what Funkenstein calls 'secular theology', and thus that theological engagement should not just be with its technical and social ramifications, but with its *own* buried or not-so-buried theology.[46] I argued that the notion of the genetic code represents an attempt to complete a *mathesis* of the human – an ordered system of knowledge which attempts to analyse its

---

[44] R.C. Lewontin, *The Doctrine of DNA: Biology as Ideology* (Harmondsworth: Penguin, 1993).

[45] Novas and Rose, 'Genetic Risk and the Birth of the Somatic Individual', remind us that 'one should not mistake the spontaneous philosophy of the scientist for the operative epistemology or ontology of scientific activity' (p. 508), and argue that the notion of the genetic code as a deep inner truth is only to be found in popular science writings, and is not characteristic of the practice of genetic science. They suggest that genetic practices such as screening and counselling *do* transform the self, but in a way in which genetic, somatized forms of personhood are hybridized with constructions of the self as autonomous, prudent and responsible, and are also embedded in networks of family members, experts and others. While their points are well made, and have helped the argument in the present chapter, nevertheless I think they underestimate the dangers posed by reductionistic genetic discourses of the human.

[46] In the chapter I have specifically focused on worries I have about the HGP; however, theological engagements of the kind I am advocating need not be solely negative.

subject matter into basic elements and to identify the logic and mechanism of their combination – by attempting to materialize the human essence on to the chromosomes in a way that parallels the embodiment of God in the seventeenth century. By trying to reduce the human to a *mathesis* the HGP can only accept features of the human that are describable in an unequivocal reference language referring to a self-identical referent. By giving the human essence a location, by stretching it out on the chromosomes, by mapping and plotting it, it may be all the more easy to destroy it.

Bibliography

Arendt, H., *The Human Condition* (Chicago: University of Chicago Press, 1998).

Bodmer, W. and McKie, R., *The Book of Man: The Quest to Discover Our Genetic Heritage* (London: Abacus, 1994).

Brooke, J.H., *Science and Religion: Some Historical Perspectives* (Cambridge: Cambridge University Press, 1991).

Deason, G.B., 'Reformation Theology and the Mechanistic Conception of Nature', in D.C. Lindberg and R.L. Numbers (eds), *God and Nature: Historical Essays on the Encounter between Christianity and Science* (Berkeley: University of California Press, 1986), pp. 167–91.

Dobbs, B.J.T., *The Janus Face of Genius: The Role of Alchemy in Newton's Thought* (Cambridge: Cambridge University Press, 1992).

Dobbs, B.J.T., 'Newton as Final Cause and First Mover', in M.J. Osler (ed.) *Rethinking the Scientific Revolution* (Cambridge: Cambridge University Press, 2000), pp. 25–39.

Duffy, E., *The Stripping of the Altars: Traditional Religion in England, c.1400–c. 1580* (New Haven: Yale University Press, 1992).

Foucault, M., *The Order of Things: An Archaeology of the Human Sciences* (London: Tavistock, 1970).

Frye, N., *The Great Code: The Bible and Literature* (London: Ark, 1983).

Fukuyama, F., *Our Posthuman Future: Consequences of the Biotechnology Revolution* (London: Profile Books, 2002).

Funkenstein, A., *Theology and the Scientific Imagination from the Middle Ages to the Seventeenth Century* (Princeton, NJ: Princeton University Press, 1986).

Giddens, A., *The Consequences of Modernity* (Cambridge: Polity Press, 1990).

Harrison, P., *The Bible, Protestantism, and the Rise of Natural Science* (Cambridge: Cambridge University Press, 1998).

Heelas, P. and Lock, A. (eds), *Indigenous Psychologies: The Anthropology of the Self* (London: Academic Press, 1981).

Hobbes, T., *Leviathan* (London: Dent, 1914).

Lewontin, R.C., *The Doctrine of DNA: Biology as Ideology* (Harmondsworth: Penguin, 1993).

Macpherson, C.B., *The Political Theory of Possessive Individualism: Hobbes to Locke* (Oxford: Clarendon Press, 1962).

McMullin, E., *Newton on Matter and Activity* (Notre Dame: University of Notre Dame Press, 1978).

Merchant, C., *The Death of Nature: Women, Ecology, and the Scientific Revolution* (San Francisco: Harper and Row, 1980).

Nelkin, D. and Lindee, M.S., *The DNA Mystique: The Gene as a Cultural Icon* (New York: W.H. Freeman, 1995).

Novas, C. and Rose, N., 'Genetic Risk and the Birth of the Somatic Individual', *Economy and Society* 29.4 (2000), pp. 485–513.

Peters, T., *Playing God* (London: Routledge, 1997).

Pickstock, C., *After Writing: On the Liturgical Consummation of Philosophy* (Oxford: Blackwell, 1998).

Reiss, T.J., *The Discourse of Modernism* (Ithaca, NY: Cornell University Press, 1982).

Shapiro, B.J., *Probability and Certainty in Seventeenth-Century England: A Study of the Relationships between Natural Science, Religion, History, Law, and Literature* (Princeton, NJ: Princeton University Press, 1983).

Shea, W.R., 'Galileo and the Church', in D.C. Lindberg and R.L. Numbers (eds), *God and Nature: Historical Essays on the Encounter between Christianity and Science* (Berkeley: University of California Press, 1986), pp. 114–35.

Sloan, P.R., 'Introductory Essay: Completing the Tree of

Descartes', in P.R. Sloan (ed.), *Controlling Our Destinies: Historical, Philosophical, Ethical and Theological Perspectives on the Human Genome Project* (Notre Dame: University of Notre Dame Press, 2000), pp. 1–28.

Taylor, C., *Sources of the Self: The Making of the Modern Identity* (Cambridge: Cambridge University Press, 1989).

Thomas, K., *Man and the Natural World: Changing Attitudes in England 1500–1800* (Harmondsworth: Penguin, 1984).

8

The Human Genome Project as Soteriological Project

Robert Song

Introduction

A number of common themes recur in standard critiques of the new molecular genetics as applied to human beings. These centre on its propensity, or at least the propensity of the philosophy often associated with it, towards reductionism, biological determinism, and the geneticization of human identity.[1] Critics who pursue this line have in their sights ideas such as the following: that all traits and behaviour can be explained largely or even solely in genetic terms, and do not require much, if any, reference to environmental explanations; that an individual's behaviour can be understood as a product of his or her genes; that the behaviour of a group or collectivity can be interpreted by reference to the genes of the individuals

---

[1] For such criticisms see, for example, Steven Rose, R.C. Lewontin and Leon J. Kamin, *Not in Our Genes: Biology, Ideology and Human Nature* (Harmondsworth: Penguin, 1984) ('the twin philosophical stances with which this book is concerned' are 'reductionism' and 'biological determinism' (pp. 5–6)); Ruth Hubbard and Elijah Wald, *Exploding the Gene Myth: How Genetic Information Is Produced and Manipulated by Scientists, Physicians, Employers, Insurance Companies, Educators, and Law Enforcers* (Boston, MA: Beacon Press, 1993) (focuses on 'geneticization' and 'reductionism' (pp. 2–3)); R.C. Lewontin, *The Doctrine of DNA: Biology as Ideology* (London: Penguin, 1993) (criticizes 'the ideology of biological determinism' (p. 23)); and Dorothy Nelkin and M. Susan Lindee, *The DNA Mystique: The Gene as a Cultural Icon* (New York: Freeman, 1995) (argues that popular culture conveys 'genetic essentialism' (p. 2)). For a theological critique of the 'gene myth', see Ted Peters, *Playing God? Genetic Determinism and Human Freedom* (New York: Routledge, 1997).

that comprise it; that if a trait or behaviour can be described as genetic, it is therefore immutable; and that the role of DNA in the make-up of a person can be depicted as a 'blueprint', 'master molecule', or through other implicitly deterministic metaphors. Ideas like these, the critics note, reinforce the ideological power of genetic categories within a technological-scientific culture. In medicine, for example, they contribute to the expanding notion of genetic disease, in which the genetic component is singled out for especial prominence. In terms of personal self-understanding, they underwrite the increasing emphasis on genetic identity as the key to people's interpretation of their psychology and physiology, their successes and failures, their past and future. Socially, they emerge in the sociobiological legitimation of patriarchal gender relations, racial discrimination, and opposition to welfare handouts or egalitarian approaches to education.

These misgivings are surely justified. As Evelyn Fox Keller has written, 'Most responsible advocates are of course careful to acknowledge the role of *both* nature and nurture, but rhetorically, as well as in scientific practice, it is "nature" that emerges as the decisive victor.'[2] The reductionist tendency of the programme always appears to end up giving biology the explanatory priority. The potency of the gene as a cultural symbol has reinforced leanings towards a genetic essentialism that equates people with their genetic make-up, thereby squeezing out the manifold historical and cultural complexities of their formation. Under the spell of such a mentality it is easy for biological difference to become definitive of social identity, in relation to gender, class, race, intelligence, bodily health, sexuality, and the various traits and behaviours putatively associated with genetic influence. Equally, in such a context recognition of genetic factors runs the risk of a fatalist mindset which forgets that it is the degree of malleability of traits which is critical, not the fact of their genetic inheritance. And such determinism consorts well with the social and political pressures towards programmes of genetic improvement that reached their nadir in Nazi Germany, only to reappear in a very different

[2] Evelyn Fox Keller, 'Nature, Nurture, and the Human Genome Project', in Daniel J. Kevles and Leroy Hood (eds), *The Code of Codes: Scientific and Social Issues in the Human Genome Project* (Cambridge, MA: Harvard University Press, 1992), pp. 281–99 at p. 282.

form in subsequent decades in the consumerist eugenics that is exemplified by pre-natal testing leading to abortion.[3]

I entirely concur with these critics, therefore. Indeed in what follows I will take the general thrust of their criticisms for granted. However, in my view their understanding of the phenomenon of the new genetics is incomplete. They fail to give a sufficiently plausible account of its appeal not only to scientists and corporate biotechnology interests, but to the ordinary inhabitants of modern Western culture as a whole. They do not explain why anybody should be attracted to the reductionist project or should be inclined towards under-standing human beings in these etiolated terms. In this chapter I want to explore some of the cultural commitments that have given rise to the new genetics, and ultimately to the Human Genome Project. In particular I will attempt to draw some connections between its roots on the one hand in seventeenth-century scientific and technological aspirations, and an underlying quality of motivation on the other which I will argue should be seen as quasi-religious in nature. Only once this has been acknowledged, I shall claim, will we be free to ask the question whether the Human Genome Project is a project which human beings might properly embark on.

The reductionist project

According to the critics we are considering, the programme of the new genetics which has given birth to the Human Genome Project should be criticized for its reductive philosophical stance: it understands human beings solely, or at least pre-dominantly, in terms of their genetic inheritance. As I have indicated, I share these concerns, and think that it is open to criticism at least to the extent that it shares in such a stance. However, of itself such a style of critique is inadequate, for a variety of reasons. By appreciating these, I hope that we may work towards a fuller understanding and perhaps more adequate critique of the new genetics.

The first problem with the critique of the new genetics as reductive is that the new genetics is not necessarily committed

---

[3] Robert Song, *Human Genetics: Fabricating the Future* (London: Darton, Longman & Todd, 2002), pp. 41–56, 81–95.

to this philosophical stance. While the science may often have proceeded under the impress of a reductive imperative, for reasons we shall discuss later, there is a plausible case for saying that the new genetics is not itself intrinsically reductive. It would be quite possible for a researcher to argue that the only way of understanding the relative contributions and mutual implications of genetic and environmental factors is to obtain a more precise comprehension of each, and that on the genetic side this requires the detailed knowledge that is being provided by gene mapping and sequencing that has been undertaken by the Human Genome Project, together with the exploration of protein structure and interaction and all the other developments in understanding which it is hoped will emerge during the next decades and beyond. Greater knowledge here would imply no prejudgement in favour of genetic explanations; indeed it might thwart the pretensions of reductive approaches by showing precisely what genetics is incapable of accounting for. In other words, to the extent that the philosophical commitments and broader cultural representations of the new genetics are guilty of reductionism or determinist essentialism, they should be rejected, but it should not be presumed that these errors are somehow intrinsic to the science itself.

The second problem with the critique is that by itself it does not complete the critical task. It is one thing to show the intellectual and moral errors of reductionism as a philosophical stance, another to give an account of what gave rise to it in the first place. To criticize a philosophy of genetics simply for being reductive leaves unexplained why anybody should be attracted to such a view, a difficulty which is made the more severe, the more obviously absurd the reductionist position can be shown to be. We can elucidate this point by developing the critique in a little more depth.

The reductionist approach to genetics, we might elaborate the critics' argument, compromises a true understanding of human persons. This is achieved by down-playing or even analysing out the role of environmental factors, or by neglecting the inward, self-constituting nature of agents, or both. In doing so, it aligns the study of human genetics with the modernist project of attempting to explain the properties of larger and more complex entities in terms of the properties of the units out of which they are composed. This project can in turn be seen as a consequence of the new approach to the science of nature that was articulated in the seventeenth century,[4] an account which (in Amos Funkenstein's portrayal) united four previously separate ideals: the drive for unequivocation in language, which required the abandonment of the picture of the natural world as itself symbolic and referential, with a view to ensuring that only language could designate; the drive to regard nature as homogeneous, such that the laws of nature should be presumed to apply uniformly throughout the universe; mathematization, that nature could be understood in the language of mathematics; and mechanization, that final causes should be discarded in favour of the complete explanatory adequacy of efficient causes alone.[5] These ideals paved the way for the considerable success of the physical sciences from the seventeenth century. But they were also increasingly applied to the study of human beings, and formed a framework of thought which has given rise to a family of theories that have recurred in a variety of forms, from mechanistic approaches to anatomy in the late eighteenth century to psychological behaviourism and attempts to create artificial intelligence in the twentieth century and beyond.

The specific ebbs and flows of this process of applying the methods and assumptions of the natural sciences to the study of human beings are of less concern to me here[6] than the question of the motivation of this naturalist programme. We need to uncover the nature of the appeal it has had.

In answer to this it is of course possible to see a number of intellectual attractions: it would be disingenuous to deny the enormous advances in scientific understanding made on the basis of such an approach, not just in relation to the ostensibly 'hard' sciences of the physical body, but also in relation to 'softer' sciences such as psychology.[7] But given the manifest

---

[4] Rose *et al.* refer the origins of the reductive view of human nature to the emergence of bourgeois society in the seventeenth century and Hobbes's view that (in their words) 'it was biological inevitability that made humans what they were' (*Not in Our Genes*, p. 5).

[5] Amos Funkenstein, *Theology and the Scientific Imagination from the Middle Ages to the Seventeenth Century* (Princeton: Princeton University Press, 1986), pp. 28–31.

[6] Though for some insightful elaboration of this see Bronislaw Szerszynski's piece in the present volume.

[7] For an account of what mechanistic models can and cannot explain in psychology, see Charles Taylor, 'Peaceful Coexistence in Psychology', in *Philosophical Papers*, 2

unpersuasiveness of the thoroughgoing reductive project, even starker in some fields than it is in genetics, the question arises compellingly for all but true believers how such an approach could ever have come to seem plausible.

In searching for the motivations behind reductive accounts of the human sciences, we might take a cue from conventional explanations for the appeal of their equivalents in the physical sciences, namely the search for a certain kind of knowledge. This might be expressed in terms of the increased powers of prediction and control over nature. If this were applied by analogy to the social sciences, it might illuminate how their naturalist desire for overarching laws of the social world could be explained by reference to greater capacities for organization and administration of populations. But it could also throw some light on the case we are concerned with, that of human genetics. For the early history of the attraction towards genetic determinism is inseparable from the rise of eugenic ambitions. Most geneticists in the early decades of the twentieth century regarded it as the proper role of science to improve the human race, and the prevalence of eugenic beliefs among those working in the field both informed and was informed by their belief in the decisive role of heredity in the formation of intellectual and moral traits.[8] Their confidence in eugenics grew because their belief in determinism made it possible; their confidence in determinism grew because their eugenic ideals made it desirable.

Yet even this kind of explanation only takes us so far. In relation to genetics, it does not account for the continuing appeal of genetic essentialism in an era which has repudiated all overt eugenic intentions. Nor does it explain the continuing presence of the reductive mentality even in areas – such as the geneticization of identity – which have prima facie rather little to do with eugenics, even in its new consumerist form. There is an element in the explanation which is missing.

---

vols (Cambridge: Cambridge University Press, 1985), vol. i: *Human Agency and Language*, pp. 117–38. Much of Taylor's *oeuvre* has been devoted to explaining the appeal of reductive naturalisms in the human sciences. In addition to both volumes of *Philosophical Papers*, see also esp. *Sources of the Self: The Making of the Modern Identity* (Cambridge: Cambridge University Press, 1989).

[8] Diane Paul, *Controlling Human Heredity: 1865 to the Present* (Atlantic Heights, NY: Humanities Press, 1995), pp. 121–5.

What we are searching for, therefore, is a critical explanatory account of the phenomenon of the new genetics as a whole which will do justice to the critique of the reductive tendencies that we have been discussing, but will also set it in a broader framework. More specifically, we may conclude from our discussion so far, such an account will do at least four things. First, it should be able to furnish an explanation of the coming-to-be of the new genetics, and not just assume its facticity as something to be subject to a posteriori criticism. Rather than taking the genetic phenomenon as a brute given, it should be able to provide a narrative of the causal dynamics that have given rise to the new genetics in such a way that some light will be shed on its possible future trajectories. This is not the same as asking it to predict the future, of course, but merely to give a deeper understanding of the forces that have created the present and will shape the future.

Second, this critique will not presume that the genetic phenomenon is necessarily reductive in nature. It will not lose all critical power if it were to be shown that the Human Genome Project is not inherently committed to a reductive programme. Third, on the other hand, it must be able to explain the temptation to reductionism with which genetics has rightly been connected. If the relation between genetics and reductionism is contingent, as I have suggested, the two still display a mutual affinity, and this needs illumination. Fourth, it must be able to give a full account of the motivations which might be associated with the reductive tendencies of the new genetics which goes beyond those which we have examined so far. In particular, we need to consider not merely the intellectual and socio-political attractions of determinism in genetics, but also the moral and even existential appeal of it.

The seventeenth-century project

As a first step towards this account, we should note something insufficiently recognized by commentators on the Human Genome Project, namely that it is a public, social act. At one level it is a highly complex endeavour of scientific research, for which spending has had to be argued over against other funding priorities, but at another level it is also a social act with a high degree of ownership by the wider public. Evidence of this public interest can be found in the massively disproportionate media coverage devoted to new discoveries in genetics compared with other areas of science, as well as in the active support and vociferous advocacy of genetic research by interest groups and others. While those who undertake or fund genome research may do so for their own scientific or commercial (or charitable) reasons, they do so to a significant extent on behalf of society as a whole. No doubt there is a process of legitimation at work in order to render publicly plausible the genetics project as a whole (through rhetorical expansion of the notion of genetic disease, of the potential of genomic research, and so on), but even so the role of the public is still better depicted as knowing complicity rather than passive or innocent acquiescence.[9]

What then is the cause of the public obsession with the new genetics? At least at the level of presenting reasons, the most palpable attraction is of course the promise of benefits. These benefits include increased human self-understanding – the role of genes in behaviour, for example. But their main appeal is surely in relation to health and the potential they are perceived to hold for improved diagnosis and ultimately treatment of disease, from highly penetrant single-gene disorders such as Huntington's disease in which environmental factors play a minimal role, to cancers at the other extreme where the presence even of several alleles acting in concert may contribute only an incremental increase in susceptibility. Indeed, so intuitively plausible is the notion that human medical benefit is outstandingly the most compelling reason for undertaking genomic research that an official HGP website courts absurdity when it lists molecular medicine as just one of six potential benefits of human genome research, of which the others are 'microbial genomics; risk assessment; bioarchaeology, anthropology, evolution, and human migration; DNA forensics (identification); agriculture, livestock breeding, and bioprocessing' – as if bioarchaeology were on a par in the public mind with a cure for cancer.[10]

---

[9] David F. Noble assumes wrongly that the religion of technology was always 'in essence an elitist expectation, reserved only for the elect' (*The Religion of Technology: The Divinity of Man and the Spirit of Invention* (New York: Knopf, 1997), p. 201).

[10] 'Potential Benefits of Human Genome Project Research', <http://www.ornl.gov/hgmis/project/benefits.html> (accessed 28 June 2002).

Scientists also have a fundamental interest in the medical benefits of genetic research, whatever else may motivate them. Even if individual researchers may be moved by the joy of knowledge alone, effective arguments for funding the Human Genome Project have been very largely based on the putative clinical outcomes. Thus Nancy Wexler, as chair of the working group on the Ethical, Legal and Social Implications of the Project: 'those of us who have been working in the field of genetic disease for a long time and who are engrossed in efforts towards finding treatments and cures, feel strongly that the question is not whether we can afford to do this project but whether we can afford *not* to do this project'.[11] Or James D. Watson, as co-discoverer of the structure of DNA and first director of the Human Genome Project: '[w]hen you ask a supporter of the project "Why do you want to do it?" the overriding reason is that it will let us get handles on genetic disease much more efficiently'.[12] The interests of corporate pharmaceutical and biotechnological interests likewise are not far removed from diagnostic and therapeutic success. While of course they may benefit from creating medical needs where none had existed previously (for example – in a currently non-genetic field – in the case of aesthetic surgery), in the vast majority of cases long-term commercial success will be dependent on satisfactorily meeting human medical need. At least in relation to human genomic research, therefore, there is a case for seeing the attractions of pure research and the pressures of the market economy as secondary levels of explanation compared with the potential for medical benefit.

Any reasonable interpretation of the whole phenomenon of the new genetics will therefore give a prima facie priority to the motivation of freedom from disease. How might this fit into the broader account we are attempting to construct? To answer

[11] In a round-table discussion held in 1990, 'An Invitation to Genetics in the Twenty-First Century', in Necia Grant-Cooper (ed.), *The Human Genome Project: Deciphering the Blueprint of Heredity* (Mill Valley, CA: University Science Books, 1994), pp. 314–29 at p. 318.

[12] James D. Watson, 'The Human Genome Initiative', in Barry Holland and Charalambos Kyriacou (eds), *Genetics and Society* (Wokingham: Addison-Wesley, 1993), pp. 13–26 at p. 19. Watson opines that this is the majority position of older scientists who find their minds turning to questions of disease; younger scientists by contrast are more fascinated by the HGP's 'intrinsic benefits to pure science' (ibid.).

this, we need to revisit the seventeenth century, this time interested in the period not just as the origin of mechanizing and reductivist motifs in the human sciences, but as the source of a particular kind of motivation.

The Human Genome Project is best seen, I suggest, as the latest avatar of a set of aspirations which were most influentially formulated in their distinctively modern form in seventeenth-century England. These ambitions, which I shall term 'the Baconian project', following Gerald McKenny,[13] centre on the effort to deny the necessity of suffering, achieved by the instrumental control of nature. Francis Bacon's project centred on the reconstruction of philosophy with a view to the discovery of nature's secrets and improvements in the conditions of human life. At his most visionary, these improvements included 'the prolongation of life, the restitution of youth in some degree, the retardation of age, the curing of diseases counted incurable, the mitigation of pain'.[14] Although he was not a Puritan, his emphasis on practical betterment over against sterile scholasticism ('the knowledge that we now possess will not teach a man even what to *wish*'),[15] set within a biblical framework, rendered him an instinctively congenial philosopher in Puritan eyes. They in turn busied themselves with exploitation of the fruits of the earth in the service of God, a process that would be eased by the mechanistic rejection of the teleological ordering of nature and the adoption of reductive modes of explanation.[16]

---

[13] Gerald P. McKenny, *To Relieve the Human Condition: Bioethics, Technology and the Body* (Albany, NY: State University of New York Press, 1997), pp. 17–21, drawing on the work of Charles Taylor. The term is used by synecdoche, and should not be taken to imply that Bacon himself was responsible for the larger project to which I have attached his name.

[14] Francis Bacon, 'Magnalia Naturae', in *The Advancement of Learning and New Atlantis*, ed. Arthur Johnston (Oxford: Clarendon Press, 1974), p. 249. Strikingly, in view of the new genetics, the list also includes 'The altering of statures; The altering of features ... Making of new species; Transplanting of one species into another'.

[15] Preface to *De Interpretatione Naturae*, quoted by Johnston, p. x.

[16] For the influence of the Puritans on the development of early modern science and medicine, see Charles Webster, *The Great Instauration: Science, Medicine and Reform, 1626–60* (London: Duckworth, 1975), esp. pp. 1–31, 324–42, 484–520. Note however that the millenarianism and this-worldly utopianism that Webster sees as motivating technological development was relatively uncommon compared with more conventional eschatological beliefs: see John Henry, 'Atomism and Eschatology: Catholicism and Natural Philosophy in the Interregnum', *British Journal for the History of Science* (1982), pp. 211–39.

In subsequent centuries the goals would be furthered while the thought was slowly secularized. The early utilitarians of the radical Enlightenment reduced moral value to the net utility of pleasure over pain, thereby reducing suffering to a mere negative in a felicific calculus. Similarly, deist questioning of God's action in the world turned providence into impersonal fate, making unnecessary the spiritual discipline of finding meaning in suffering. Combined with an Enlightenment and Romantic emphasis on individual autonomy, and the increased mastery of nature afforded by nineteenth- and twentieth-century technological developments, the Baconian project has consequently bequeathed to modern medicine its animating ideals: namely, the elimination of suffering and the maximization of individual choice.

It is important to note that these twin ideals do not merely address the infirmities of bodily existence. They also implicitly raise the hope of freedom from subjection to the necessities of the human condition. Shorn of the limitations imposed by religion, the promise of modern medicine is not just of therapy for disease, but of therapy for the existential anxieties of finitude and mortality. The conquest of nature has become the conquest of fate, and it is this desire for domination which we should see as motivating the project of modern technological medicine, of which the Human Genome Project itself is but one part. The quest for an instrumentalized, reductive understanding of human beings is in other words the outworking of a desire for freedom from necessity.

This gives us in brief compass the elements of a theory in which reductionism has a role, but one that is secondary to a certain kind of motivation. Support for this interpretation of the direction of seventeenth-century thinking might also be argued from the case of Descartes. It is tempting to portray his philosophy as fundamentally motivated by epistemological concerns about the possibility of certainty, which in turn carried implications for his dualist metaphysics of mind–body relations. But, as Drew Leder has suggested,[17] it is at least arguable that his metaphysics was driven by existential concerns about disease and death. This may be seen from his own discussions about the

---

[17] Drew Leder, *The Absent Body* (Chicago: University of Chicago Press, 1990), pp. 138–41, as discussed by McKenny, *To Relieve the Human Condition*, pp. 190–2.

motivations for his philosophy. Towards the end of the *Discourse on Method* he talks of 'the possibility of gaining knowledge which would be very useful in life, and of discovering a practical philosophy which might replace the speculative philosophy taught in the schools', through which we might 'make ourselves, as it were, the lords and masters of nature'. The most important reason he gives for this is 'the maintenance of health, which is undoubtedly the chief good and the foundation of all the other goods in this life', and includes freedom from 'innumerable diseases, both of the body and of the mind, and perhaps even from the infirmity of old age, if we had sufficient knowledge of their causes and of all the remedies that nature has provided'.[18] And beyond this, he claims, arguments for the distinct substances of body and mind are needed 'to show that the decay of the body does not imply the destruction of the mind' and 'to give mortals the hope of an after-life', such that 'while the body can very easily perish, the mind is immortal by its very nature'.[19] The mechanization of the body is therefore not just a propaedeutic to its yielding physiological knowledge, but part of a strategy of evading existential threats to the self by ensuring that the pure substance of the soul can never be contaminated by the accidents of the body.

The Baconian project, echoed by Descartes, provides us with the elements of a theory of modern technological medicine as a whole. But in relation to the Human Genome Project, we can go a step further in learning from the seventeenth century by looking further at Bacon's own philosophy of science. Antonio Pérez-Ramos, in an influential study, has argued that Bacon should not be understood in broad categories such as 'inductivism', 'utilitarianism', and the like.[20] Rather, underlying his thought is the notion of 'maker's knowledge', that knowledge of the truth of the thing is knowledge of the way it is constructed and could be reconstructed. The epistemological guarantee of one's understanding of nature is the ability to

---

[18] René Descartes, *Discourse on Method* (1637), Part Six, in *The Philosophical Writings of Descartes*, trans. John Cottingham, Robert Stoothoff and Dugald Murdoch, 3 vols (Cambridge: Cambridge University Press, 1985-91), vol. i, pp. 142–3.

[19] Descartes, *Meditations on First Philosophy* (1641), Synopsis, in *The Philosophical Writings of Descartes*, vol. ii, p. 10.

[20] Antonio Pérez-Ramos, *Francis Bacon's Idea of Science and the Maker's Knowledge Tradition* (Oxford: Clarendon Press, 1988).

produce it and the interiorization of the skills to enable one to reproduce it. This analysis of the nature of knowledge cuts across the categories of pure/applied and theory/practice: since maker's knowledge is not simply knowledge as the capacity for making but also knowledge as the ability to conceptualize the practice, it reconfigures the terms.

One implication of this is that we should distinguish the broader 'Baconian project', extending over centuries, from the more precise understanding of Bacon's own philosophy of science. In the strict sense, Pérez-Ramos maintains, 'no recognizable artefact or technique can be identified as approximately bespeaking Baconian desiderata in the sense advanced here until, say, the development of the chemical or pharmaceutical industry in the nineteenth century, or the rise of genetic engineering in our own'.[21] Appreciating this enables us to refine our understanding of the Human Genome Project in relation to the broader account of technological medicine. Not only does the HGP share in all the broader features of the project of eliminating suffering and maximizing choice, it does so in a particular way. It radicalizes the search for causes, not just by driving them back to their molecular basis, but by implicitly thinking of true knowledge of the body as the ability to construct it. And in this model, knowledge of the 'basic building blocks' of the body is not just knowledge of how it is constructed, but at once also knowledge of how it might be reconstructed.

The soteriological project

I have suggested therefore that the desire for reductionist explanations and for instrumental approaches to the body should be seen as secondary to and derivative from the motivation of freedom from necessity. But it has also been evident that this motivation cannot be divested of an existential dimension: the Baconian project has been not just a matter of healing of particular infirmities, but a more radical freedom from the burdens of finitude. This quasi-religious dimension needs to be explored more directly.

The Puritans of course handled their thinking about science and medicine within the matrix of the biblical narrative. It was

---

[21] Ibid., pp. 294–5.

not possible, they agreed, to be too well studied in the book of God's word or the book of God's works. 'To know the secrets of nature, is to know the works of God' was a common tag of the period, while a particular favourite of Bacon's had been Proverbs 25.2: 'The glory of God is to conceal a thing: the glory of the King to search it out.'[22] This knowledge of the workings of nature was interpreted as a restoration of Adam's former knowledge, a recapitulation of the lost condition of creation.

However, for them such knowledge was always bounded by religion. In answer to the question how knowledge could be a godly pursuit if the fall itself was the result of the desire for knowledge, Bacon had answered that 'all knowledge is to be limited by religion, and to be referred to use and action'.[23] And so the Puritans had guarded against the potential for moral corruption and social exploitation through the discipline afforded by the virtues and precepts of Christian morality, and had sought to control the distribution of the fruits of knowledge through careful oversight by the godly parliament.[24] Far from detracting from their service of God, the investigation of nature to advance learning and provide benefit for humankind was one of its highest expressions.

But it was not clear that the quest for knowledge of nature could always be limited in this way. This can be seen from Funkenstein's commentary on the seventeenth-century project. He argues that the constructivist understanding of knowledge, the theory which I earlier attributed to Bacon as 'maker's knowledge', was in fact characteristic of the new epistemological project of the seventeenth century as a whole.[25] In the medieval period, he suggests, the identity of truth with doing had been a characteristic mark of the divine knowledge of the Creator alone. In so far as it was a property of human knowledge, it was confined to machines and other human artefacts. Human knowledge of the universe as a whole, by contrast, whether it was conceived as a matter of illumination, introspection or abstraction from sense impressions, was fundamentally a passive or receptive knowledge. However, in the seventeenth century the active, constructionist epistemology was extended to human

---

[22] Webster, *The Great Instauration*, pp. 105, 329.
[23] Ibid., p. 22.
[24] Ibid., pp. 517–18.
[25] Funkenstein, *Theology and the Scientific Imagination*, pp. 290–9.

knowledge of the universe as well, threatening a disintegration
of the barrier between divine and human knowledge so radical
that many baulked at its implications. As Funkenstein writes:
'applying knowledge-through-construction to the whole world
was as inevitable as it was dangerous. It was dangerous because
it makes mankind be "like God, knowing good and evil".'[26] The
new epistemology had a transgressive potential that could
breach the ultimate of boundaries.

If the new epistemological commitments of the seventeenth
century were to give human beings access to previously
forbidden divine knowledge, so the trajectory of the Baconian
project was to take the new learning far beyond the bounds
placed on it by the Puritans. As millenarianism waned in the
latter part of the century and gave way to a secularized faith in
progress, so the theological framework for addressing the issues
was also gradually dismantled. But the repudiation of the
explicit theology did not mean the disappearance of religious
functions or the loss of religious needs. Rather as God was first
made a function of the new scientific knowledge and then
abandoned as unnecessary, so the existential nature of
suffering changed, and the effort to eliminate it began to
absorb the weight of soteriological expectation. Instead of
suffering being an opportunity for receiving God's grace,
through which endurance, character, and hope might come, in
which one might participate in the sufferings of Christ, it began
to be interpreted as brute, unreferential pain whose only value
lay in being eradicated. In this new religious project, behind
the relief of individual bodily infirmities lay the hope of
freedom from the burdens and randomness of finitude and
mortality.

So the Baconian project becomes a surrogate form of
salvation, its religious significance and doctrinal commitments
occluded from many of its proponents because of their self-
conscious secularism. It develops, for example, a doctrine of
creation, which conceives nature as raw material available for
technological manipulation, while its anthropology defines
human beings in terms of self-defining freedom above the
contingencies of bodily life. It espouses an eschatological hope,
which lies in the dream of escape from finitude, and locates the

---

[26] Ibid., p. 327.

means of salvation to that end in the application of technical reason and the 'power of modern science'. It has generated its own ethics, in which both utilitarian and Kantian lineages of standard philosophical bioethics share an allegiance to the instrumentalization of the nature and alienation of the self from the body.

Modern technological medicine, in its obsession with the elimination of suffering and its fetishization of health, can therefore be seen as soteriological in nature. But this dimension is most pointed in the case of molecular genomics, not just because of its potentially central role in the medicine of the future, nor because it requires the intensive application of high technology, but because of the conception of knowledge that it embodies: knowledge of construction which, as we have seen, is at once also knowledge of reconstruction and therefore of transformation. 'For the first time in all time,' as Robert Sinsheimer declared after an initial conference about launching a genome sequencing project, 'a living creature understands its origin and can undertake to design its future.'[27] And at least something of the same goal is implied in James Watson's talk of the need for 'the courage to make less random the sometimes most unfair courses of human evolution'.[28]

We have become familiar with the religious resonances of many of the pronouncements about the potential of the Human Genome Project, from Walter Gilbert's early talk of the Grail,[29] to President Clinton's statement on announcing the completion of the first draft of the human genome: 'Today we are learning the language in which God created life.'[30] But their soteriological nature stems not from the fact that their authors felt compelled to reach for religious language to describe their feelings of awe at what might be and (partly) has been achieved, as that they represent the tip of the iceberg of a much profounder set of allegiances which are often only partly acknowledged, and which it is certainly blasphemous to

---

[27] Quoted in Noble, *The Religion of Technology*, p. 189.

[28] James D. Watson, 'Viewpoint: All for the Good – Why Genetic Engineering Must Soldier On' (1999), in *A Passion for DNA: Genes, Genomes and Society* (Oxford: Oxford University Press, 2000), pp. 227–9 at p. 229.

[29] Cf. Walter Gilbert, 'A Vision of the Grail', in Kevles and Hood, *The Code of Codes*, pp. 83–97.

[30] *The Times*, 27 June 2000, p. 1.

question. And at this altar many comments which do not use religious language – 'the most important and the most significant project that humankind has ever mounted',[31] comparisons to the invention of the wheel,[32] and so on – are equally pinches of incense.

Because this allegiance to the elimination of suffering and the escape from the toils of finitude through the application of technological reason is a soteriological quest which is never quite acknowledged as such, a large number of questions which could be put to the Human Genome Project are hidden from sight and never receive the attention they deserve. Some of these are questions of priorities. For example, can money spent on this project finally be justified in a world where many are suffering and dying of diseases or other causes which are already much more easily treatable? Who is likely to benefit most in the short, medium and long terms – and how should we ensure equitable distribution of the benefits of the research?

Other questions focus on the idolatry of the technological fix. Should we be committing ourselves to a medicine of heavily technological intervention and cure when other kinds of medical practice might be more appropriate? Does the mentality behind the project not end up marginalizing even those with genetic diseases who might be expected to be among the first to benefit, reducing their needs merely to a cure at all costs?[33] Indeed, given the time span between the discovery of diagnostic techniques and possible clinical therapies (which may in many cases extend to several decades), as well as the daunting sense of the tiers of complexity in functional genomics that are now emerging subsequent to the sequencing of the genome, are we allowed to ask whether it was ever responsible to promote this entire line of research?

Following on from this, there are questions about esteeming technological enterprises above other valuable human undertakings. For example, why is this so much greater a project for

---

[31] Francis Collins, quoted in Noble, *The Religion of Technology*, p. 191.
[32] Mike Dexter, Director of the Wellcome Trust, quoted in *New Scientist*, 1 July 2000, p. 4. Cf. also John Sulston and Georgina Ferry, *The Common Thread: A Story of Science, Politics, Ethics and the Human Genome* (London: Bantam Press, 2002), p. 202.
[33] See Alan Stockdale's discussion of cystic fibrosis research: 'Waiting for the Cure: Mapping the Social Relations of Human Gene Therapy Research', in Peter Conrad and Jonathan Gabe (eds), *Sociological Perspectives on the New Genetics* (Oxford: Blackwell, 1999), pp. 79–96.

human beings to embark on than concerted efforts to address global poverty or seek for reconciliation in situations of conflict? Should we really be so proud to belong to a culture which has prized all of this but has not had the wit or political will to address the threat of global warming?

And there are many other questions in different areas. In relation to the 'yuk factor' and talk of 'playing God', does the earlier discussion about knowledge by construction not suggest that concerns about these have a rather more illustrious pedigree and greater intellectual integrity than dismissing them as merely vacuous emotionalism would suggest? In relation to the only 'therapy' available now in the case of most genetic diseases, namely abortion, should we be happy to endorse James Watson's blithe expectation that 'over the next several decades we shall witness an ever-growing consensus that humans have the right to terminate the lives of genetically unhealthy fetuses'?[34] (One might also ask how our technical capacities influence our moral judgements here.) And with regard to suffering, do we not have to agree with Ivan Illich that the technological mentality is removing one of the functions of traditional cultures, namely to 'equip the individual with the means for making pain tolerable, sickness or impairment understandable, and the shadow of death meaningful'?[35]

Conclusion

These are not the only questions which could be put to the Human Genome Project or the broader project of the new genetics, but they give an indication. In putting them, I am not suggesting that the anti-reductivist critics I discussed earlier could not make them; on the contrary, they could – and many do. But they do so in separation from their views on the reductivist nature of modern genetics, whereas I have argued that the questions point to an overarching pattern of thought, only part of which is correctly diagnosed by the critique of reductionism.

---

[34] James D. Watson, 'Ethical Implications of the Human Genome Project' (1994), in *A Passion for DNA*, pp. 169–77 at p. 176.

[35] Ivan Illich, *Limits to Medicine: Medical Nemesis – The Expropriation of Health* (London: Marion Boyars, 1976), pp. 127–8. See in general his discussion of cultural iatrogenesis, according to which professionalized medicine leads people no longer to have the will to 'suffer their reality' (pp. 127–54).

This pattern of thought, which for shorthand I have labelled the Baconian project, answers the four criteria I laid down earlier. It gives an explanation of the coming-to-be of the new genetics in terms of the desire to eliminate suffering and address the condition of human disease and death, an explanation which (in the fuller setting I have pointed to) should not be neglected in any understanding of likely future trajectories. Since it shows that reductionism is secondary to this primary motivation, it allows the reductive tendencies of the new genetics to be a contingent part of its identity. But on the other hand, the desire to escape the burdens of finitude does go naturally with an objectifying mentality, which suggests an explanation for the natural affinity genetics has for reductive approaches. And in talking about a quality of motivation that is quasi-religious in nature, it gives a fuller account of the appeal of the new genetics which does not exclude or diminish the significance of socio-political and other factors.

It should not however be taken as another totalizing narrative which in one neat theory encapsulates the reality behind all the phenomena. The world is too complex to be hospitable to such accounts. Not all medicine currently practised bears the marks of the Baconian technological medicine that I have criticized: many doctors, patients and scientists have more limited and sober expectations, and have learned to place their ultimate hopes elsewhere. Rather this is intended to delineate a pattern of thought, a characteristic quality of motivation that has taken up residence in the modern world and which leads us to ignore or misunderstand important questions.

Nor do these questions, some of which I have just mentioned, form part of an effort to demonstrate the wrongness of the Human Genome Project or the new genetics as a whole. They arise because we have invested hopes in a set of aspirations whose quasi-religious nature we dare not avow. It is only when we acknowledge these that we will be able to answer the questions truthfully and freely. And it is only when we are genuinely free to answer that the Human Genome Project might after all be wrong, that we will be free to think that it might after all be right.

Bibliography

Bacon, F., *The Advancement of Learning and New Atlantis*, ed. Arthur Johnston (Oxford: Clarendon Press, 1974).

Conrad, P. and Gabe, J. (eds), *Sociological Perspectives on the New Genetics* (Oxford: Blackwell, 1999).

Descartes, R., *The Philosophical Writings of Descartes*, trans. John Cottingham, Robert Stoothoff and Dugald Murdoch, 3 vols (Cambridge: Cambridge University Press, 1985–91).

Funkenstein, A., *Theology and the Scientific Imagination from the Middle Ages to the Seventeenth Century* (Princeton, NJ: Princeton University Press, 1986).

Grant-Cooper, N. (ed.), *The Human Genome Project: Deciphering the Blueprint of Heredity* (Mill Valley, CA: University Science Books, 1994).

Hubbard, R. and Wald, E., *Exploding the Gene Myth: How Genetic Information Is Produced and Manipulated by Scientists, Physicians, Employers, Insurance Companies, Educators, and Law Enforcers* (Boston, MA: Beacon Press, 1993).

Illich, I., *Limits to Medicine: Medical Nemesis – The Expropriation of Health* (London: Marion Boyars, 1976).

Kevles, D.J. and Hood, L., (eds), *The Code of Codes: Scientific and Social Issues in the Human Genome Project* (Cambridge, MA: Harvard University Press, 1992).

Lewontin, R.C., *The Doctrine of DNA: Biology as Ideology* (London: Penguin, 1993).

McKenny, G.P., *To Relieve the Human Condition: Bioethics, Technology and the Body* (Albany, NY: State University of New York Press, 1997).

Nelkin, D. and Lindee, M.S., *The DNA Mystique: The Gene as a Cultural Icon* (New York: Freeman, 1995).

Noble, D.F., *The Religion of Technology: The Divinity of Man and the Spirit of Invention* (New York: Knopf, 1997).

Paul, D., *Controlling Human Heredity: 1865 to the Present* (Atlantic Heights, NY: Humanities Press, 1995).

Pérez-Ramos, A., *Francis Bacon's Idea of Science and the Maker's Knowledge Tradition* (Oxford: Clarendon Press, 1988).

Peters, Ted, *Playing God? Genetic Determinism and Human Freedom* (New York: Routledge, 1997).

Rose, S., Lewontin, R.C. and Kamin, L.J., *Not in Our Genes: Biology, Ideology and Human Nature* (Harmondsworth: Penguin, 1984).

Song, R., *Human Genetics: Fabricating the Future* (London: Darton, Longman & Todd, 2002).

Sulston, J. and Ferry, G., *The Common Thread: A Story of Science, Politics, Ethics and the Human Genome* (London: Bantam Press, 2002).

Taylor, C., *Philosophical Papers*, 2 vols (Cambridge: Cambridge University Press, 1985).

Taylor, C., *Sources of the Self: The Making of the Modern Identity* (Cambridge: Cambridge University Press, 1989).

Watson, J.D., 'The Human Genome Initiative', in Barry Holland and Charalambos Kyriacou (eds), *Genetics and Society* (Wokingham: Addison-Wesley, 1993), pp. 13–26.

Watson, J.D., *A Passion for DNA: Genes, Genomes and Society* (Oxford: Oxford University Press, 2000).

Webster, C., *The Great Instauration: Science, Medicine and Reform, 1626–60* (London: Duckworth, 1975).

PART V

Rethinking Bioethics

Introduction to Part V

This section turns to the issue of how to consider bioethical issues and whether currently available ethical models are adequate for such a task. Julie Clague's chapter explores the specific use of the term 'beneficence', as it has come to dominate discussion in biomedical texts, as well as the burgeoning field of what she calls 'genomorality', that is, moral and ethical issues associated with questions arising out of genetics. The dominant mode of ethical assessment has been in terms of medical progress and human benefits, a point raised by a number of different authors throughout this volume. She reviews the different possible Christian responses to moral dimensions of genetic intervention, contrasting those who align themselves with scientific dominance and those who appeal to fixity in theological traditions, such as natural law. More specifically, her critique leads into a discussion of the way medical ethics has turned away from wider considerations about human dignity. Instead, the emphasis has been placed on respect for autonomy, which is linked in turn with professional obligations couched in terms of risks and benefits. She argues that a wider conception of genomorality is now needed that develops the ideal of the common good, consistent with Roman Catholic social teaching. She argues that the results of the HGP need to be publicly available to all so that the benefits are shared.

My own chapter begins with a discussion of genetic science, arguing that by its nature any sense of absolute predictability and certainty implicit in earlier claims are being subtly challenged, from within genetic science itself. The earlier portrayal of science in salvific language helped to establish moral acceptability with the public, but I suggest that the time has come for a more honest appraisal of goals and concerns, instead of cloaking the issue in purported risks and benefits. One reaction may be to resort to deontological theological language, but this, I suggest, can be alienating in a secular context. A possible alternative is through exploration of a virtue ethic approach that appeals not primarily to consequences alone, but also scrutinizes the motivation of those who make certain claims. I argue, in particular, for a recovery of the four cardinal virtues of prudence, justice, temperance and fortitude, alongside the three theological virtues of faith, hope and charity. All are orientated towards the goodness of God. Such an approach takes its bearing from the thought of Thomas Aquinas, where prudence, or practical wisdom, is the mother of the virtues. I consider in specific ways how such development of character might contribute to decision-making in genetics. In particular, the virtue of justice is needed to ensure fair access and accountability. I then move on to discuss the particular virtue of wisdom and how this is related to the idea of wisdom as gift of God's grace. Such a trait leads to a further consideration of the importance of peacemaking, embedded, as it is, in the birth of wisdom in charity.

9

Beyond Beneficence: The Emergence of Genomorality and the Common Good

Julie Clague

The benefits of the Human Genome Project

On the historic day of the announcement of the completion of the international effort to create a working draft sequence of the human genome (26 June 2000), President Bill Clinton, flanked by Francis Collins and Craig Venter, the American scientists who led the genome sequencing efforts, remarked:

> Without a doubt this is the most important, most wondrous map ever produced by humankind ... Today we are learning the language in which God created life. We are gaining ever more awe for the complexity, the beauty, the wonder of God's most divine and sacred gift. With this profound new knowledge, humankind is on the verge of gaining immense new power to heal. Genomic science will have a real impact on all our lives, and even more on the lives of our children. It will revolutionise the diagnosis, prevention and treatment of most, if not all, human diseases. In coming years, doctors increasingly will be able to cure diseases like Alzheimer's, Parkinson's, diabetes and cancer by attacking their genetic roots ... We must ensure that new genome science and its benefits will be directed towards making life better for all citizens of the world, never just a privileged few.[1]

---

[1] Verbatim transcript from BBC website, Monday, 26 June 2000, 'Scientists crack human Code' <http://news.bbc.co.uk/hi/english/sci/tech/newsid_805000/805803.stm>. (All webpages cited were accessed at the time of going to press.)

The Clinton speech outlined the considerable medical benefits expected as a consequence of the completion of the Human Genome Project. It is beyond dispute that the genetic knowledge gained will help humans to understand better how to safeguard health, and how to tackle disease. The immediate value of the sequence data lies in its use to identify disease-causing genes that will eventually lead to the improved diagnosis, prevention and treatment of a variety of maladies. The long-term goal is the medical treatment of the vast array of disorders that have a genetic component. More immediately, newly identified biochemical target sites in the body are already emerging as suitable for the pharmaceutical equivalent of precision-bombing. The trial and error involved in the one-size-fits-all approach to prescribing drug therapies should give way to a bespoke tailoring of drug and dosage to the genetic make-up of patients, thereby improving effectiveness and minimizing side-effects. Genetic testing for inherited disorders and predisposition will become commonplace, allowing individuals and families to discover whether they or their offspring risk developing disease. In combination with appropriate genetic counselling, this can provide such individuals with the opportunity to minimize risks – for instance, by modifying diet, by taking preventative drugs or by changing harmful lifestyle patterns – and help them to understand, prepare for and manage diseases for which there is no existing treatment. Those couples who risk passing diseases to their offspring but who wish to have children may be able to utilize the technique of pre-implantation genetic diagnosis as a means of selecting healthy embryos. Ultimately, application of the knowledge gained from the Human Genome Project is expected to transform the practice of medicine, lead to the eradication of many diseases and improve the life expectancy of many. Death will not be put out of business, but he will lose far more poker games.

The emergence of genomorality

Inevitably, this rapidly expanding branch of medicine is bringing with it complex and various ethical questions. There are concerns over the distressful effects of disclosure of adverse health information to patients about diseases for which no treatment is available, and the role such knowledge might play in their life choices. Issues of confidentiality are raised when patients are provided with information about a genetic disorder that also affects the well-being or interests of third parties. Are there circumstances in which there might be a duty to disclose information to family members, or to insurance providers, or to employers? As the power to predict, prevent, treat and cure disease increases one might expect subtle shifts in cultural attitudes to health, disease and death. New genetic knowledge gained could be misused to discriminate against or stigmatize certain individuals or social groups unfairly. As genetic therapies gradually become available, consideration will have to be given to whether it is appropriate to use public funds to correct certain sorts of disorder: which count as medical and which count as enhancement? To what extent is germ-line gene therapy justifiable, in which future generations inherit the genetic modification? Will such changes to the genome exert as-yet-unknown harmful long-term effects on populations? And, given that biotechnology and pharmaceutical companies have to invest huge sums of money in the research and development of new drugs and treatments, how might an equitable balance be struck between providing incentives to and protecting the interests of commercial investors through copyright and patent laws, while at the same time ensuring both that there is healthy competition, and that the benefits of research are made widely available to patients at a fair price?

The moral questions that have emerged as a result of the genetic revolution have been and continue to be the subject of important and legitimate public scrutiny, and have given rise to extensive scholarly discussion within biomedical ethics and related disciplines for over thirty years. The scale and scope of the 'ethical pile-up' in genetics is vividly portrayed in Warren T. Reich's magisterial *Encyclopedia of Bioethics*. All the entries under 'G' in the first edition of 1978 relate to ethical questions in genetics. The additional entries under 'G' in the revised edition of 1995 all relate to genetics, except for Timothy Murphy's article on 'Gender Identity and Gender-Identity Disorders'![2] Indeed, one could say that the proliferation of concerns created

---

[2] W.T. Reich (ed.), *The Encyclopedia of Bioethics* (New York: Free Press, 1978); W.T. Reich (ed.), *The Encyclopedia of Bioethics*, rev. edn (New York: Simon & Schuster/Macmillan, 1995).

by new genetic knowledge and technologies has given rise to a whole new sub-discipline of ethics, which I would term 'genomorality'. The significance of and justification for coining the neologism would be that genomorality is more than a simple sub-set of medical ethics or bioethics – since the questions put to humanity by the ability to manipulate genes extend beyond the questions normally addressed within these traditional categories. Their scope incorporates the social, economic and political as well as the biological and personal realms. More than any other medical issue, genetics reminds us that morality is intimately linked to polity.

Consider, for example, the vast commercial promise of genetics to the biotechnology industry. According to the US government, the revenue from DNA-based technologies and products is projected to exceed $45 billion by 2009.[3] This makes the $3 billion cost of the HGP appear modest and illustrates the enormous significance of so-called genomics to the global economy – not least in further increasing the wealth of the industrialized nations of the northern hemisphere.[4] In the context of the transformative effects of the industrial revolution on the world's political, economic and social landscape, the term 'genetic revolution' is also wholly appropriate and should be understood to carry a similarly transformative resonance. Genomorality must therefore be understood to include questions related to the economic and political order, such as: how humans can create and distribute wealth fairly; to what extent the mechanisms of liberal democracy are sufficient to deliver social justice; whether the free reign of market forces and consumer choice alone should determine which genetic therapies are made available; how to widen access to genetic technologies; and so on. Genomorality would also encompass questions of ultimate human meaning. Humankind's ability to

[3] The White House, 'Press Release on the Human Genome Project', 14 March 2000 <http://usinfo.state.gov/topical/global/biotech/00031402.htm>.
[4] For further discussion of the moral implications of the commercial exploitation of genetics see T. Caulfield and B. Williams-Jones (eds), *The Commercialization of Genetic Research: Ethical, Legal, and Policy Issues* (New York: Kluwer Academic/Plenum Press, 1999); J. Clague, 'Genetic Knowledge as a Commodity: The Human Genome Project, Markets and Consumers', in M. Junker-Kenny and L.S. Cahill (eds), *The Ethics of Genetic Engineering, Concilium* (April 1998), pp. 3–12; S. Holm, 'Genetic Engineering and the North–South Divide', in A. Dyson and J. Harris (eds), *Ethics and Biotechnology* (London: Routledge, 1999), pp. 47–63.

control nature and increase longevity will be greatly extended perhaps leading to changes in our understanding of the human condition, including more ambitious expectations concerning the drawing up of life-plans and in the assessment of what constitutes a successful human life. As a result, the assumptions that lie at the heart of our value systems and philosophies of life will need to be interrogated and reassessed. As will be seen through discussion of the notion of beneficence, it is the convergence in genomorality of this complex nexus of concerns that gives rise to disquiet concerning the adequacy and efficacy of conventional ethical terminology that forms the mainstay of bioethical writing.

The coordinated international effort to map and sequence the genome accelerated the genetic revolution, and brought to light the enormity of the ethical, legal and social issues to be faced. Recognition of the urgent need for public debate into the implications of the growth of genetic medicine, and of the need to establish national guidelines for practice, gave rise to the largest injection of public funding there has ever been into the discipline of bioethics. The genome organizations in Europe and North America devoted fixed percentages of their budgets to the ethical, legal and social issues raised by the Human Genome Project. Since the formal inception of the Genome Project, in October 1990, hundreds of millions of dollars have been dedicated to research and education programmes investigating all areas of genomorality.

Weighing the benefits of genetic research

For all the important ethical, legal and social challenges that accompany the development of genetic medicine, there is no serious suggestion that research and its application to medicine should not proceed. The dominant mode of assessing the genetic revolution is in terms of medical progress and human benefit. The justification for the Human Genome Project and the possibilities arising as a result derive from the vast benefits that humankind will reap from genetic research. It is an article of faith: there really will be jam tomorrow. In this context, the resolution of moral quandaries concerning how to promote both public medicine and private enterprise, how to balance confidentiality with truth-telling, and so on, comes to seem like no more than a second-order activity: necessary, but with no overall power of veto. Nothing will stop the impetus behind the genetic revolution: its driving force maps perfectly on to the overall aim of medicine: it is the unimpeachable goal of human benefit. Whether it be genetic medicine or any other potential medical advance – such as the use of human stem cells to replace diseased and damaged tissue, or the prospects for xenotransplantation – its beneficial contribution to humankind is the desired outcome against which any objections, problems, risks and costs ultimately must be measured.

This is not to say that everything which appears to be beneficial should be permitted. Universal moral abhorrence would rightly accompany any suggestion that it were permissible to kill a healthy child in order to harvest organs for transplantation purposes. Perhaps the 'murder one, save five' types of scenario that ethics students have endured in the interests of learning about unnuanced utilitarianism might also count as abuse; but there is little need to employ such hypothetical cases. Sadly, instances from history and contemporary medical practice abound which provide ample evidence of medical practitioners disregarding human rights in pursuit of a misguided notion of the social good. The sorry history of the eugenic aim of social engineering illustrates the dangers of conceiving of beneficence apart from personal autonomy. Many research subjects have been abused by medical personnel in the supposed interests of research, and there is a well-documented history of physician involvement in the maltreatment of detainees.[5]

Suffice it to say that it would be wrong to assume that the benefits promised by a new medical advance will always trump the objections. For instance, some people believe that the destruction of human embryos that is necessarily involved in embryonic stem cell research rules out such stem cell techniques as a morally permissible means of repairing diseased and damaged human tissue. Similarly, although the desperate shortage of human organs for transplantation might be ameliorated by the use of animal organs, any putative benefit to individual patients must be weighed against various factors

---

[5] Cf. British Medical Association, *Medicine Betrayed: The Participation of Doctors in Human Rights Abuses* (London: Zed Books, 1992); British Medical Association, *The Medical Profession and Human Rights: Handbook for a Changing Agenda* (London: Zed Books, 2001).

including the risk of introducing a deadly or dangerous virus into the human population.[6] In the case of embryo research the objection is of the deontological 'some things should never be done despite the benefits' sort of argument. In the xenotransplantation example, the fear of transmission of xenozoonoses is of the consequentialist 'we could do more harm than good' variety. As genetic medicine develops further, only the careful assessment of risks, combined with the fastidious application of the ethical ground-rules that have shaped the international and national codes of medicine – the Kantian notion of respect for persons, the requirement that human rights be respected, that informed consent be obtained and so on – will guarantee that the benefits of genetic medicine are truly humanizing. Thus, the World Medical Association *Declaration on the Human Genome Project*, September 1992, states: 'we can assess the ethical outcomes with the same parameters that guide us whenever we examine a new diagnostic or therapeutic method. The main criteria remain the evaluation of risk versus advantage, the respect of a person as a human being and the respect of autonomy and privacy.'[7] Similarly, Unesco's *Universal Declaration on the Human Genome and Human Rights*, 1997 (which will be discussed in more detail later) recognizes 'that research on the human genome and the resulting applications open up vast prospects for progress in improving the health of individuals and of humankind as a whole', but emphasizes 'that such research should fully respect human dignity, freedom and human rights, as well as the prohibition of all forms of discrimination based on genetic characteristics'.[8]

---

[6] For a discussion of this issue see F.H. Bach *et al.*, 'Uncertainty in Xenotransplantation: Individual Benefit Versus Collective Risk', *Nature Medicine* 4.2 (1998), pp. 141–4.

[7] World Medical Association, *Declaration on the Human Genome Project* (adopted by the 44th World Medical Assembly, Marbella, Spain), September 1992, 'Recommendations', p. 3 <www.wma.net/e/policy/17-s-1_e.html>.

[8] Unesco, *Universal Declaration on the Human Genome and Human Rights*, 1997, Introduction (Unesco Document 27V/45, adopted by the General Conference of Unesco at its 29th session, Paris, 11 November 1997) <www.unesco.org/human_rights/hrbc.htm>.

Christian responses to the genetic revolution

> 'I will praise thee; for I am fearfully and wonderfully made; marvellous are thy works'.
>
> Psalm 139.13–15

President Clinton chose to describe the scientific achievement of mapping the genome in rich theological terms. He invoked the *sensus divinitatis* in order to powerfully convey the miracle of life and the inherent value of humankind. Genetics has always had the power to capture the human imagination, prompting recourse to the sort of transcendent language that can express both the truth of individual uniqueness and humanity's collective power to transform itself. Perhaps it is no coincidence that the modern academic discipline of bioethics began to establish itself (in the 1950s and 1960s) at the same time that the field of human genetics first promised to transform the human condition. In any case, it is noteworthy that Christian writers were the first to respond to the moral dimensions of the genetic revolution. The first documented religious response to genetics was Pope Pius XII's Address to the First International Symposium of Genetic Medicine in September 1953, less than five months after Crick and Watson presented their double-helix model of DNA to the world. With the atrocities of the Second World War still at the forefront of the collective consciousness, the Pope described 'racialism' and 'eugenic sterilization' as 'contrary to morality'. However, invoking the common good of humanity, he found no reason to disapprove of the beneficial aims of genetics:

> Genetics has not merely a theoretical interest; it is eminently practical as well. It aims at contributing towards the good of individuals and of the community – towards the common good ... The fundamental tendency of genetics and eugenics is to influence the transmission of hereditary factors in order to promote what is good and eliminate what is injurious. This fundamental tendency is irreproachable from the moral viewpoint ... The practical aims being pursued by genetics are noble and worthy of recognition and encouragement.[9]

---

[9] Pius XII, 'Moral Aspects of Genetics', *Address to the First International Symposium of Genetic Medicine*, 7 September 1953 (AAS 44 (1953), 605).

Thirty years later, Pope John Paul II, in his Address to the World Medical Association, employed the same line of moral argumentation to justify genetic medicine:

> A strictly therapeutic intervention, having the objective of healing various maladies – such as those stemming from chromosomic deficiencies – will be considered in principle as desirable, providing that it tends to real promotion of the personal well-being of man, without harming his integrity or worsening his life conditions. Such intervention actually falls within the logic of the Christian moral tradition ... And since, in the order of medical values, life is man's supreme and most radical good, there is need for a fundamental principle: first prevent any damage, then seek and pursue the good.[10]

John Paul reiterated this basic position in 1995. He acknowledged that 'the biomedical sciences are currently experiencing a period of rapid and marvellous growth, especially with regard to new discoveries in the area of genetics'. In this regard, scientific research must respect personal dignity and support human life, but must also endeavour 'to promote the true good of human beings as individuals and as a community. This happens when efforts are made to eliminate the causes of disease by putting real prevention into practice, or whenever more effective therapies are sought for the treatment of serious illnesses.'[11]

This positive attitude towards genetics may suprise those who are inclined to view Roman Catholicism as the church that likes to say 'No'. It is true that there are a number of medical interventions that are considered illicit in official Roman Catholic teaching, but which gain widespread approval within all other mainstream Christian denominations. Examples include: direct sterilization, artificial contraception, artificial insemination by husband (AIH), *in-vitro* fertilization (IVF), abortion to save a woman's life, and non-therapeutic embryo research. In these cases – apart from the last two, that are deemed to be direct attacks on innocent human life – the chief ground for Catholic disapproval is the sense that the action constitutes a

---

[10] John Paul II, 'The Ethics of Genetic Manipulation', *Address to the World Medical Association*, 29 October 1983 (AAS 76 (1984), 389–402).

[11] John Paul II, *Address to the Pontifical Academy for Life*, 20 November 1995 (AAS 88 (1996), 668–71).

dehumanizing intervention into the God-given natural order. More specifically, it is said to do so by separating the procreative and unitive meanings of sex from their proper locus in the conjugal bonding of man and woman. By contrast, in the case of genetic interventions, the underlying Catholic attitude is more positive. These sorts of interventions into nature, provided that they respect human rights, are justified because of their humanizing contribution to the common good. Similar teleological arguments lead to the approval in principle (i.e. provided the risks are not great) of xenotransplantation[12] and the use of adult stem cells for diseased and damaged tissue replacement.[13]

Prescinding from discussion of the so-called 'inseparability principle' in Catholic natural law ethics (a topic that has been subjected to exhaustive scrutiny for several decades), it is clear that there are two different attitudes to 'nature' and what is 'natural' at work in these moral teachings. They can be considered as two basic outlooks or world-views that often characterize Christian (and non-Christian) responses to medical interventions.[14] The first describes certain sorts of actions as unnatural and therefore immoral because they interfere with the given order, the structure of which constitutes either a 'design classic' that cannot be improved upon by human manipulation, or a finely tuned organism that will be knocked out of kilter by human tampering. To interfere disrupts the way things should be and frequently leads to harmful consequences. The second approach takes a more optimistic view of humankind's ability to apply God-given intelligence to the task of transforming and humanizing the world. Pius XII appealed to this line of argument in order to justify the use of anaesthetics and analgesics in the medical treatment of

---

[12] Cf. John Paul II, *Address to the 18th International Congress on Organ Transplants*, 29 August, 2000, n. 7 (AAS 92 (2000) 822–6); Pius XII, *Address to the Italian Association of Cornea Donors and to Clinical Oculists and Legal Medical Practitioners*, 14 May, 1956 (AAS 48 (1956)).

[13] Cf. John Paul II, *Address to the 18th International Congress on Organ Transplants*, 29 August 2000, n. 8 (AAS 92 (2000) 822–6); Pontifical Academy for Life, *Declaration on the Production and the Scientific and Therapeutic Use of Human Embryonic Stem Cells*, 25 August 2000, n. 5.

[14] For an excellent discussion of these contrasting attitudes to nature see L. Woodhead, 'Human Genetics: A Theological Response', in I. Torrance (ed.), *Bio-Ethics for the New Millennium* (Edinburgh: Saint Andrew Press, 2000) (on behalf of the Church of Scotland Board of Social Responsibility), pp. 82–96.

pain: 'Man preserves, even after the Fall, the right of dominating the forces of Nature, of using them in his service, and of employing the resources so offered to him to avoid or suppress physical suffering.'[15] The same fundamental attitude to humanity's place in God's creation is at work in papal approval of genetic medicine. It goes without saying that the Catholic Church would reject the suggestion that this line of argument could fruitfully be applied to those medical interventions already identified that are ruled out by appeal to natural law. By contrast, it is precisely the application of such logic that has led to their approval by the rest of mainstream Christianity. In summary, though the Catholic Church rules out some medical interventions on the basis of their supposed unnaturalness, it approves of genetic interventions that respect human rights on the basis of their beneficial contribution to both individuals and society.

Two Protestant theologians, instrumental in founding the discipline of bioethics and early influential writers on genomorality, were the Episcopalian Joseph Fletcher and the Methodist Paul Ramsey. Their writings now appear somewhat dated, and both frequently had recourse to rhetorical overkill stylistically. However, the underlying theological visions that inspired these writers remain of interest. Joseph Fletcher was an exponent of the view of the human being as in essence 'a maker and a selecter and a designer',[16] who acts morally when he or she controls the genetic slings and arrows of outrageous fortune; but his conclusions were extreme and his consequentialist argumentation notoriously weak:

> Not to control, not to weigh one thing against another, would be subhuman... It used to be that we had no way of knowing which couples were carrying a common gene defect or which pregnancies were positive for it. But now we *can* know; we have lost that excuse for taking genetic risks... Screening by one means or another is the obvious way to fulfill our obligation to potential children, as well as to the community which has to suffer when defectives are born.[17]

---

[15] Pius XII, *Allocution on the Relief of Pain*, 24 February 1957, n. 13 (AAS 49 (1957), 135).

[16] J. Fletcher, 'Ethical Aspects of Genetic Controls: Designed Genetic Changes in Man', *New England Journal of Medicine* 285.14 (1971), pp. 776–83, p. 780.

[17] J. Fletcher, *The Ethics of Genetic Control: Ending Reproductive Roulette* (New York: Prometheus, 1988), pp. 159–60, p. 181 (first published New York: Doubleday, 1974).

In his essay 'Ethical Aspects of Genetic Controls', Fletcher goes so far as to suggest that laboratory reproduction is more human than sexual intercourse on the basis that: 'the more rationally contrived and deliberate anything is, the more human it is'.[18] In contrast to what Linda Woodhead describes as the 'masters of the universe' approach to genetic interventions that is represented in almost parodic form by Fletcher,[19] Paul Ramsey rejected any optimistic confidence concerning humankind's ability to intervene wisely in the created order. Thus, in somewhat purple prose, Ramsey poses the rhetorical question: '. . . are we then to say that man is let loose here [on earth] with the proper task of disassembling his own "courses of action," making himself and his species wholly plastic to ingenious scientific interventions and alterations? . . . it follows that thereafter human nature has to be wrought by Predestinators in the Decanting and Conditioning Rooms of the East London Hatchery and in commercial firms bearing the name "Genetic Laboratories, Inc." in all our metropolitan centres.'[20]

Ramsey believed the technological age was one 'in which "progressives" are in the saddle and ride mankind – ahead if not forward'.[21] Instead of Fletcher's 'bend nature to human purposes' approach, Ramsey's appeal was to the inherent wisdom of God's created order and God's ultimate control of history. The manufacturing of progeny pays disrespect to God's design and intentionality: 'Men ought not to play God before they learn to be men, and after they have learned to be men they will not play God.'[22] As Gordon Dunstan observed, Ramsey's attitude to medical research was 'a literally protestant "thus far and no further"'.[23] His objection to the supposed severing of procreation from its context in conjugal love in IVF gained support from a deontological appeal to the scriptural theme of covenantal fidelity based on readings of the prologue of John's Gospel and Ephesians 5.[24] However, Ramsey's deep

---

[18] 'Ethical Aspects of Genetic Controls', p. 780.

[19] Woodhead, 'Human Genetics', p. 83.

[20] P. Ramsey, 'Shall We "Reproduce"? ii. Rejoinders and Future Forecast', *Journal of the American Medical Association* 220.11 (1972), pp. 1480–5, p. 1484.

[21] P. Ramsey, *Fabricated Man: The Ethics of Genetic Control* (New Haven: Yale University Press, 1970), p. 55.

[22] *Fabricated Man*, p. 138

[23] G. Dunstan, *The Artifice of Ethics* (London: SCM Press, 1974), p. 60.

[24] *Fabricated Man*, pp. 32–9.

pessimism regarding fallen humankind's capacity to act morally extended also to a sense of impending disaster: many proposals for 'man's radical self-modification and control of his evolutionary future ... must simply be described as a project for the suicide of the species'.[25] Ramsey believed that humanity's attempts to play God are likely to unleash a Pandora's box of uncontrollable forces. Thus, his deontological-sounding theological appeals function to give support to what are ultimately consequentialist concerns.[26] Nevertheless, despite his pessimistic predictions of humankind's fate, it was Ramsey's teleological argumentation based on the promotion of human benefit that shaped his response to genetics and allowed him – along with Fletcher – to approve of certain interventions such as genetic screening:

> Should the practice of such medical genetics become feasible at some time in the future, it will raise no moral questions at all – or at least none that are not already present in the practice of medicine generally ... [Although] The science of genetics (and medical practice based on it) would be obliged both to be fully informed of the facts and to have a reasonable and well-examined expectation of doing more good than harm by eliminating the genetic defect in question ... In making genetic decisions to be effected by morally acceptable means, the benefits expected from a given course of action must be weighed against any risk (or loss of good) incurred.[27]

These writings, Catholic and Protestant, represent two recurring tendencies in Christian approaches to genomorality based on differing visions of the legitimate scope of human interaction with the world.[28] Nevertheless, all remain open to the new genetic possibilities because of their positive contribution to human well-being. Theological colourings are often applied to these outline sketches of nature in order to enrich

---

[25] Ibid., p. 159.

[26] Cf. Ibid., pp. 52–9.

[27] Ibid., pp. 44–5, 57–8.

[28] A typically Protestant 'created order' approach in the tradition of Ramsey is found in O. O'Donovan, *Begotten or Made?* (Oxford: Clarendon, 1994). Karl Rahner's positive theological anthropology informs his interventionist approach in 'Experiment: Man', *Theology Digest*, February 1968, pp. 57–69 (the essay was first delivered in September 1965). His later essay 'The Problem of Genetic Manipulation', *Theological Investigations*, vol. ix (New York: Crossroad, 1972), pp. 244–52, is less naively optimistic.

the vision. Oliver O'Donovan reminds Christians of the need to 'confess their faith in the providence of God as the ruling power of history'.[29] Humans show respect for God's dominion through attentive obedience to the immanent laws of creation.[30] Positive attitudes to technological intervention into nature are expressed through the theological idea of humans as free co-creators with God, participating in the work of bringing the earth to fulfilment. This theme is invoked by the Protestant theologian Ronald Cole-Turner, who argues that humans restore creation and act as participants in redemption when they use medicine to overcome genetic defects.[31] More frequently, the language of humans as stewards or viceroys is employed to impart the idea of humanity's ongoing care for and maintenance of creation. This performs a useful mediating role between the non-interference 'natural order' and inter-ventionist 'masters of the universe' approaches. The stewardship theme is usefully deployed in a Church of Scotland report on the use of genetically modified animals, and it functions as a means of placing limits on the extent to which humans can exploit their fellow creatures.[32]

The selection of writings presented here comprises only a tiny fraction of the Christian responses to genetics. They have been chosen in order to indicate the pervasiveness of the two main overarching narratives of nature that inform Christian judgements on any number of scientific and technological innovations that call for moral evaluation. Yet, they also show that Christians of all hues tend to greet genetic medicine favourably, while acknowledging both its challenges and the proper limits of medical research in terms of respect for human rights. In other words, Christians, on the whole, believe that the benefits of genetic medicine outweigh the objections. This is not to say that Christians might not also perceive a role for themselves in witnessing to an alternative set of values and priorities to those of either the 'herd' or the 'superman',

---

[29] *Begotten or Made?*, p. 13.
[30] Ibid., p. 5.
[31] R. Cole-Turner, *The New Genesis: Theology and the Genetic Revolution* (Louisville, KY: Westminster/John Knox Press, 1993).
[32] Society, Religion and Technology Project, 'GM Animals, Humans and the Future of Genetics', Appendix V, *Board of National Mission Deliverance to the General Assembly of the Church of Scotland*, May 2001, para. 2.

thereby challenging prevailing societal norms about normality and perfectibility. Neither is it to exclude the important insights and traditional wisdom that Christians can bring to bear on the life experiences of suffering and death, and the offering of hope, compassion, companionship and so on – thus providing a more sober and less materialistic appreciation of the medical goals of longevity, preservation of life and quality of life.

The goals of medicine and biomedical research

The Clinton speech indicated the important contribution that genetic technologies are making to the transformation of twenty-first-century medicine. The benefits gained for genetic research through the Human Genome Project are benefits that will accrue to humanity as such through the improvements that will be made to the practice of medicine. Medicine is geared towards the well-being of patients: to the restoration and maintenance of health. Medical research and treatments are undertaken in order to achieve a proportionate human benefit, and medical progress is measured by the degree to which it delivers improvements in human well-being. This humanitarian impetus is enshrined in the foundation codes of medicine. The World Medical Association's version of the Hippocratic Oath, the *Declaration of Geneva*, 1948 (amended 1968, 1983, 1994), establishes in its opening statement the humanitarian goal of medicine. It includes the promise that as a member of the medical profession: 'I solemnly pledge myself to consecrate my life to the service of humanity.'[33] This is echoed in the WMA's ethical guidelines for research on human subjects, the *Declaration of Helsinki*, 1964 (amended 1975, 1983, 1989, 1996, 2000), which opens as follows: 'It is the duty of the physician to promote and safeguard the health of the people.'[34]

A similar sentiment used to be expressed in the American Medical Association's *Principles of Medical Ethics* (amended 1980,

---

[33] World Medical Association, *Declaration of Geneva* (adopted by the 46th WMA General Assembly Stockholm, Sweden, September 1994), <www.wma.net/e/policy/17-a_e.html>.

[34] World Medical Association, *Declaration of Helsinki, Ethical Principles for Medical Research Involving Human Subjects* (adopted by the 18th WMA General Assembly, Helsinki, Finland, June 1964 and amended by the 52nd WMA General Assembly, Edinburgh, Scotland, October 2000), <www.wma.net/e/policy/17-c_e.html>.

2001), which sets out standards of conduct for physicians. These were first outlined in 1957 in the form of ten principles. The first of these states: 'The principal objective of the medical profession is to render service to humanity with full respect for the dignity of man.'[35] Interestingly, however, explicit mention of the humanitarian goal and meaning of medicine that provides the context for the duties of physicians in the 1957 code is absent from the revised *Principles of Medical Ethics* of 1980[36] and the further revised version of June 2001.[37] Instead, since the revisions of 1980, there has been explicit commitment to the physician's duty to respect the rights of patients. Thus, the first of the nine principles outlined in the 2001 code states: 'A physician shall be dedicated to providing competent medical care, with compassion and respect for human dignity and rights.' Despite mention of the physician's responsibility to participate in activities that contribute to 'the betterment of public health' in Principle VII of the *Principles* (2001), the sense of the overall purpose of medicine remains, at best, implicit. It is not that there exists confusion or dispute about the aims of medicine. Rather, the focus has shifted from the concept of the profession's service to humanity as such, to a description of the duties of individual physicians in their dealings with particular patients.

The development that has taken place in the AMA's articulation of the profession's duties over the half-century is instructive. The expression of respect for human dignity in terms of the language of human rights specifies the physician's responsibilities and protects patient autonomy more fully and less ambiguously than the 1957 *Principles*. However, the amended statement of *Principles* also reflects the tendency to assume rather than to state explicitly the importance of the notion of human benefit as the justificatory and defining *telos* of medicine and medical research. This shift in emphasis is also evident in the bioethical literature in discussions of beneficence and, as we will see, has led to an unfortunate narrowing of the moral meaning of medicine.

[35] American Medical Association, *Principles of Medical Ethics*, June 1957, Section 1.

[36] American Medical Association, *Principles of Medical Ethics*, Revised version, 1980 <www.ama-assn.org/ama/pub/print/article/4256-4928.html>.

[37] American Medical Association, *Principles of Medical Ethics*, Revised version, 17 June 2001 <www.ama-assn.org/ama/pub/category/2512.html>.

Beneficence in bioethics

Thus far it has been suggested that the chief justificatory paradigm of the Human Genome Project be understood in terms of its beneficial role within medicine. Similarly, it has been seen that medicine's goal is to benefit humankind through the health promotion of individuals and communities. In the bioethical literature, discussion of the promotion of human benefit within medicine is conceptualized in terms of 'beneficence', which is variously described as an obligation or principle to do good. For example, Larry Churchill's article 'Beneficence' in the revised *Encyclopedia of Bioethics* states: '"Beneficence" denotes the practice of good deeds. In contemporary ethics, the principle of beneficence usually signifies an obligation to benefit others or to seek their good.'[38] The classic Beauchamp and Childress text, *Principles of Biomedical Ethics*, describes beneficence as: 'an action done to benefit others', and the principle of beneficence as: 'a moral obligation to act for the benefit of others'.[39] Beauchamp and Childress identify the principle of beneficence as one of four clusters of moral principles that are considered basic for biomedical ethics (the others being respect for autonomy, non-maleficence and justice). As such, beneficence constitutes: 'a group of norms for providing benefits and balancing benefits against risks and costs'.[40] They distinguish their principle of beneficence from classical utilitarianism on the grounds that it is to be construed as: 'one among a number of prima facie principles' rather than an absolute requirement.[41]

Beauchamp and Childress pioneered the now familiar strategy of codifying the tasks of bioethics in terms of key principles.[42] Over the last twenty-five years they have refined and developed their articulation of the principles of bioethics.

---

[38] L. Churchill, 'Beneficence', in W.T. Reich (ed.), *The Encyclopedia of Bioethics*, rev. edn (New York: Simon & Schuster/Macmillan, 1995), vol. i, pp. 243–7. Note that there is no article on beneficence in the first edition of Reich's *Encyclopedia of Bioethics*, published in 1978.

[39] T. Beauchamp and J. Childress, *Principles of Biomedical Ethics*, 5th edn (Oxford: Oxford University Press, 2001), p. 166 (first published 1979).

[40] Ibid., p. 12.

[41] Ibid., p. 166.

[42] Other instances of principles-based approaches include: R. Veatch, *A Theory of Medical Ethics* (New York: Basic Books, 1981); T. Engelhardt, *The Foundations of Bioethics* (Oxford: Oxford University Press, 1986).

Theirs is the most comprehensive and integrated presentation of the principles-based approach to biomedical ethics and is therefore worthy of close scrutiny. The principles-based approach has undoubted value, though perhaps more often at the level of pedagogy than practice: it provides a convenient conceptual framework through which to understand the discipline of bioethics, rather than reflects the actual means by which practitioners resolve bioethical dilemmas.[43] Particularly in the last decade, the principles approach has come to be viewed as one among a number of valuable conceptual models for thinking about the scope and tasks of bioethics (other notable – and some would say overlapping – approaches include rights-based, virtue ethics, care ethics, and case-based approaches). Typical lists of bioethical principles or physician obligations might include the duties of non-maleficence, beneficence, respect for personal autonomy, veracity, confidentiality, respect for privacy, fidelity, and contract-keeping. The requirement that physicians obtain informed consent from patients or research subjects is usually also included within such lists.

However, it is suprising how seldom principles-based expressions of the duties of healthcare professionals set these out as norms that necessarily follow from the more fundamental requirement of respect for the dignity of the human person as a *conditio sine qua non*. This contrasts with the approach generally adopted within professional medical codes and guidelines – as the brief survey of the WMA and AMA declarations has indicated. Although it might be assumed that Beauchamp and Childress believe the starting point and basis for the development of all bioethical obligations and principles is that human persons possess an inherent dignity and value that requires absolute respect, no such commitment is ever established or expressed. Thus the physician's duties are simply

---

[43] For more detailed discussion and critiques of principles-based approaches to bioethics see e.g.: 'Special Issue: Theories and Methods in Bioethics: Principlism and Its Critics', *Kennedy Institute of Ethics Journal* 5.3 (1995); E.R. DuBose, R.P. Hamel and L.J. O'Connell (eds), *A Matter of Principles? Ferment in U.S. Bioethics* (Valley Forge, PA: Trinity Press International, 1994); S. Holm, 'Not Just Autonomy: The Principles of American Biomedical Ethics', *Journal of Medical Ethics* 21.6 (1995), pp. 332–8; and Raanan Gillon's editorial response, 'Defending "The Four Principles" Approach to Biomedical Ethics', pp. 323–4 in the same issue.

asserted as self-evident premises, detached from the moral vision of the person that provides their meaning and justification: a somewhat remarkable omission. The result of this oversight is that the concept of respect for persons is merely subsumed within the important but more anthropologically impoverished notion of personal autonomy. A notable exception to this tendency is found in the Belmont Report issued by the US National Commission for the Protection of Human Subjects of Biomedical and Behavioral Research in 1978.[44] The Report – which could be regarded as the American equivalent of the Declaration of Helsinki – identifies and discusses the ethical principles that should underlie research involving human subjects. It has been widely employed to form the basis of the mandatory statement of principles required of all the federally funded research programmes in the United States. Belmont identifies three ethical principles as fundamental in biomedical research: respect for persons, beneficence and justice. In this instance, the duty to respect persons as autonomous agents and protect those whose autonomy is diminished is explicitly understood to be included within the broader and more comprehensive principle of respect for persons.

The Belmont Report also offers one of the more successful treatments of beneficence, which is understood as an obligation to secure the well-being of another. It interprets beneficence broadly to include the duty to do no intentional harm (non-maleficence) in addition to the duty to maximize benefit. The important 'justifying role' that beneficence plays in determining the ethical acceptability of biomedical research is identified. The ethical task is: 'to decide when it is justifiable to seek certain benefits despite the risks involved, and when the benefits should be foregone because of the risks ... In the case of scientific research in general, members of the larger society are obliged to recognize the longer term benefits and risks that may result from the improvement of knowledge and from the development of novel medical, psychotherapeutic, and social procedures.'[45]

[44] National Commission for the Protection of Human Subjects of Biomedical and Behavioral Research, *The Belmont Report: Ethical Principles and Guidelines for the Protection of Human Subjects of Research*, OPRR Reports (Washington, DC: US Government Printing Office, 1978).
[45] *The Belmont Report*, Part B, 'Basic Ethical Principles'.

There necessarily follows the need to examine and assess potential risks and benefits of research, both in terms of their probability and magnitude. The assumption is that some degree of comparative measuring of the risks and benefits is possible, in order to judge whether there is a proportionate benefit in research programmes. The Report's explicit commitment to respect for persons as a non-negotiable principle prevents any crass utilitarian interpretation of the sort that subordinates individuals to the so-called 'greater good' of society. Nevertheless, it is acknowledged that the knowledge and understanding gained through biomedical research stands to benefit society in general, but not always the research subjects.

Most bioethics texts discuss beneficence as they do non-maleficence: they generally assume the context of the physician–patient relationship in which the doctor's duty is to pursue the good of his or her individual patient. The focus of discussion is therefore that of the healthcare professional's obligations, in which one's role carries responsibilities for health promotion and standards of care. This sense is to be distinguished from (though need not preclude) beneficence understood as acts of virtue and works of supererogation (such as expressions of kindness, compassion, charity and altruism). In terms of the duties of healthcare personnel, key questions concerning the nature of beneficence involve: how to determine what is in a person's best interests; how to balance individual interests against those of society (and future generations); and the difficulty of carrying out risk–benefit assessments. However, discussion is usually dominated by questions of potential conflicts of duty between beneficence and the principles of respect for autonomy and justice. Controverted issues include: whether one has a duty to help those who do not wish to be helped; how to proceed when physician and patient (and possibly family) disagree on what is in the patient's best interest; and how to distribute benefits fairly. It is probably the case that, in the first half of the twentieth century, medicine focused on the physician's beneficence to the detriment of the patient's autonomy. This risked either over-idealized portrayals of medicine in terms of philanthropy and altruism, or over-confident gestures of paternalism. In recent debate, patient autonomy has taken centre stage.

The greater emphasis that is now placed on the concept of patient autonomy (or right to self-determination) acts as an important corrective to the overly paternalistic understanding of beneficence ('doctor knows best') that has constantly dogged the practice of medicine.[46] Paternalism stems from an obscuring of the distinction between the notion of being an authority (in terms of expertise) and having authority over someone (in terms of leadership or responsibility). The result is the paternalistic belief that the physician knows what is in the patient's best interests and believes the physician's responsibility lies in pursuing that good, even if this would mean overriding the wishes of the patient. The history of paternalism in medicine and the neglect of patient self-determination indicate why the notion of beneficence alone is an insufficient measure and expression both of the physician's duties and of the requirements of bioethics.[47]

While medical ethics at the turn of the twentieth century tended to view medicine predominantly in terms of the ideals of beneficence, this was later to be supplemented within medical codes of ethics by explicit commitment to the underlying prerequisite of respect for the dignity of the human person (from whence the duty of beneficence derives). This commitment is usually expressed in terms of respect for patient autonomy or in terms of respect for human rights. The effect of this has been to reduce the likelihood of paternalistic abuses in medicine. However, in the bioethical literature preoccupation with the theme and scope of autonomy has, perhaps inadvertently, led to the one-to-one exchange between patient and doctor being the chief context for articulating the notion of 'doing good' in healthcare. The physician–patient relationship is obviously an important focus in bioethical discussion. Nevertheless, the concept of beneficence is too narrowly

[46] For an illustration of a more paternalistic understanding of the duties of physicians see T. Percival, *Medical Ethics: A Code of Institutes and Precepts, Adapted to the Professional Conduct of Physicians and Surgeons* (Manchester: S. Russell, 1803), which greatly influenced the composition of both the British and American Medical Associations' codes of conduct.

[47] Edmund Pellegrino and David Thomasma argue for the primacy of beneficence, but include within its scope respect for autonomy. Cf. E.D. Pellegrino and D.C. Thomasma, *For The Patient's Good: The Restoration of Beneficence in Health Care* (Oxford: Oxford University Press, 1988). Their position is analysed in Beauchamp and Childress, *Principles of Biomedical Ethics*, 5th edn, pp. 176–7.

framed when understood and explored solely within this context. This tends to obscure questions concerning beneficence as it relates to the communal benefits of biomedical research and as it relates to the overarching and defining goal of medicine – both of which (as we have seen) are important for consideration of genetic medicine.

Beneficence as an expression of the common good

A modest attempt is made to relate explicitly the source of the principle of beneficence to the overall goal of medicine in the fourth edition of Beauchamp and Childress: 'the principle of beneficence derives, in part, from long-standing, professional role obligations in medicine to provide medical benefits to patients'.[48] Similarly, in the fifth edition we find: 'In an inchoate form, the idea that beneficence expresses the primary obligation in health care is ancient. Throughout the history of health care, the professional's obligations and virtues have been interpreted as commitments of beneficence.'[49] Beauchamp and Childress address the question of social benefit under the heading 'general beneficence', distinguishing obligations that arise from specific relationships (e.g. to family, friends and patients) from those directed to unspecified others.[50] This discussion takes them into territory concerning the line between requirements to help and supererogatory actions. The basis on which they choose to defend the existence of a duty to help unspecified others is that of 'reciprocity': social interaction requires a return of benefit by proportional benefit. Thus, they state:

> obligations of beneficence to society (as distinct from those to identified individuals) are typically derived from some form of reciprocity ... many physicians and health care professionals are today deeply indebted to society (e.g., for education and privileges) and to patients, past and present (e.g., for research and practice). Because of this indebtedness, the medical profession's role of beneficent care of patients is misconstrued if modeled primarily on philanthropy, altruism, and personal commitment ... Such

---

[48] T. Beauchamp and J. Childress, *Principles of Biomedical Ethics*, 4th edn (Oxford: Oxford University Press, 1994), p. 37.
[49] *Principles of Biomedical Ethics*, 5th edn, p. 176.
[50] Ibid., pp. 168–76.

reciprocity creates an obligation of general beneficence both to patients and to society, although the precise terms of the obligation are rarely specified (and are very difficult to specify).[51]

These writers are correct to indicate that a supererogatory notion of charity is insufficient to carry the weight of the obligations of beneficence that fall on healthcare personnel (irrespective of whether those obligations are conceived as directed to specified individuals or to society more generally). In settling on the notion of reciprocity they begin to capture something of the mutuality of social living. However, they concede that the concept of reciprocity cannot exhaust all a person's obligations to do good (such as the duty to help strangers unable to reciprocate).[52] Their use of the illustration of helping strangers is instructive. It shows how the concept of reciprocity alone cannot carry the weight of all a person's moral obligations. Such a minimalistic *quid pro quo* morality could too easily collapse into mere self-interest. Surely, a more comprehensive expression than that of reciprocity (though not unrelated to it), capable of uniting individual and social understandings of promotion of the good along with the receipt of benefits, is to be found in the notion of the common good.[53]

At its most basic, the term 'common good' (or 'commonweal') connotes those collective goods that are held in common (shared) by a group or community. As such, it is broadly synonymous with the terms 'public interest' or 'general welfare'. As a philosophical term it is best understood as a piece of pre-Enlightenment wisdom preserved within the Aristotelian and Thomistic strands of political philosophy, both of which stress the social nature of human living. This communitarian focus has led to its being retained as a fundamental element of post-Enlightenment Christian (and particularly Roman Catholic) social doctrine. We have already encountered the use

[51] Ibid., pp. 174–75.

[52] Ibid., p. 174.

[53] For discussion of the common good see D. Hollenbach, 'Common Good', in J. Dwyer (ed.), *The New Dictionary of Catholic Social Thought* (Collegeville, MN: Liturgical Press, 1994); M. Novak, *Free Persons and the Common Good* (Lanham, MD: Madison Books, 1989); L. Dupré, 'The Common Good and the Open Society', in R. Bruce Douglass and D. Hollenbach (eds), *Catholicism and Liberalism: Contributions to American Public Policy* (Cambridge: Cambridge University Press, 1994), pp. 172–95.

of the term in Pope Pius XII's 1953 approval of genetic
medicine in which it functions to describe the good which is
proper to both the community and its individual members who
share in it. More recently, the common good has been
described succinctly by Pope John Paul II as 'the good of all and
of each individual'.[54] In such usages, the common good
expresses the inherently social and interdependent nature of
human living and therefore of moral obligations. As social
beings we are immediately and inescapably in a position of both
benefiting from and contributing to the good of others. This
occurs directly in terms of one's social exchanges with others
(where reciprocity might apply). It occurs indirectly from the
multitude of beneficial aspects of life in community. Examples
might include the benefits gained from the accumulation of
knowledge and development of technology, from the establishment of infrastructure that builds up the social fabric, from
the provision of national healthcare programmes, from pension
schemes and so on. Therefore, the common good can be
considered the mutual benefit that redounds to all (not merely
a minority, nor even the majority), when each participates in
and contributes to the good of all, rather than privately
pursuing self-interest. Thus, the common good is best realized
when there is a commitment to inclusive solidarity of the sort
summarized in the motto of Alexandre Dumas's Three
Musketeers: 'All for one. One for all.'

The common good is not a precise term, but one that seeks
to encapsulate a number of moral concerns in social ethics.
First, where aspects of communal living are involved, there is
always a social good or public interest to be pursued and
protected as well as the good of particular individuals. Second
(and just as importantly), the common good (precisely as the
good of all and of each) is not best served when individual
rights and freedoms are not protected. The common good does
not equate to a form of the 'greatest good of the greatest
number' in which individuals and their interests are sacrificed
for a greater good that excludes them. That is to say, the
common good is not served when some flourish at the expense
of other members of the community of those who have an

---

[54] Pope John Paul II, Encyclical Letter *Sollicitudo Rei Socialis*, 30 December 1987, n.
38 (AAS 80 (1988), 513–86).

interest. Third, as a consequence of the idea of a good that is common because it is shared by all, there is the assumption of an equitable distribution of the benefits that accrue in societies.

In this examination of the various beneficial aspects of the Human Genome Project, it has been seen that the promotion of benefit can be understood in three ways. These are: the beneficial *telos* of healthcare (health as a human good to be promoted), the benefits of biomedical research (including the scientific investigations that comprised and will arise from the Human Genome Project), and the physician's duty to benefit the patient (the focus of most bioethical writing). It has become apparent that these three aspects of the same idea have tended to be treated in a rather fragmentary way within the bioethical literature and medical codes, with no sense of any underlying or unifying features. Furthermore, bioethical discussion of beneficence in the sense of social benefit and professional obligations to unspecified others has tended to be eclipsed by focus on the one-to-one doctor–patient exchange, in which client autonomy is (rightly) given legal priority over claims of beneficence. A more 'joined-up' approach to thinking about medical benefit is required. It is suggested that the supple notion of the common good can provide a more coherent and unified understanding of the various aspects of 'doing good' that are relevant for the Human Genome Project in a way that more adequately integrates communal benefits with individual gain.

Genetic medicine and the common good

The common-sense morality that is the common good tells us that the genetic diseases that afflict humans can only be tackled cooperatively, but the benefits of so doing are shared globally – there is a communal dividend in medicine's progress. The same spirit of cooperation (as opposed to competition) characterized the public genome sequencing initiative. The international collaboration and sharing of genetic data speeded up the sequencing work, thereby demonstrating the benefits to be gained by working jointly rather than disparately. Similarly, a commitment to the common good lay at the heart of the conviction that the genetic knowledge gained should be freely and readily available to all as a means of maximizing the benefit of the sequencing work and distributing it as widely as possible. These principles were brokered at a crucial strategy meeting sponsored by The Wellcome Trust in 1996, representing participants of the publicly funded project (European, Japanese and US researchers).[55] The so-called Bermuda statement agreed: 'that all human genomic sequence information, generated by centres funded for large-scale human sequencing, should be freely available and in the public domain in order to encourage research and development and to maximise its benefit to society'.[56] It went on: 'these principles should apply for all human genomic sequence generated by large-scale sequencing centres, funded for the public good, in order to prevent such centres establishing a privileged position in the exploitation and control of human sequence information'.[57]

On 14 March 2000, UK Prime Minister Tony Blair and US President Bill Clinton endorsed the Bermuda principles in a joint statement: 'To realize the full promise of this research, raw fundamental data on the human genome, including the human DNA sequence and its variations, should be made freely available to scientists everywhere . . . We applaud the decision by scientists working on the Human Genome Project to release raw fundamental information about the human DNA sequence and its variants rapidly into the public domain, and we commend other scientists around the world to adopt this policy.'[58] The effect of this support of the public genome initiative was to send the share prices of the biotech companies – including that of Craig Venter's Celera Genomics, the private genome sequencing initiative – into a slump.[59] It was the threat of gene sequence data being held entirely in a commercial 'pay-to-view' database that mobilized the scientific and political communities into supporting the public initiative.[60]

[55] Human Genome Organisation (HUGO), 'Summary of Principles Agreed at the International Strategy Meeting on Human Genome Sequencing', Bermuda, 25–28 February 1996 <www.hugo-international.org/hugo/bermuda.htm>.

[56] Ibid., p. 1.

[57] Ibid.

[58] The White House, 'Joint Statement on Human Genome by President Clinton and Prime Minister Tony Blair of the U.K.', 14 March 2000 <http://usinfo.state.gov/topical/global/biotech/00031401.htm>.

[59] G. Ferry, 'The Whole Thing', *Wellcome News Supplement* 4: *Unveiling the Human Genome* (London: The Wellcome Trust, 2001), pp. 5–9, p. 8.

[60] For further discussion of the controversy surrounding the public versus private genome initiatives, see Ferry, 'The Whole Thing', pp. 8–9.

Nevertheless, patenting by commercial biotechnology companies will be the chief means by which the benefits of genetic research filter through to medical practice. There is ongoing ambivalence concerning the extent to which the patenting of genes and gene products will serve or hinder the promotion of the common good. The fear that some gene patenting could be detrimental to the common good was expressed in HUGO's *Statement on the Patenting of DNA Sequences*: 'HUGO (The Human Genome Organisation) is worried that the patenting of partial and uncharacterized cDNA sequences will reward those who make routine discoveries but penalize those who determine biological function or application. Such an outcome would impede the development of diagnostics and therapeutics, which is clearly not in the public interest.'[61] Similar reservations about the public interest are expressed about the disclosure of personal genetic information to insurance providers, since those who stand to benefit most from health insurance will find their premiums prohibitively expensive. The nature and extent of ownership of personal genetic information is further called into question by its inter-generational and familial value. The ramifications of genetic testing and therapy for present and future blood relations indicates why a purely individualistic account of moral interests and obligations is insufficient when considering genetic data.

The relevance and importance of the notion of the common good for genomorality is clearly seen in some of the inter-national statements on the genome. The key text is Unesco's commendable *Universal Declaration on the Human Genome and Human Rights*, 1997 – the first international instrument in the field of biology – which successfully harmonizes both a concern for the rights of the individual with a commitment to social responsibility. Its communitarian credentials are established in the opening section, which recalls that one of the founding aims of the United Nations Organization was to promote 'the common welfare of mankind'.[62] Article 1 of the *Declaration* announces: 'In a symbolic sense, [the human genome] is the heritage of humanity.' This expresses the shared value of

---

[61] Human Genome Organisation (HUGO), *Statement on the Patenting of DNA Sequences,* January 1995, p. 1 <www.gene.ucl.ac.uk/hugo/patent.htm>.
[62] Unesco, *Universal Declaration on the Human Genome and Human Rights*, 1997, Introduction.

the genome, in which humans have a common interest and for which humans have a collective responsibility. In other words, the human genome can be understood, in and of itself, as a good that is held in common, worthy of special protection. However, whatever the symbolic associations and meanings that can be extracted from human DNA, the use of the phrase 'in a symbolic sense' surely minimizes the *de facto* material value of the genome as humanity's common property – simultaneously both a state-of-the-art instruction manual/database, and an ancestral archive. Article 12 directs attention to the universal destination of the goods of genetic medicine: 'Benefits from advances in biology, genetics and medicine, concerning the human genome, shall be made available to all, with due regard for the dignity and human rights of each individual ... The applications of research, including applications in biology, genetics and medicine, concerning the human genome, shall seek to offer relief from suffering and improve the health of individuals and humankind as a whole.' Having indicated the communal benefit of genetic research, articles 17 and 19 point to the responsibility of nation states in ensuring that no individuals or groups are intentionally excluded from participating in the common good of genetic medicine. Thus, article 17 reads: 'States should respect and promote the practice of solidarity towards individuals, families and population groups who are particularly vulnerable to or affected by disease or disability of a genetic character.' Article 19 (a) (iii) highlights society's obligations towards poorer countries that are usually the last to benefit from the trickle-down effect of medical progress: 'States should seek to encourage measures enabling developing countries to benefit from the achievements of scientific and technological research so that their use in favour of economic and social progress can be to the benefit of all.'

The influence of the Unesco *Declaration* is evident in the subsequent *Statement on Benefit-Sharing* published in 2000 by the Ethics Committee of the international interest group, the Human Genome Organization (HUGO) which promotes genomic research and comprises scientists and researchers from industry, academic and government bodies.[63] The HUGO

---

[63] HUGO Ethics Committee, *Statement on Benefit-Sharing*, 9 April 2000 <www.gene.ucl.ac.uk/hugo/benefit.html>.

Statement offers a socially concerned discussion employing the terms: community, common heritage (described as 'common shared interest in the genetic heritage of mankind'), justice and solidarity in order to argue that the benefits of genetic research should be fairly distributed between research participants, researchers and the wider community. The *Statement* recommends 'that all humanity share in, and have access to, the benefits of genetic research'. Echoing the Unesco *Declaration*, it is observed that:

> there is a great inequality between the rich and poor nations in the direction and priorities of research and in the distribution and access to the benefits thereof ... research efforts should promote health universally and so include developing countries ... It is in everyone's best interest that wealthy and powerful nations as well as commercial entities foster health for all humanity.[64]

The seriousness with which the concept of benefit-sharing is taken by HUGO can be seen from the final recommendation of the *Statement*: that a small fixed percentage of profits from genetic technologies be redistributed to invest in humanitarian aid and healthcare.

Despite the socially responsible discussion that characterizes both the Unesco *Declaration* and the HUGO Ethics Committee *Statement*, it is difficult to disagree with the remark of Lisa Cahill that: 'considerations of the common good have been minimal in debating the ethics of human genetics in the era of globalization'.[65] There is little doubt that the attention to issues of social justice in both these documents is due to the philosophical input of Bartha Maria Knoppers, who chairs the HUGO Ethics Committee and was a member of the Unesco Bioethics Committee that drafted the *Universal Declaration on the Human Genome and Human Rights*.[66] International statements on the genome certainly exhibit a greater social concern than that demonstrated in the autonomy-led academic bioethics literature. Like Cahill, Knoppers argues that in this respect

---

[64] Ibid., Parts E and F.

[65] Lisa Sowle Cahill, 'Genetics, Individualism, and the Common Good', in Adrian Holderegger and Jean-Pierre Wils (eds), *Interdisziplinäre Ethik Grundlagen, Methoden, Bereiche: Festgabe für Dietmar Mieth zum sechzigsten Geburtstag* (Fribourg: Universitätsverlag, 2001), pp. 378–91, p. 384.

[66] Cf. Bartha Maria Knoppers, 'From Medical Ethics to "Genethics"', *The Lancet* 356 Supplement (December 2000), p. S38.

there has been a 'general failure to develop and include an ethics of public interest, public health, and the notion of civic participation in genetic research for the welfare of the community or for the advancement of science'.[67] She hopes that through genetic research there will be 'a rekindling of the ethic of solidarity' since 'we need to encourage, not prevent, civic participation for the public welfare' and 'force medical ethics towards an ethic of care and concern beyond that of individual autonomy and private interest'.[68] Due to the efforts of Knoppers a socially responsible attitude has emerged in international statements on the human genome. These, in turn, have shaped the political rhetoric. The challenge is to ensure that worthy words – such as President Clinton's appeal that the benefits of genome science be directed to all humanity, never just the privileged few[69] – influence public policy and shape the activities of commercial enterprise. This is particularly pressing since private investment in genomics far outstrips that of government and charitable funding.

Summary

The many and various ethical and social issues raised by the emergence of genetic technologies (genomorality) challenge humanity. They also challenge the conventional bioethical frameworks designed to respond to them. This study has argued that the questions which fall under the heading of genomorality require a broader social and political compass than bioethics has tended to afford them. In particular, the bioethical category of beneficence can be situated within a more comprehensive vision of social obligation using the philosophical concept of the common good, which offers a more versatile and robust means to discuss the social questions that genetics poses.

With characteristic flourish, John Mahoney closes *Seeking the Spirit* with the following epigram: 'In the old maps one might have come across uncharted areas where an uninformed but imaginative cartographer would fill in the occasional empty

---

[67] Ibid.
[68] Ibid.
[69] Cf. Clinton speech in note 1 above <http://news.bbc.co.uk/hi/english/sci/tech/newsid_805000/805803.stm>.

space with the legend "here be dragons". What we have tried to explore is whether our best preparation for venturing into such areas as our biological and genetic future is to equip ourselves with the best available fire-fighting apparatus, or at least with a good life of Saint George, or whether in fact the dragons will turn out to be not too unfriendly.'[70] There will undoubtedly be fierce challenges that face humanity as it pursues the good amid the new genetic territory; but new terrain – however dramatic – soon appears familiar, and dragons – whether metaphorical or otherwise – can be avoided and occasionally tamed. However, lest we grow complacent, perhaps an alternative Saint might be Margaret of Antioch, another dragon killer and patron of women in childbirth, who promised that those who honoured her would (in modern parlance) bear genetically healthy children.[71]

Bibliography

American Medical Association, *Principles of Medical Ethics*, June 1957.

American Medical Association, *Principles of Medical Ethics*, revised version, 1980, <www.ama-assn.org/ama/pub/print/article/4256-4928.html>.

American Medical Association, *Principles of Medical Ethics*, revised version, 17 June, 2001, <www.ama-assn.org/ama/pub/category/2512.html>.

Bach, F.H. *et al.*, 'Uncertainty in Xenotransplantation: Individual Benefit Versus Collective Risk', *Nature Medicine* 4.2 (1998), pp. 141–4.

Beauchamp, T. and Childress, J., *Principles of Biomedical Ethics*, 4th edn (Oxford: Oxford University Press, 1994).

Beauchamp, T. and Childress, J., *Principles of Biomedical Ethics*, 5th edn (Oxford: Oxford University Press, 2001).

British Medical Association, *Medicine Betrayed: The Participation of Doctors in Human Rights Abuses* (London: Zed Books, 1992).

---

[70] J. Mahoney, *Seeking the Spirit: Essays in Moral and Pastoral Theology* (London: Sheed & Ward, 1981), p. 252.

[71] For an account of her life see C. Pearce, 'The Cult of St Margaret of Antioch', *Feminist Theology* 16 (September 1997), pp. 70–85.

British Medical Association, *The Medical Profession and Human Rights: Handbook for a Changing Agenda* (London: Zed Books, 2001).

Cahill, L.S., 'Genetics, Individualism, and the Common Good', in A. Holderegger and J.-P. Wils (eds), *Interdisziplinäre Ethik Grundlagen, Methoden, Bereiche: Festgabe für Dietmar Mieth zum sechzigsten Geburtstag* (Fribourg: Universitätsverlag, 2001), pp. 378-91.

Caulfield, T. and Williams-Jones, B. (eds), *The Commercialization of Genetic Research: Ethical, Legal, and Policy Issues* (New York: Kluwer Academic/Plenum Press, 1999).

Churchill, L., 'Beneficence', in W.T. Reich (ed.), *The Encyclopedia of Bioethics*, rev. edn (New York: Simon & Schuster/Macmillan, 1995), vol. i, pp. 243–7.

Clague, J., 'Genetic Knowledge as a Commodity: The Human Genome Project, Markets and Consumers', in M. Junker-Kenny and L.S. Cahill (eds), *The Ethics of Genetic Engineering, Concilium* (April 1998), pp. 3–12.

Cole-Turner, R., *The New Genesis: Theology and the Genetic Revolution* (Louisville, KY: Westminster/John Knox Press, 1993).

DuBose, E.R., Hamel, R.P. and O'Connell, L.J. (eds), *A Matter of Principles? Ferment in U.S. Bioethics* (Valley Forge, PA: Trinity Press International, 1994).

Dunstan, G., *The Artifice of Ethics* (London: SCM Press, 1974).

Dupré, L., 'The Common Good and the Open Society', in R. Bruce Douglass and D. Hollenbach (eds), *Catholicism and Liberalism: Contributions to American Public Policy* (Cambridge: Cambridge University Press, 1994), pp. 172–95.

Engelhardt, T., *The Foundations of Bioethics* (Oxford: Oxford University Press, 1986).

Ferry, G., 'The Whole Thing', *Wellcome News Supplement* 4: *Unveiling the Human Genome* (London: Wellcome Trust, 2001), pp. 5–9.

Fletcher, J., 'Ethical Aspects of Genetic Controls: Designed Genetic Changes in Man', *New England Journal of Medicine* 285.14 (1971), pp. 776–83.

Fletcher, J., *The Ethics of Genetic Control: Ending Reproductive*

Roulette (New York: Prometheus, 1988; first published New York: Doubleday, 1974).

Gillon, R., 'Defending "the Four Principles" Approach to Biomedical Ethics', *Journal of Medical Ethics* 21.6 (1995), pp. 323–4.

Hollenbach, D., 'Common Good', in J. Dwyer (ed.), *The New Dictionary of Catholic Social Thought* (Collegeville, MN: Liturgical Press, 1994).

Holm, S. 'Not Just Autonomy: The Principles of American Biomedical Ethics', *Journal of Medical Ethics* 21.6 (1995), pp. 332–8.

Holm, S., 'Genetic Engineering and the North–South Divide', in A. Dyson and J. Harris (eds), *Ethics and Biotechnology* (London: Routledge, 1999), pp. 47–63.

Human Genome Organisation (HUGO), *Statement on the Patenting of DNA Sequences,* January 1995, <www.gene.ucl.ac.uk/hugo/patent.htm>.

Human Genome Organisation (HUGO), 'Summary of Principles Agreed at the International Strategy Meeting on Human Genome Sequencing', Bermuda, 25–8 February 1996, <www.hugo-international.org/hugo/bermuda.htm>.

Human Genome Organisation (HUGO), Ethics Committee 'Statement on Benefit-Sharing', 9 April 2000, <www.gene.ucl.ac.uk/hugo/benefit.html>.

John Paul II, 'The Ethics of Genetic Manipulation', *Address to the World Medical Association,* 29 October 1983 (*Acta Apostolicae Sedis* 76 (1984), 389–402).

John Paul II, Encyclical Letter *Sollicitudo Rei Socialis,* 30 December 1987 (*Acta Apostolicae Sedis* 80 (1988), 513–86).

John Paul II, *Address to the Pontifical Academy for Life,* 20 November 1995 (*Acta Apostolicae Sedis* 88 (1996), 668–71).

John Paul II, *Address to the 18th International Congress on Organ Transplants,* 29 August 2000 (*Acta Apostolicae Sedis* 92 (2000), 822–6).

Knoppers, B.M., 'From Medical Ethics to "Genethics"', *The Lancet* 356 Supplement (December 2000), p. S38.

Mahoney, J., *Seeking the Spirit: Essays in Moral and Pastoral Theology* (London: Sheed & Ward, 1981).

National Commission for the Protection of Human Subjects of Biomedical and Behavioral Research, *The Belmont Report: Ethical Principles and Guidelines for the Protection of Human Subjects of Research*, OPRR Reports (Washington, DC: US Government Printing Office, 1978), <http://ohsr.od. nih.gov/mpa/belmont.php3>.

Novak, M., *Free Persons and the Common Good* (Lanham, MD: Madison Books, 1989).

O'Donovan, O., *Begotten or Made?* (Oxford: Clarendon Press, 1994).

Pearce, C., 'The Cult of St Margaret of Antioch', *Feminist Theology* (September 1997), pp. 70–85.

Pellegrino, E.D. and Thomasma, D.C., *For the Patient's Good: The Restoration of Beneficence in Health Care* (Oxford: Oxford University Press, 1988).

Percival, T., *Medical Ethics: A Code of Institutes and Precepts, Adapted to the Professional Conduct of Physicians and Surgeons* (Manchester: S. Russell, 1803).

Pius XII, 'Moral Aspects of Genetics', *Address to the First International Symposium of Genetic Medicine*, 7 September 1953 (*Acta Apostolicae Sedis* 44 (1953), 605).

Pius XII, *Address to the Italian Association of Cornea Donors and to Clinical Oculists and Legal Medical Practitioners*, 14 May 1956 (*Acta Apostolicae Sedis* 48 (1956)).

Pius XII, *Allocution on the Relief of Pain*, 24 February 1957 (*Acta Apostolicae Sedis* 49 (1957), 135).

Pontifical Academy for Life, *Declaration on the Production and the Scientific and Therapeutic Use of Human Embryonic Stem Cells*, 25 August 2000.

Rahner, K., 'Experiment: Man', *Theology Digest* (February 1968), pp. 57–69.

Rahner, K., 'The Problem of Genetic Manipulation', *Theological Investigations*, vol. ix (New York: Crossroad, 1972), pp. 244–52.

Ramsey, P., *Fabricated Man: The Ethics of Genetic Control* (New Haven: Yale University Press, 1970).

Ramsey, P., 'Shall We "Reproduce"? ii: Rejoinders and Future

Forecast', *Journal of the American Medical Association* 220.11 (1972), pp. 1480–5.

Reich, W.T. (ed.), *The Encyclopedia of Bioethics* 1st edn (New York: Free Press, 1978).

Reich, W.T. (ed.), *The Encyclopedia of Bioethics*, rev. edn (New York: Simon & Schuster/Macmillan, 1995).

Society, Religion and Technology Project, 'GM Animals, Humans and the Future of Genetics', Appendix V, *Board of National Mission Deliverance to the General Assembly of the Church of Scotland*, May 2001.

'Special Issue: Theories and Methods in Bioethics: Principlism and Its Critics', *Kennedy Institute of Ethics Journal* 5.3 (1995).

Unesco, *Universal Declaration on the Human Genome and Human Rights*, 1997.

Unesco Document 27V/45, adopted by the General Conference of Unesco at its 29th session, Paris, 11 November 1997, <www.unesco.org/human_rights/hrbc.htm>.

Veatch, R., *A Theory of Medical Ethics* (New York: Basic Books, 1981).

Woodhead, L., 'Human Genetics: A Theological Response', in I. Torrance (ed.) (on behalf of the Church of Scotland Board of Social Responsibility), *Bio-Ethics for the New Millennium* (Edinburgh: Saint Andrew Press, 2000), pp. 82–96.

World Medical Association, *Declaration on the Human Genome Project* (adopted by the 44th World Medical Assembly, Marbella, Spain, September 1992), <www.wma.net/e/ policy/17-s-1_e.html>.

World Medical Association, *Declaration of Geneva* (adopted by the 46th WMA General Assembly, Stockholm, Sweden, September 1994), <www.wma.net/e/policy/17-a_e.html>.

World Medical Association, *Declaration of Helsinki, Ethical Principles for Medical Research Involving Human Subjects* (adopted by the 18th WMA General Assembly, Helsinki, Finland, June 1964 and amended by the 52nd WMA General Assembly, Edinburgh Scotland, October 2000), <www.wma.net/e/policy/17-c_e.html>.

Electronic resources

BBC website, Monday, 26 June 2000, 'Scientists Crack Human Code' <http://news.bbc.co.uk/hi/english/sci/tech/newsid_805000/805803.stm>.

The White House, 'Press Release on the Human Genome Project', 14 March 2000, <http://usinfo.state.gov/topical/global/biotech/00031402.htm>.

The White House, 'Joint Statement on Human Genome by President Clinton and Prime Minister Tony Blair of the UK', 14 March 2000, <http://usinfo.state.gov/topical/global/biotech/00031401.htm>.

10

How Might A Virtue Ethic Frame Debates In Human Genetics?

Celia Deane-Drummond

The premise of this chapter is that in order to arrive at an adequate ethical position on debates in human genetics we need to consider the particular ways in which such ethical debates are approached. The consequentialist position, which stresses the balance of risks and benefits, seems to win over even in those theological contexts where one might expect a deontological approach to be dominant. I present an argument for an alternative framing of the debates that takes its bearings from virtue ethics, but one that is rooted theologically by reference to the four cardinal virtues of prudence, justice, fortitude and temperance, and through wisdom to the three theological virtues of faith, hope and charity. While such a position takes its inspiration from the thought of Thomas Aquinas, it attempts to appropriate themes in his theological/ethical corpus in a way that I argue is of particular relevance to issues in human genetics. The theme of wisdom, in particular, becomes a way of integrating strands in deontological, consequentialist and virtue ethics, while remaining theocentric in orientation, drawing on a sophianic theology of nature.

Introduction

One of the most significant features of the discourse surrounding the Human Genome Project (HGP) is that, in the early stages at least, genes were treated as if they were discrete entities; identifying gene activity was the key for unlocking the particular 'secrets' of life at a fundamental level.[1] The idea that our genes control basic human functions is the premise behind the 'mapping' process and one of the bases for the justification of the HGP itself. The biological belief in discrete species has become undermined by the concept of the gene, so that the boundaries between species are no longer thought to be significant at the level of genetics. Such a shift has implications for philosophy and ethics, since it challenges how far and to what extent humans are definable as a distinct species.[2] Furthermore, it means that genetic studies in other species such as mice or sheep, or even more so in the case of primates, have a direct bearing on human genetics.

More recently, however, the definition of what constitutes a gene has become the subject of considerable debate among philosophers of biology and biologists themselves.[3] The difficulty consists of this, namely that gene products are subject to such considerable revision and change after transcription into the messages that relate the information to the protein-synthesizing components of the cells, that in many cases at least it is no longer possible to specify precisely what particular part of the deoxyribonucleic acid makes up the gene. As a consequence some biologists prefer to talk much more loosely in terms of regions of nucleic acid that may be activated at different times for particular functions during development.[4] The potential to manipulate this switching on and off process during development comes to prominence in techniques such as nuclear transfer or 'cloning', where the genome itself becomes reprogrammed so that the locks on deactivation are taken away and the process starts, as it were, from scratch. The fact that so many abnormalities are evident in 'cloned' animal

---

[1] See E.F. Keller, 'Is there an Organism in this Text?', in P.R. Sloan (ed.), *Controlling our Destinies: Historical, Philosophical, Ethical, and Theological Perspectives on the Human Genome Project* (Notre Dame: University of Notre Dame Press, 2000), pp. 273–8.

[2] S. Clark, *Biology and Christian Ethics* (Cambridge: Cambridge University Press, 2000), p. 234.

[3] See, for example, P. Portin, 'The Concept of the Gene: Short History and Present Status', *Quarterly Review of Biology* 68 (1992), pp. 173–223; P. Kitchner, 'Gene: Current Uses', in E.F. Keller and E. Lloyd (eds), *Keywords in Evolutionary Biology* (Cambridge, MA: Harvard University Press, 1992), pp. 128–31.

[4] Kitchner, 'Gene: Current Uses', p. 130; see also H.J. Rheinberger, 'Genes: A Disunified View from the Perspective of Molecular Biology', in P. Beurton, W. Lefevre and H.J. Rheinberger (eds) *Gene Concepts and Evolution* (Berlin; Max Planck Institut für Wissenschaftgeschichte, Preprint No. 18, 1995), pp. 7–13.

organisms demonstrates the difficulty of completing such reprogramming without serious effects. Exactly how such inactivation occurs and the processes involved in reactivation is, at the time of writing, still largely a matter of conjecture. More to the point, in the present context, is the difficulty of specifying precisely, in most cases, the multiple stages from DNA to particular protein products. The switching on and off of particular regions of DNA, the coordination with particular cellular requirements and the synergistic effects of different gene products all combine to make the possibility of extensive therapeutic applications of the discoveries of the HGP rather more remote than was first considered to be the case. Hence, the initial somewhat inflated discourse about the particular benefits of the HGP to humanity as a whole has become subverted, as it were, from the inside, namely through genetic science. In other words the challenges facing those who wish to apply knowledge gained through the HGP are as much biochemical and physiological as they are purely genetic.

What implications does this shift in genetics have on the way human genetics is perceived? First of all, claims that the HGP would lead to immediate medical benefits across a wide range of genetic diseases need to be viewed with a certain amount of caution. This is not to say that there are no attainable benefits at all, but that each claim needs to be qualified in the light of what is known precisely about the particular way gene function is regulated in particular cases. The idea that the DNA is like a predetermined 'blueprint' or 'code' for life does not do justice to the fluid nature of the way genes are expressed in particular contexts. Unravelling the complex biology of genes is, then, challenging notions of fixity that seem to have gripped the populist understanding of genetics, or 'gene myth'. There is no need to invoke theological frameworks in order to confront the ideal of genetic determinism; it is happening, as it were, from within biological science itself.

Of course this does not rule out the fact that, according to the science, there may be ways and means of developing therapeutic treatments of different genetic diseases. However, the line of approach may be equally at the level of biochemistry or physiology, rather than genetic manipulation as such. Any move towards genetic change has to be put in its proper context of its function in the whole organism. The early claims that the HGP would lead to a reduction in suffering of those who were subject to the 'lottery' of their genes needs to be reviewed, or at least reconsidered.[5] The idea that humanity has inherited genes as part of a lottery is particularly popular among genetic scientists reflecting on the public significance of their science, since now the motive becomes a moral one, namely to deliver human subjects from the threat of their 'bad' genes. The break between the gene and the person is significant, since persons themselves are not blamed for their genetic inheritance; rather it is the genes that have to be rooted out in the manner analogous to the 'war' against disease.[6] The individual person is not directly associated with having such genes, in the manner suggestive of earlier eugenic programmes; rather the task of science becomes one of liberation from such genes for the benefit of the individual. James Watson, for example, who pioneered the Human Genome Project in the USA, suggested that:

> until the decision was made to go for the whole human genome, the majority of families suffering from genetic diseases would have no reason to hope for release from the pains inflicted upon them by past errors in the copying of their families' genetic messages.[7]

Other benefits to the human condition include the idea of 'enhancement' of particular characteristics deemed to be beneficial. In the past, geneticists such as Professor Hermann J. Muller have even included character traits essential for good science on the list of those to be fostered by genetic manipulation, such as the ability to have independence of judgement and intellectual honesty![8] However, the moral basis for this aspect of genetics is harder to fathom, quite apart from the scientific difficulty of locating 'genes', if they exist, for such character traits. Watson suggests that this kind of enhancement

---

[5] See, for example, P. Frossard, *The Lottery of Life; The New Genetics and the Future of Mankind* (London and New York: Bantam Press, 1991).

[6] See A. Domurat Dreger, 'Metaphors of Morality in the Human Genome Project', in P.R. Sloan (ed.), *Controlling Our Destinies; Historical, Philosophical, Ethical, and Theological Perspectives on the Human Genome Project* (Notre Dame: University of Notre Dame Press, 2000), p. 169.

[7] J. Watson, *A Passion for DNA: Genes, Genomes and Society* (Oxford: Oxford University Press, 2001) p. 171.

[8] H.J. Muller, 'The Guidance of Human Evolution' (1959), cited in P. Ramsey, *Fabricated Man: The Ethics of Genetic Control* (London and New Haven: Yale University Press, 1970), p. 7.

is permissible, as it would be immoral not to pursue a 'good' where it is technically possible to do so. He cites examples such as raising human intelligence, though the genetic basis for intelligence is itself highly controversial.[9] In addition, Watson suggests that while the risks to human health should be taken into account, they should not be allowed to stem the tide of research. He looks back with regret to a time when early DNA recombinant research was delayed because of public concerns about safety. He is much more cavalier in his approach to genetics in the light of this experience:

> Never postpone experiments that have clearly defined future benefits for fears of dangers that can't be quantified. Though at first sight it might sound uncaring, we can react rationally only to real (as opposed to hypothetical) risks. . . .
> When they are finally attempted, germ-line genetic manipulations will probably be done to change a death sentence into a life verdict by creating children who are resistant to a deadly virus, for example, much the same way we can protect plants from viruses by inserting anti-viral DNA segments into their genomes.[10]

The way HGP has been portrayed in salvific language is significant, as it served to bolster public support for the project. The concept that research into human genetics should be restricted is dismissed through reference to the basic ideal of human freedom as practised in science.[11] Of course the appeal to freedom and the notion of the HGP as a frontier to be crossed chimes with the American cultural values that approve and foster pioneer mentality. It is doubtful that political support from Congress could have been achieved for the HGP if it had been couched in a different kind of language that did not draw on these particularly powerful images that are rooted in the American culture.[12] In addition to the moral and scientific worth of the project, those considering funding had to consider whether it would draw in economic benefits. The HGP

---

[9] He suggests this, 'If your life is going nowhere, shouldn't you seize the chance of jump-starting your children's future', Watson, *Passion for DNA*, p. 208. For a critique of the view that intelligence is inherited, see R. Lewontin, *The Doctrine of DNA: Biology as Ideology* (London: Penguin, 1993), pp. 17–37; for a critique of the strident claims for the HGP, see pp. 61–83.

[10] Watson, *Passion for DNA*, pp. 228–9.

[11] Domurat Dreger, 'Metaphors of Morality', p. 170.

[12] Ibid., p. 157.

now is couched in terms of a 'real estate', something to be traded with other countries and developed as a 'fertile land', subject to exploitation for human financial rewards. The scientific and moral language becomes a cover for what is at root a business enterprise. In this respect genetics is no different from other forms of biotechnology. As Phillipe Frossard, a practising scientist who has worked for many years in the biotechnology industry, suggests:

> I have always had the uneasy feeling that the potential of a drug to treat human disease is a fortuitous side effect, a marketable commodity that helps win over media attention while the primary goal concerns two of the strongest human motivating factors; greed and ambition.[13]

Uncovering the real motivation behind research is an important aspect in disentangling various claims for or against what is possible through human genetic discoveries. Alice Domurat Dreger has suggested, correctly in my view, that appraising the history of the way the HGP has unfolded points to a need for much more open discussion by scientists and the public alike:

> not only should HGP proponents and participants be much more explicit about their values, interests, etc., so should non-scientists ... this model would make life much easier for genome scientists. It would give them the opportunity to speak frankly about their goals, needs and concerns – instead of having to cloak these in metaphors and myths – and it would require non-scientists to listen and to respond with equally frank discussion of their goals, needs and concerns. Such a genuine 'cultural' exchange, one that would occur because of a common value of good knowledge and responsible behaviour, would surely be better for all concerned.[14]

Such a discussion points to an alternative way of conceiving ethical issues in human genetics, one that does not simply take its bearings from purported risks and benefits, but rather looks to the *motivation* of those making such claims.

---

[13] Frossard, *The Lottery of Life*, p. 225.
[14] Domurat Dreger, 'Metaphors of Morality', p. 184.

Styles of practical Christian ethics

Discussion of ethical issues in genetics from a Christian perspective has tended to follow the secular debate by portrayal of these issues in terms of a consequentialist assessment of the relative risks and benefits of the various genetic interventions.[15] The limitations of consequentialism have been recognized by a number of other scholars writing on the ethics of genetic intervention.[16] James Gustafson, in a book *Theology and Christian Ethics*, which has now become something of a classic, suggested that there are two broad styles of practical ethics when it comes to consideration of human genetic engineering.[17] The first style is where there is a fixed view of what consists of human nature and genetic changes are judged in relation to this particular view. While he does not name specific Christian traditions, he stresses that this view is to accept the absolute authority of a tradition from the 'outside' as it were, and then apply this to specific examples. In this case:

> One would define the licit and illicit kinds of experiments in the light of an *a priori* definition of what man is, and everything done both in learning and in doing from what has been learned would have to conform to these determinations.[18]

Another style, one that he prefers, is that humanity 'has assumed and seized the right to intervene in nature, including his own nature'.[19] Yet the discovery of self-creativity is not without any limits, but premised on the basis of whether or not it is for the 'well-being' of the human community. Such a discovery, he suggests, does not come from the idea of fixed limits, itself deriving from a fixed understanding of what it is to be human, but 'he discovers the direction in which development ought to go as it is consistent with or abrasive upon, the

---

[15] See C. Deane-Drummond, *Biology and Theology Today: Exploring the Boundaries* (London: SCM Press, 2001), pp. 119–43.

[16] See C. Deane-Drummond and B. Szerszynski (eds), *Re-Ordering Nature: Theology, Society and the New Genetics* (London: T & T Clark, 2002).

[17] J. Gustafson, *Theology and Christian Ethics* (Cleveland, OH: Pilgrim Press, 1974). It is noteworthy that his subsequent major books, namely *Theology and Ethics* (Oxford: Blackwell, 1981) and *Ethics from a Theocentric Perspective* (Chicago: University of Chicago Press, 1984), did not discuss specifically ethical issues in genetics.

[18] Gustafson, *Theology and Christian Ethics*, p. 284.

[19] Ibid., p. 285.

moral requisites for human life and community'.[20] The moral requisites become the 'guidemarks' for ethical practice. However, it is not clear exactly what these requisites might be, how they are to be applied to genetic engineering, or the extent to which they are predicated in any way on a particular understanding of anthropology. What does it mean, for example, to say that a particular development is for the well-being of the human community? How might this differ from the purely secular analysis of risks and benefits, normally couched in terms of particular risks to human welfare? He hints at his own distinctive position in those passages where he insists on an integration of the spiritual and moral life. He suggests that certain senses in human experience are developed in the spiritual life, including a sense of radical dependence, a sense of gratitude, a sense of repentance, a sense of obligation and a sense of direction.[21] Such qualities are based not so much on a particular fixed view of anthropology, but a theology of God, namely God as creator, beneficent, judge, orderer and end of creation. His own particular view of God, according to the liberal Protestant tradition, especially Schleiermacher, turns out to be reflected in how to perceive human being and becoming. How and in what sense this might apply to particular examples in the case of genetic engineering is left obscure. However, it seems to me that Gustafson is arguing for a different style of Christian deontological ethics, one that draws particularly on his own perception of who God is, rather than primarily in terms of risks and benefits. Moreover, as becomes apparent in his later work, he argues that ethics needs to move away from an anthropocentric orientation towards a more holistic approach based on the relationship between God and creation.[22]

A similar conception of the current debate in Christian ethics of genetics comes through reflection on papal statements about human nature in contrast with the idea of

---

[20] Ibid.

[21] Ibid., p.166.

[22] See especially Gustafson, *Theology and Ethics*, pp. 99–113. It should be noted that I am in agreement with Gustafson that ethics needs to be viewed in theocentric perspective, and thus becomes inclusive of all creatures. However, the manner in which the ethics is then elaborated is somewhat different, as will be clear below.

Arthur Peacocke that human characteristics are 'emergent' in human evolution.[23] In the Pope's traditional message for Lent in 2002 he issued a new warning about genetic manipulation, suggesting that 'man' would be tempted to modify the 'tree of life', treating it as 'private property' instead of accepting it as a 'gift from God'.[24] However, if we examine other documents that have been published by the Pontifical Academy for Life, it is clear that the kind of ethics that might be predicated by such a position is not always taken up in practice.[25] Many of the authors contributing to the latter volume were scientists, and a number of them discussed the particular ethical issues in human genetics primarily in terms of risks and benefits.[26] The official church statements on human nature were set alongside the more scientific papers, but a proper integration between the deliberations was harder to decipher. One senses a real struggle between the practical demands of the working scientist and the demands of traditional Roman Catholic faith.[27] Kevin Fitzgerald, for example, believes that a simple reliance on philosophical/theological accounts of human nature in order

---

[23] For a comparison of these views see E. McMullin, 'Biology and the Theology of the Human', in P. Sloan (ed.), *Controlling Our Destinies; Historical, Philosophical, Ethical, and Theological Perspectives on the Human Genome Project* (Notre Dame; University of Notre Dame Press, 2000), pp. 367–93.

[24] Vatican City, 'Pope Warns Scientists about Genetic Manipulation', Deutsche Presse-Agentur, 5 February 2002.

[25] J. de Dios Vial Correa and E. Sgreccia (eds), *Human Genome, Human Person and the Society of the Future, Proceedings of Fourth Assembly of the Pontifical Academy for Life*, Vatican City, 23–5 February 1998 (Vatican: Libreria Editrice Vaticana, 1999).

[26] See, for example, W.M. O'Connor Moore, 'Gene Therapy: Clinical Aspects', pp. 244–54; H. Watt, 'Human Gene Therapy: Ethical Aspects', pp. 255–69. The way the science, understood as analysis of risk and benefit, influences the ethics becomes clear in statements such as the following: 'Recent progress in the field of genetics has made it possible to obtain a greater knowledge of the human genome and the nature of genetic disorders, as well as recognizing the risks and benefits of these techniques not only for the individual, but also for relatives and for the population as a whole. In this light, many governments and national and international organizations have begun to issue guidelines with both an ethical and political value in order to prepare for the passing of specific laws.' The interjection of some papal comments on the sanctity of life sat rather uneasily with this approach. See A.G. Spagnolo, 'Predictive and Presymptomatic Genetic Testing: Service or Sentence', pp. 212–34.

[27] G. Herranz, 'Medical-Ethical Problems in Prenatal and Pre-implantation Genetic Diagnosis', pp. 190–211. In this case faith categories seem to win out, so that prenatal genetic diagnosis is described as 'a wolf in sheep's clothing', p. 210.

to frame ethics 'creates heuristic frameworks often at odds with contemporary scientific knowledge'.[28]

The question now arises, are there ways of framing theocentric ethics in a way that does not necessarily rely on a particular liberal Protestant understanding of God, that is distinctive in terms of theological insight, but which avoids the dilemma of two parallel worlds that seems to appear once theology becomes remote from scientific practice? The argument of this chapter is that there *is* another possibility worth exploring, namely through consideration of the virtues.

I have argued elsewhere for inclusion of a virtue ethic approach in relation to issues in the new genetics.[29] Rediscovery of wisdom draws on a particular way of understanding who God is in sophianic language.[30] The idea that there could be a distinctive Christian ethic is somewhat controversial among Roman Catholic theologians, who have tended to be deeply suspicious of any attempt to claim that Christian ethics is anything more than simply reason informed in some sense by faith.[31] While this approach has served to develop a natural law tradition, authors sensitive to the Grisez-Finnis school have tried, through philosophical reflection, to free interpretations of natural law from any fixed casuistry that dominated earlier interpretations.[32] As a counter-reaction to this trend there have been attempts to reinstate the priority of theology, to call for a morality 'out of the middle of the revelation'.[33] Counter-reactions to this move in favour of an entirely autonomous ethic are not particularly helpful, except insofar as they rebutted an uncritical appeal to scripture.

---

[28] K. Fitzgerald, 'Do We Know Ourselves Well Enough to be Engineering Humans?', in G. Stock and J. Campbell (eds), *Engineering the Human Germline: An Exploration of the Science and Ethics of Altering the Genes we Pass On to Our Children* (Oxford and New York: Oxford University Press, 2000).

[29] See, for example, 'Aquinas, Wisdom Ethics and the New Genetics', in Deane-Drummond and Szerszynski, *Re-Ordering Nature*, pp. 293–311.

[30] C. Deane-Drummond, *Creation Through Wisdom: Theology and the New Biology* (London: T & T Clark, 2000).

[31] For a useful discussion of different possible positions, see V. MacNamara, 'The Distinctiveness of Christian Morality', in B. Hoose (ed.), *Christian Ethics: An Introduction* (London: Cassell, 1998), pp. 149–60, esp. pp. 157–8.

[32] For discussion of this trend in natural law, see N. Biggar and R. Black (eds), *The Revival of Natural Law: Philosophical, Theological and Ethical Responses to the Finnis-Grisez School* (Aldershot: Ashgate, 2000).

[33] MacNamara, 'The Distinctiveness of Christian Morality', p. 157.

The acid of postmodern deconstruction could easily dissolve any claim for a theological basis for ethics, or even a philosophical basis through natural law. Yet even those conscious of postmodern sensibilities have to admit the diversity that exists and needs to be respected. I suggest that the language of virtue, in particular wisdom, invites reflection in such a way that a space is opened up for dialogue between those of different presuppositions, including scientists. This is not the same as imposing a rigid scheme based on particular 'foundations'; rather, by being eschatological in orientation, it explores, through a particular theological telos, what might be the good end for humanity. Taken on its own, postmodern deconstruction could ultimately lead to the isolated individual or even simply consciousness and then despair, along with nihilism. I suggest that virtue ethics is particularly suggestive in as much as it mediates between the extreme of a Kantian deontology and postmodern deconstruction and also lends itself to a resonance of shared concern across the wider human community, including those of no religious persuasion. However, this does not mean that Christian ethics has *nothing* distinctive to add to the debate, as is often assumed by Catholic moral philosophers. The ways and forms of ethical reflection are grounded in a particular story and tradition.

The four cardinal virtues

My intention in this section is to show the relevance of the four cardinal virtues to consideration of issues in genetics. I suggest that by giving priority to prudential understanding Aquinas pointed to a way of developing ethics that is of particular relevance in the present context of human genetic engineering, where decisions have to be made and action has to be taken. Prudence is necessary for the expression of the other virtues and also includes discernment. Moreover, secular philosophers, working within a virtue ethics approach, recognize the priority given to the first cardinal virtue, or practical wisdom. James Gustafson resisted any understanding of the link between the moral and spiritual life in terms of the theological virtues or gifts of the Spirit, but he did not explain why he rejected such a view, except insofar as for him such ideas seemed to carry the connotation of fixity of being.[34] However, rather than encourage any sense of fixity, I hope to show that consideration of the four cardinal virtues alongside theological virtues evokes a dynamic concept of human nature, as well as providing clear moral requisites for human action in the case of the genetic engineering of humans that will eventually become possible through the discoveries emerging from the HGP. Romanus Cessario has consistently argued for the recovery of the theological virtues of faith, hope and charity as the basis for developing what he calls the theological life.[35] By this he means the vocation of Christians to act in specific ways according to the virtues of faith, hope and charity. While he does recognize the importance of wisdom, he does not develop the theme in the way I am suggesting here or apply it to genomorality.[36]

Developing a virtue ethic has certain advantages compared with other conceptual frameworks for ethics, since it takes the pressure off just thinking about particular ethical dilemmas or quandaries.[37] By looking at the character of the agent primarily, the question of *What should I do?* breaks into subsidiary ones of *Who am I?*, *Who shall I become?* and *How am I to get there?*[38] Developing prudential understanding, for example, does not *avoid* questions of practical decision-making in ethics; rather it shows how developing a particular character will foster particular decisions. Such decisions are like an 'overflow' of the particular habits of virtue or character developed. Hence the decision-making is arrived at in a rather different way from the usual focus on the dilemma in and of itself. James Keenan has also pointed out the particular advantage of a virtue ethic approach as applied to questions surrounding genetic engineering, for it offsets the tendency in genetics to objectify the subject.[39] The focus away from the problem towards the agent is

---

[34] Gustafson, *Theology and Christian Ethics*, p. 166.

[35] R. Cessario, *Christian Faith and the Theological Life* (Washington: Catholic University of America Press, 1996). See also R. Cessario, *Introduction to Moral Theology* (Washington: Catholic University of America Press, 2001).

[36] I am borrowing this term from Julie Clague's chapter in this volume.

[37] E.L. Pincoffs, *Quandaries and Virtue: Against Reductionism in Ethics* (Lawrence: University of Kansas Press, 1986).

[38] This scheme is taken from James Keenan's typology of virtue ethics. For a summary of his views, see J.F. Keenan, 'Virtue Ethics', in Hoose, *Christian Ethics*, pp. 84–94.

[39] J.F. Keenan, 'What is Morally New in Genetic Manipulation?', *Human Gene Therapy* 1 (1990), pp. 289–98.

not something that will necessarily come easily to practising scientists, who are used to viewing issues from an 'objective' perspective by rarifying the issue at hand and applying reasoning powers in order to develop a 'solution'. This is, perhaps, one reason why bioethics is dominated by a risk/benefit type of analysis, since it seems to find echoes in the premises behind scientific practice.[40] As Gregory Jones and Richard Vance point out, one of the most significant aspects of virtue approaches is that they are more easily recognized as being socially embedded in a particular tradition.[41]

Prudence, or practical wisdom, is the 'mother' of all the other cardinal virtues.[42] For the occidental Christian view Being precedes Truth and Truth precedes Goodness. In colloquial use prudence 'carries the connotation of timorous, small minded self-preservation, of a rather selfish concern about oneself', hence those who shun danger do so by an appeal to 'prudence'.[43] Instead, Aquinas links prudence specifically with *goodness,* moreover there is no justice or fortitude without the virtue of prudence. Instinctive inclinations towards goodness as set through natural law become transformed through prudence, so that prudence gives rise to a perfected ability to make choices. Free activity of humanity is good insofar as it corresponds to the pattern of prudence. As such prudence is the 'cause, root, mother, measure, precept, guide and prototype of all ethical virtues, it acts in all of them, perfecting them to their true nature, all participate

---

[40] For discussion of this point, see Michael Banner, *Christian Ethics and Contemporary Moral Problems* (Cambridge: Cambridge University Press, 1999), pp. 1–46. There are other authors who have explored the use of a virtue ethic approach to bioethics; this may either be through a supplement to what is basically a principles approach, as in Beauchamp and Childress, or, a more radical rejection of such principles of obligation. See T.L. Beauchamp and J.F. Childress, *Principles of Biomedical Ethics* (Oxford: Oxford University Press, 2001), pp. 26–55. James Drane adopts a similar position to this: see 'Character and the Moral Life: A Virtue Approach to Biomedical Ethics', in E.R. Du Bose, R.P. Hamel and L.J. O'Connell (eds), *A Matter of Principles? Ferment in US Bioethics* (Valley Forge: Trinity Press International, 1994), pp. 284–309.

[41] L. Gregory Jones and R.P. Vance, 'Why the Virtues are Not Another Approach to Medical Ethics: Reconceiving the Place of Ethics in Contemporary Medicine', in P.F. Camenisch (ed.), *Religious Methods and Resources in Bioethics* (Dordrecht: Kluwer Academic, 1994), pp. 203–25.

[42] See, for example, Deane-Drummond, *Creation Through Wisdom*, p. 99.

[43] J. Pieper, *Prudence*, trans. R. Winston and C. Winston (London: Faber and Faber, 1959), p. 11.

in it, and by virtue of this participation they are virtues'.[44] Hence truly human action is the inward shaping of volition and action by reason perfected in truth. However, reason is not understood in a narrow sense analogous to mathematical reasoning, often assumed in modernity; rather, for Aquinas it is 'regard for and openness to reality'.[45] Reality includes *both* supernatural and natural reality, so that realization of goodness presupposes knowledge of reality – simply good intentions are not sufficient. Josef Pieper, in a book written long before virtue ethics became popular among philosophers, summarizes the work of prudence in Aquinas's thought in the following way:

> It holds within itself the humility of the silent, that is to say, of unbiased perception, the trueness to being of memory, the art of receiving counsel, alert, composed readiness for the unexpected. Prudence means studied seriousness and, as it were, the filter of deliberation, and at the same time the brave boldness to make final decisions. It means purity, straightforwardness, candour and simplicity of character, it means standing superior to the utilitarian complexities of mere 'tactics'.[46]

It is worth fostering such attitudes in order to develop the capacity to make decisions in difficult circumstances, whatever these might be. The priority for an ethic of prudence remains one that focuses on the character of the agent, but it also points to particular ways of how such a character could be formed. However, I suggest that the different facets of prudence that he mentions are worth considering carefully in the light of proposals for genetic intervention in humans. The first trait, namely the 'humility of the silent', relates to the ability to contemplate carefully the truth in any given situation, related, as he suggests, to 'unbiased perception'. The way the Human Genome Project was portrayed in its earlier history shows how biases were introduced in order to win public support. It coheres with Alice Dreger's call for greater intellectual honesty among all parties, both scientists and public alike. This quality sets the stage, as it were, for fruitful dialogue and public deliberation of the issues. The characteristic of 'trueness to being of

---

[44] Ibid., p. 16.
[45] Ibid., p. 17.
[46] Ibid., p. 36.

memory' reflects the ability to consider the implications in the light of past experiences. Europeans have been far more reluctant to approve patenting of human genes compared to those in the USA, partly because, according to Otmar Kloiber of the German Medical Association:

> The substance patents now being given to the human genome are inappropriate and endanger research and medicine. Information about the human genome can't be invented. It is the common heritage of all humans.[47]

Kloiber was referring specifically to the patent for the breast cancer gene, BRCA1 held by Myriad Genetics. While American users have paid the patent fee for use in breast cancer screening programmes, Europeans have generally been defiant. I suggest that behind this feeling of defiance there is a memory of the way genetics was abused as part of a programme of social control in the eugenic philosophy of the Nazi regime. Contemporary geneticists are anxious to distance themselves from such eugenic practices and speak much more in terms of genetics as a way of alleviating individual suffering.[48] However, I suggest that the memory of such abuses of genetics is strong enough to act like a precautionary principle in any development that shows a trend towards the use of genetic information as a means of power over others.

The art of receiving counsel is also worth pondering, partly because of the resistance to open dialogue from all sides of the debate. Alice Dreger makes the point that it is not just the scientists who dismiss the value of public forums in genetics, rather non-specialists have much to learn as well, especially about the scientific possibilities inherent in human genetic technologies.[49] The ability to have composed readiness for the unexpected is also particularly important in consideration of the rapid expansion of knowledge in human genetics. The possibility of human reproductive cloning, for example, was not even considered prior to the cloning of Dolly the sheep. Some of the reactions to this possibility have been over-reactions

---

[47] Cited in M. Wadman, 'Testing Time for Gene Patent as Europe Rebels', *Nature* 413 (2001), p. 443.
[48] J. Gilliot, 'Screening for Disability: A Eugenic Pursuit?', *Journal of Medical Ethics* 27 (2001) Supplement 11, pp. 1121–3.
[49] Domurat Dreger, 'Metaphors of Morality', p. 184.

stemming from an inability to take stock of what is realistically likely to be the case. The difficulty of finding suitable donor human eggs for use in therapeutic cloning, for example, has curbed the development of this technique that a few years before was heralded as a breakthrough for clinical practice.[50]

The way choices are made through a filter of deliberation alongside the ability to be decisive applies not just to the decisions of scientists – for example, what priority to give competing claims in the search for therapeutic tools in human genetic disease – but also at the level of political decision-making. For example, government policy will need to be in place in order to give guidelines about the access to the information gained from the Human Genome Project. If the use of genetic 'fingerprinting' becomes affordable, how far and to what extent will insurance companies or employers have access to this information? What restrictions, if any, should apply to patenting either parts of the human genome or products of DNA activity?

Ideals of 'purity, straightforwardness, candour and simplicity of character' as well as 'standing superior to the utilitarian complexities of mere "tactics"' are particularly challenging goals for those intent on a particular mission, whether it be a 'passion for DNA' or a drive to make political decisions that lead to the greatest public support. Yet, I suggest that these aspects of prudence are worth pursuing if a genuine ethic of genetic intervention is to be achieved. Of course there may be failures, and the Christian message has much to say about the ability to have charity towards those who, for one reason or another, are not as honest as they might be. Yet if the good of humanity is the goal to be achieved, then these prudential qualities of character are part of this process. One could argue that a good goal might be achieved even if the motivation of the agents is not all that it should be. This kind of argument is commonly made against a virtue ethic approach. However, it seems to me that once we simply accept dishonesty as part of human nature, then the ability to perceive the good itself becomes distorted. The goal towards goodness needs to be realistic in as much as it admits to human frailties, but the challenge of an ethic is to find ways and means of encouraging

[50] P. Aldhous, 'Can They Rebuild Us?', *Nature* 410 (2001), pp. 622–5.

behaviour that will lend itself to the overall good of the human community as a whole.

The virtue closely aligned with prudence in Aquinas's scheme and one that is commonly not given due weight by virtue ethicists is that of justice. Justice 'is the habit whereby a person with a lasting and constant will renders to each his due'.[51] If each is given his or her due, given equality in dignity of humans, this implies a movement towards equality in relationships. This idea is then formalized in legal frameworks, hence human will establishes laws that are commensurate with 'natural justice', based on natural law. Legal justice between the individual and state can be compared with distributive justice between the state and the individual, and with commutative justice between individuals. The ideal of equality is not possible in practice because of the social and political divisions in society. In this scenario we need to ask the question: What is due and to whom? How do we work out what is due? Aquinas is realistic about the place of human laws. Such laws do not restrain all vice or enjoin every act of virtue that is found even in natural law. They restrain only those vices which 'the average man can avoid' and foster those virtues that bring actions in order to 'serve the common good'.[52] The legal aspects of human genetic engineering in the UK are bound up with a number of regulatory committees, including, for example, the Human Genetics Advisory Committee (HGAC) and the Human Fertilisation and Embryology Authority (HFEA). The 1990 Human Fertilisation and Embryology Act has served to restrict work on human embryos up to fourteen days old. Within this time frame only certain medical experiments are permissible, and following a controversial debate in both the House of Commons and the House of Lords, such experimentation now includes the use of human embryos for cell nuclear transfer and stem cell research.[53] Those lobbying against such a move, led by Lord Alton, failed to win sufficient support. After the House of Lords debate the government put a moratorium in place while a Lords select committee gathered material on the ethical

---

[51] Aquinas, *Summa Theologiae*, vol. 37, *Justice*, trans. T. Gilby (London: Blackfriars, 1974), 2a2ae Qu. 58.1.

[52] Aquinas, *Summa Theologiae*, vol. 37, *Justice*, 2a2ae Qu. 96.2, 96.3.

[53] For discussion, see C. Davis, 'Lords Back Broader Stem Cell Research', *The Times Higher Educational Supplement*, 26 January 2001.

issues. The problem with such a decision is that the vote to agree on the technology was taken *prior* to ethical deliberation. It is a good example of imprudence, where insufficient time was taken for the sake of pacifying a particular group of scientists. Such hasty decisions do not work in favour of winning over public support for science. As human genetic technology becomes more and more sophisticated, we can expect similar political and public debates. The issue of justice will apply not only to who has access to genetic screening, but also who has access to the information once it is available.

Fortitude, loosely translated as 'courage', is informed by prudence insofar as it presumes a correct evaluation of things. Fortitude is a willingness to suffer, but only in the light of knowledge of goodness. It is needed in order to preserve the good that is perceived by prudence and established by justice. In its traditional sense it included the willingness to be a martyr for the sake of Christ. A radical willingness to act in courageous ways, even to the point of death, seems too extreme for modern ears. A modified way we could think of fortitude in the context of the HGP is a readiness to speak out. The awareness that we live in a pluralistic culture has encouraged many ethicists to dissolve their ethical reflection into forms of relativism. While we need not go as far as what Michael Banner calls 'dogmatic ethics', I suggest that being prepared to witness from within the Christian tradition is part of the Christian vocation.[54] The nature of justice, for example, according to Christian tradition, means a particular concern for the poor and oppressed. We need to ask: Who is going to be disadvantaged as well as advantaged by the new technological developments?

Fortitude is also linked with the fourth cardinal virtue, temperance. Popular understanding could imply restriction, or just not acting in excess. While any interpretation of temperance includes such a meaning, in a classical sense it pointed to a real awareness and sense of the ordered unity of the human person. Out of this inner unity a serenity of spirit arises, and it is this that fills the inner recesses of the human being.[55] However, in order that such a turning in towards self is

---

[54] Banner, *Christian Ethics*, pp. 1–46.

[55] J. Pieper, *The Four Cardinal Virtues* (Notre Dame: University of Notre Dame Press, 1966), pp. 147–7.

really demonstrative of the virtue of temperance, it must be *selfless*, rather than *selfish*. Intemperance is the misdirection of the desires for self-preservation in actions that are selfish, and ultimately self-destructive. Temperance implies, further, a self-restraint that is governed by reason. Such self-restraint can degenerate in a sophisticated way in the search for knowledge itself, so that 'inquisitiveness' or more accurately *curiositas* itself becomes a negative force, associated with a compulsive greed. It is an obsessive addiction to seeing, a 'concupiscence of the eyes', leading to a form of obsessive addiction, a 'roaming unrest of spirit'.[56] Is the almost obsessive drive to clone human beings or patent sections of the human genome for commercial gain a form of this *curiositas,* demonstrating a lack of the real desire to know what is true according to *studiositas?*

Wisdom and the theological virtues[57]

Prudence, as practical wisdom, is one of the two virtues of practical reason together with art. In addition, as discussed above, it is the foremost of the four cardinal virtues. The pivotal role for wisdom in relation to the virtues has been noted by secular philosophers. Rosalind Hursthouse, for example, suggests that 'the only virtue term we have which is guaranteed to operate as a virtue term – that is to pick out something that always makes its possessor good – is "wisdom"'.[58] Yet from a theological perspective wisdom is not simply prudence. Rather, according to Aquinas, wisdom is one of the three intellectual virtues of theoretical reason, alongside *scientia* and understanding.[59] Wisdom is distinct from science in that while knowing what one ought to believe is, according to Aquinas, the gift of science, 'relating to the realities in themselves through being united with them, this is for the Gift of Wisdom.

---

[56] Ibid., pp. 199–201.

[57] A lower case initial is used for 'wisdom' when referring to human wisdom, or created wisdom; upper case is used when referring to divine Wisdom, or Wisdom endowed by the Holy Spirit on human beings.

[58] R. Hursthouse, *On Virtue Ethics* (Oxford University Press, 1999), p. 13. It is worth noting that Hursthouse, along with many advocates of virtue ethics, does not treat justice as a virtue term. I am adopting the classical approach, following Aquinas, that does argue for justice as a virtue. Wisdom, or prudence, is, nonetheless, prior to justice.

[59] See discussion in Deane-Drummond, *Creation Through Wisdom*, p. 99.

Accordingly, the Gift of Wisdom corresponds more to charity which conjoins man's mind to God.'[60] For Aquinas, science is about human or created things, while wisdom includes reference to God as well. Any sense that Wisdom is referred to God has to presuppose the virtue (and gift) of faith, which is the necessary first step in the development of a theological life.[61] Aquinas links the virtue of wisdom specifically with the virtue of charity. However, other theological virtues accompany wisdom, such as joy and peace, so that 'Accordingly, spiritual peace and the resulting joy correspond directly to the Gift of Wisdom.'[62] He rejects the idea that a beatitude can come from science alone; for Aquinas human happiness comes 'not in contemplating creatures, but in contemplating God', and any such happiness is ascribed to Wisdom.[63] This renders Aquinas's scheme theocentric, the path to happiness reaches a limit in the material world; indeed he would suggest that there is no ultimate comparison between the kind of happiness that comes from God compared with that found in the material world. The goodness towards which he turns and towards which the human enterprise is directed is thus, ultimately, the goodness of God.

Wisdom, as well as being an intellectual virtue, which can be learned, is also the gift of the Holy Spirit. Wisdom can be misdirected towards evil ends, while true Wisdom considers the ultimate end in God. If the end is simply material, and fixed on external goods, this engenders a distorted form of wisdom that 'copies the pride of the devil, and of all the sons of pride, he is the King'.[64] The idea that material goals are 'devilish' sounds out of keeping with particular Christian virtues of tolerance and respect. It might also imply a rejection of the goodness of the created order, yet this is not Aquinas's intention. Yet while we might wish to modify the kind of language used, it seems to me important to show the distinctions between the kind of goals envisaged by attachment to worldly pleasures and those informed by reference to the goodness of God. I suggest that

---

[60] Aquinas, *Summa Theologiae*, vol. 32, *Consequences of Faith*, trans. Thomas Gilby (London: Blackfriars, 1975), 2a2ae Qu. 9.2.

[61] This view is also shared with Romanus Cessario: see Cessario, *Christian Faith and the Theological Life*.

[62] Aquinas, *Summa Theologiae*, vol. 32, *Consequences of Faith*, 2a2ae, Qu. 92.4.

[63] Ibid.

[64] Aquinas, *Summa Theologiae*, vol. 35, *Consequences of Charity*, trans. Thomas R. Heath (London: Blackfriars, 1972), 2a2ae Qu. 45.1.

those who argue that ethics can be derived simply from reasoning informed by faith need to take into account not only Aquinas's strong rejection of materialistic goals other than theological ones, but also the way wisdom is related to faith as a theological virtue. For Aquinas, faith is a form of assent to divine truths, whereas Wisdom, as gift, judges things according to divine truth.[65] The gift of Wisdom, as well as being rooted in charity, presupposes the theological virtue of faith. Such faith is expressed in practical ways through Christian worship, and so indirectly it is in worship that Wisdom becomes manifest. Hence:

> piety makes wisdom manifest too, and because of that we can say that piety is wisdom and for the same reason also is fear. If a man fears and worships God he shows that he has a right judgement about divine things.[66]

Aquinas believes that true Wisdom is to be fostered through the pious practice of a worshipping community. The theologian Professor Daniel Hardy has made a similar point regarding the way wisdom and worship intersect and interrelate with each other.[67]

How does the virtue of wisdom as learned relate to the gift of Wisdom as given by the Holy Spirit and engendered in the worshipping community? Aquinas suggests that the gift of Wisdom takes human participation closer to the being of God, so that 'the gift is higher than the virtue of wisdom, it gets closer to God by a certain union of soul, it is able to direct us not only in contemplation, but in action as well'.[68] Wisdom contemplates first of all the divine realities, and 'this is the vision of the source. Afterwards it directs human action according to the divine reasons.' Such a contemplative stance does not lead to a difficult practical task for ethics, rather 'This guidance of human acts by wisdom does not bring bitterness nor toil, rather by wisdom the bitter becomes sweet and the toil a rest.'[69] It is this stress on

---

[65] Ibid.
[66] Ibid.
[67] D.Hardy, 'Rationality, the Sciences and Theology', in G. Wainwright (ed.), *Keeping the Faith; Essays to Mark the Centenary of Lux Mundi* (London: SPCK, 1989), pp. 284–8. See also D. Hardy, 'The God Who Is With the World', in F. Watts (ed.), *Science Meets Faith* (London: SPCK, 1998), p. 137.
[68] Aquinas, *Summa Theologiae*, vol. 35, *Consequences of Charity*, 2a2ae Qu. 45.3.
[69] Ibid.

the way *actions* are ultimately guided through reference to the Wisdom of God and through receiving the gift of wisdom that has led me to suggest that Aquinas's ethic is a wisdom ethic.[70] I should note that this interpretation of Aquinas does not rule out other possible interpretations of his ethics, as, for example, that based on the idea of natural law. However, I suggest that this interpretation, which is my own, is not out of keeping with his own determination to claim a theological space for ethics: the thrust of the whole *Summa* is towards seeing reality through the lens of who God is, while acknowledging that knowledge of God is always provisional and incomplete. To ignore the way he works to weave together philosophical reasoning and theological speculation seems to me to be a mistake.[71]

The kind of ordering that is possible through Wisdom brings another theological virtue into view, namely the gift of peace. It is worth noting that the beatitude most closely aligned with wisdom is peacemaking.[72] The belief in the possibility for peace in spite of the diversity of opinions over, for example, the legitimacy of 'germ-line' human genetic engineering, would be impossible to achieve without consideration of the third main theological virtue in addition to charity and faith, namely the virtue of hope. For Aquinas hope comes when the human will is directed to the divine end, both in reaching out for it and in the 'movement of intention towards what is attainable'.[73] Once the will is transformed into the end itself, then this is the work of charity. I suggest that the ability to hope is an essential component of deliberations about human genetics. This is not just a positive attitude or a false sense of peace where there is none, rather it is the belief that the God-given grace towards which the human spirit searches is one that can be reflected in the practical decisions made in this life. In other words, the supernatural end of divine Goodness and Wisdom impinges in

---

[70] See, especially, Deane-Drummond, 'Aquinas, Wisdom Ethics and the New Genetics'.

[71] In this respect I am entirely in agreement with Jean Porter, who has criticized contemporary interpretations of Aquinas, in as much as they seize on isolated fragments of his thought and do not do justice to his attempt to integrate theology and philosophy. See J. Porter, *The Recovery of Virtue: The Relevance of Aquinas for Christian Ethics* (London: SPCK, 1994), pp. 13–16.

[72] Deane-Drummond, *Creation Through Wisdom*, p. 103.

[73] Aquinas, *Summa Theologiae*, vol. 23, *Virtue*, 1a2ae, trans. W.D. Hughes (London: Blackfriars, 1966), Qu. 62.3.

a real way on human existence now. Such grace is not simply a utopian blessing on human life, since it also exposes the reality of distortions in human relationships with each other and with God, in other words the reality of human sinfulness. While Aquinas's view of the relationship between God and creation was ultimately dualistic, this does not mean that there could be no signs of the work of the Holy Spirit in the practice of everyday life. It reflects the fact that the theological virtues are born in charity, which takes the form of a friendship between God and humanity. It is out of this friendship that hope becomes visible, and from this friendship that human wisdom echoes the divine Wisdom.

I have suggested elsewhere that the shape of theological Wisdom is Trinitarian in structure.[74] This reinforces the idea suggested by consideration of the ethics of wisdom, namely that wisdom as virtue and gift is also about right relationships with God and other creatures. Aquinas suggests that it is in contemplation of God that the ability to discern aright becomes fostered and developed. Once we view God in a Trinitarian way, then it is no longer possible to consider friendship with God through charity just in terms of a monist understanding of who God is. Rather, friendship informs the moral life, and as such relates specifically to a virtue ethic.[75] There is a sense in which deliberations about human genetics take place in the context of virtue ethics, but also take their bearing from a theology of God as characterized by Wisdom and Love. The dialectic between theology and ethics is also characteristic of James Gustafson's approach to ethics. The difference is that he seems to posit an understanding of God that engenders a 'sense of the divine' in everyday life, without relating this to the Trinity as such. Nonetheless, he does describe the moral life as one that is rooted in the ability to practise discernment.[76]

Conclusions

I began this chapter with a discussion of the way discoveries from research into the human genome have served to challenge

---

[74] Deane-Drummond, *Creation Through Wisdom*, pp. 126–31.
[75] For a discussion of friendship and the moral life see P. Wadell, *Friendship and the Moral Life* (Notre Dame: University of Notre Dame Press, 1989).
[76] J. Gustafson, *Theology and Ethics*, p. 327.

the view that 'genes' are fixed entities, but rather gene activation is just as important as gene action. Such a discovery has forced geneticists to look for wider and richer under-standings of gene action in the contexts of both the organism and the wider environment. Claims that the work from the HGP will eventually advance cures for a whole host of diseases need to be qualified. Those who sought to win over public support for HGP did so by appeal to particular trophs that chimed with American cultural values, even though the language used was couched in terms of risks and benefits. I suggested from this that a richer way of understanding complex issues in human genetics is to frame debates in terms of virtue ethics. A virtue ethic approach has become increasingly popular among philo-sophers, who are tired of the somewhat stale alternatives of deontology versus consequentialism. However, I have suggested in this chapter that this does not necessarily mean that no principles are relevant, or that goals should not be taken into account. Rather, through consideration of an ethical approach that takes its bearings from the writings of Thomas Aquinas, a critique of the relevant ethical issues comes into view. In particular, I have argued that prudence as the first of the cardinal virtues means more than just the secular precautionary principle. Rather, different facets of prudence impinge on the way decision-making takes place. Moreover, once justice is also reinstated as a virtue, one of the main criticisms of virtue ethics, namely that it avoids the principles of justice, is no longer an issue. The virtues of fortitude and temperance are also relevant in practical and political decision-making. Finally I considered the way that Wisdom, although deontological in the sense that it also reflects who God is in Godself, is both an intellectual virtue to be learned as well as a gift of the Holy Spirit. Once wisdom is joined to charity the fullness of the goal of Goodness towards which human life is directed becomes clarified. Such charity is premised on the basis of faith, which is presupposed, and issues in the virtue of hope, which, along with wisdom, becomes the ground of peacemaking. In the context of a worshipping community the search for Wisdom is no longer futile. While theological Wisdom may critique alternative claims for wisdom that are against the Wisdom of God, it is through the worshipping community that inspiration to work for the reign of God becomes manifest. In this the task of Christian ethics becomes first and foremost a task of instilling the virtues as scrutinized by prudence. All I have done here is to indicate some of the ways in which some virtues are relevant to problems likely to emerge as a result of the discoveries of the HGP. I have not discussed whether these virtues are, in their turn, products of genetic or biological action, i.e. the question of naturalism.[77] That would be the subject of another chapter.

Bibliography

Aldhous, P., 'Can They Rebuild Us?', *Nature* 410 (2001), pp. 622–5.

Aquinas, *Summa Theologiae*, vol. 23, *Virtue*, 1a2ae, trans. W.D. Hughes (London: Blackfriars, 1969).

Aquinas, *Summa Theologiae*, vol. 35, *Consequences of Charity*, trans. Thomas R. Heath (London: Blackfriars, 1972).

Aquinas, *Summa Theologiae*, vol. 37, *Justice*, trans. T. Gilby (London: Blackfriars, 1974).

Aquinas, *Summa Theologiae*, vol. 32, *Consequences of Faith*, trans. Thomas Gilby (London: Blackfriars, 1975).

Banner, M., *Christian Ethics and Contemporary Moral Problems* (Cambridge: Cambridge University Press, 1999).

Beauchamp, T.L. and J.F. Childress, *Principles of Biomedical Ethics* (Oxford: Oxford University Press, 2001).

Biggar, N. and R. Black (eds), *The Revival of Natural Law: Philosophical, Theological and Ethical Responses to the Finnis-Grisez School* (Aldershot: Ashgate, 2000).

Cessario, R., *Christian Faith and the Theological Life* (Washington: Catholic University of America Press, 1996).

Cessario, R., *Introduction to Moral Theology* (Washington: Catholic University of America Press, 2001).

Clark, S., *Biology and Christian Ethics* (Cambridge: Cambridge University Press, 2000).

Davis, C., 'Lords Back Broader Stem Cell Research', *Times Higher Educational Supplement*, 26 January 2001.

---

[77] For discussion, see, for example, W.B. Drees, *Religion, Science and Naturalism* (Cambridge: Cambridge University Press, 1996).

de Dios Vial Correa, J. and E. Sgreccia (eds), *Human Genome, Human Person and the Society of the Future, Proceedings of Fourth Assembly of the Pontifical Academy for Life*, Vatican City, 23–5 February 1998 (Vatican: Libreria Editrice Vaticana, 1999).

Deane-Drummond, C., *Creation Through Wisdom: Theology and the New Biology* (London: T & T Clark, 2000).

Deane-Drummond, C., *Biology and Theology Today: Exploring the Boundaries* (London: SCM Press, 2001).

Deane-Drummond, C. 'Aquinas, Wisdom Ethics and the New Genetics', in C. Deane-Drummond and B. Szerszynski (eds), *Re-Ordering Nature: Theology, Society and the New Genetics* (London: T & T Clark, 2002), pp. 293–311.

Deane-Drummond, C. and B. Szerszynski (eds), *Re-Ordering Nature: Theology, Society and the New Genetics* (London: T & T Clark, 2002).

Domurat Dreger, A., 'Metaphors of Morality in the Human Genome Project', in P.R. Sloan (ed.), *Controlling Our Destinies: Historical, Philosophical, Ethical, and Theological Perspectives on the Human Genome Project* (Notre Dame: University of Notre Dame Press, 2000).

Drane, J., 'Character and the Moral Life: A Virtue Approach to Biomedical Ethics', in E. R. Du Bose, R.P. Hamel and L.J. O'Connell (eds), *A Matter of Principles? Ferment in US Bioethics* (Valley Forge: Trinity Press International, 1994), pp. 284–309.

Drees, W.B., *Religion, Science and Naturalism* (Cambridge: Cambridge University Press, 1996).

Fitzgerald, K., 'Do We Know Ourselves Well Enough to be Engineering Humans?', in G. Stock and J. Campbell (eds), *Engineering the Human Germline: An Exploration of the Science and Ethics of Altering the Genes we Pass On to Our Children* (Oxford and New York: Oxford University Press, 2000).

Frossard, P., *The Lottery of Life: The New Genetics and the Future of Mankind* (London and New York: Bantam Press, 1991).

Gilliot, J., 'Screening for Disability: A Eugenic Pursuit?', *Journal of Medical Ethics* 27 (2001) Supplement 11, pp. 1121–3.

Gustafson, J., *Theology and Christian Ethics* (Cleveland: Pilgrim Press, 1974).

Gustafson, J., *Theology and Ethics* (Oxford: Blackwell, 1981).

Gustafson, J., *Ethics from a Theocentric Perspective* (Chicago: University of Chicago Press, 1984).

Hardy, D., 'Rationality, the Sciences and Theology', in G. Wainwright (ed.), *Keeping the Faith: Essays to Mark the Centenary of Lux Mundi* (London: SPCK, 1989), pp. 284–8.

Hardy, D., 'The God Who Is With The World', in F. Watts (ed.), *Science Meets Faith* (London: SPCK, 1998), p. 137.

Hoose, B. (ed.), *Christian Ethics: An Introduction* (London: Cassell, 1998).

Hursthouse, R., *On Virtue Ethics* (Oxford: Oxford University Press, 1999).

Jones, L.G. and R.P. Vance, 'Why the Virtues are Not Another Approach to Medical Ethics: Reconceiving the Place of Ethics in Contemporary Medicine', in P.F. Camenisch (ed.), *Religious Methods and Resources in Bioethics* (Dordrecht: Kluwer Academic, 1994), pp. 203–25.

Keenan, J.F., 'What is Morally New in Genetic Manipulation?', *Human Gene Therapy* 1 (1990), pp. 289–98.

Keenan, J.F., 'Virtue Ethics', in B. Hoose (ed.), *Christian Ethics: An Introduction* (London: Cassell, 1998), pp. 84–94.

Keller, E.F., 'Is There an Organism In This Text?', in P.R. Sloan (ed.), *Controlling our Destinies: Historical, Philosophical, Ethical, and Theological Perspectives on the Human Genome Project* (Notre Dame: University of Notre Dame Press, 2000).

Kitchner, P., 'Gene: Current Uses', in E.F. Keller and E. Lloyd (eds), *Keywords in Evolutionary Biology* (Cambridge, MA: Harvard University Press, 1992), pp. 128–31.

Lewontin, R., *The Doctrine of DNA: Biology as Ideology* (London: Penguin, 1993).

MacNamara, V., 'The Distinctiveness of Christian Morality', in B. Hoose (ed.), *Christian Ethics: An Introduction* (London: Cassell, 1998), pp. 149–60.

McMullin, E., 'Biology and the Theology of the Human', in P. Sloan (ed.), *Controlling Our Destinies: Historical, Philosophical, Ethical, and Theological Perspectives on the Human Genome Project* (Notre Dame: University of Notre Dame Press, 2000), 367–93.

Pieper, J., *Prudence*, trans. R. Winston and C. Winston (London: Faber and Faber, 1959).

Pieper, J., *The Four Cardinal Virtues* (Notre Dame: University of Notre Dame Press, 1966).

Pincoffs, E.F., *Quandaries and Virtue: Against Reductionism in Ethics* (Lawrence: University Press of Kansas, 1986).

Porter, J., *The Recovery of Virtue: The Relevance of Aquinas for Christian Ethics* (London: SPCK, 1994).

Portin, P., 'The Concept of the Gene: Short History and Present Status', *Quarterly Review of Biology* 68 (1992), pp. 173–223.

Ramsey, P., *Fabricated Man: The Ethics of Genetic Control* (London and New Haven: Yale University Press, 1970).

Rheinberger, H.J., 'Genes: A Disunified View from the Perspective of Molecular Biology', in P. Beurton, W. Lefevre and H.J. Rheinberger (eds), *Gene Concepts and Evolution* (Berlin: Max Planck Institut für Wissenschaftgeschichte, Preprint No. 18, 1995), pp. 7–13.

Vatican City, 'Pope Warns Scientists about Genetic Manipulation', Deutsche Presse-Agentur, 5 February 2002.

Wadell, P., *Friendship and the Moral Life* (Notre Dame: University of Notre Dame Press, 1989).

Wadman, M., 'Testing Time for Gene Patent as Europe Rebels', *Nature* 413 (2001), p. 443.

Watson, J., *A Passion for DNA: Genes, Genomes and Society* (Oxford: Oxford University Press, 2001).

PART VI

Identifying Social and Political Goods

Introduction to Part VI

While the previous chapters explored theoretical possibilities of a Christian approach to ethical issues in genetics, the following chapters are more explicitly rooted in ecclesial, social and political practice. Donald Bruce's chapter deals with questions about whether the human genome should be patented, tracing the religious and ethical problems that arise when the idea of intellectual property is applied to the living world. He considers the responses by the European churches to the European Commission Biotechnology Patent Directive. In particular he asks if patents are justifiable theoretically, hence could human genes ever be said to be 'invented'?, or practically, so that some financial compensation needs to be made to those investing in genetic research. He also asks us to consider the practical outcomes of patenting in terms of research and attitudes to human genomics. Esther Reed's chapter is a direct response to Donald Bruce, exploring more fully the theological and ethical claims behind the current debate on patenting in the European churches. Echoing Szerszynski's concern about language, she uses liturgical thinking as a device against which to measure comments about patenting and patenting rights. She is confident in the ability of particular theological statements, such as the Ten Commandments, to deliver the necessary framework for a discussion of the ethical issues. For her, human dignity is dependent on a prior conception of redemption, and we can assess the appropriateness of a given action by analogy with particular scriptural references, such as

Jesus's cleansing of the temple. Her discussion widens into a consideration not just of human genetics, but of the dignity of all creatures, so that genetic manipulation has to be seen in the context of how far it contributes to each creature's destiny as given by God.

Peter Scott, like Reed, is also conscious of the sacramental nature of human identity, and he links this specifically with ideas about redemption. He suggests that the elimination of contingency is a false desire, echoing Junker-Kenny. The goodness of God is expressed socially through the Church, in other words it is worked out in a sacramental and eucharistic way. He comments, as I did earlier, on the 'frontier' mentality inherent in the initial conceptions of the HGP. He argues that it is not only essential, but also imperative to situate genetic technologies in the historical and social contexts that inform such enterprises if they are to be evaluated in an appropriate way. He argues that the HGP is embedded in a particular political goal of liberal democratic polity that is individualistic in orientation. Instead, he invites us to consider another, more socially responsible alternative, one that considers goodness in terms of hospitality. Such a shift would invite greater consideration of the ambiguous nature of the technology as such, as well as an appraisal of the distribution of possible benefits.

11

Whose Genes Are They? Genetics, Patenting and the Churches

Donald Bruce

1 Introduction

The mapping of the human genome has been widely portrayed as one of the greatest international scientific endeavours, with researchers working together across the globe to unravel our genetic code for human benefit. While this may be true, it also has elements of a modern-day gold rush which has at times resembled the Wild West more than a sophisticated twenty-first-century scientific investigation. Once the enormous commercial prospects of charting all the genes in the human body were appreciated, it created a worldwide drive to secure exclusive rights over parts of the map. Companies and governments have fought ruthlessly to be the first to stake out their claim to the intellectual property rights for particular genes.

The situation is exemplified by a race to identify the breast cancer genes BRCA1 and 2. Many years of patient research by several groups had got close to locating the first gene. Late in the day, a US company set up for the purpose solved the last few steps and claimed the gene as their own private intellectual property, despite how little they had contributed. In the UK the Sanger Centre has a policy of publishing sequence data openly on the internet, believing it must be for the benefit of all. It was within a few hours of completing the sequence for a second breast cancer gene when the same US company stepped in and claimed the second gene also as their private monopoly. Such examples sound a note of discord against the trumpets for the

Human Genome Project. The emergence of the rival, privately funded, genome map by Celera Genomics raised concerns about information being commercially tied. This prompted Tony Blair and Bill Clinton, when announcing the genome map in January 2000, to add a belated statement to the effect that the results of the Human Genome Project should be open to humankind and not restricted to private companies.

Gene patenting has been one of the most controversial areas in genetics for over two decades, arousing remarkable passions which show no signs of diminishing. It is also the subject of much confusion and misconception. Rival campaign groups have traded slogans such as 'no patents on life' or 'no patents, no cures' which have misled policy-makers and public alike. This and the following chapter seeks to open up some of the ethical and theological questions which are posed by the use of intellectual property rights to control the information arising out of genetic research and innovation. The respective cons and pros of gene patenting have been addressed in more detail by Bruce[1] and Reiss,[2] a study by the Church of Scotland's Society, Religion and Technology Project[3] and a report of its General Assembly.[4] This chapter focuses on the practical Christian ethical engagement of the issue since 1995 by the bioethics working group of the European Ecumenical Commission for Church and Society (EECCS), and its successor group of the Church and Society Commission of the Conference of European Churches (CEC).[5] It traces the inter-action of these groups with the European Commission and Parliament over the biotechnology patenting directive 98/44/EC.[6]

---

[1] D.M. Bruce, 'Patenting Human Genes: A Christian View', *Bulletin of Medical Ethics* (January 1997), pp. 18–20.

[2] M.J. Reiss, 'Is it Right to Patent DNA?', *Bulletin of Medical Ethics* (January 1997), pp. 21–4.

[3] D. Bruce and A. Bruce (eds), *Engineering Genesis* (London: Earthscan, 1998), ch. 8.

[4] Church of Scotland, *Ethical Concerns about Patenting in Relation to Living Organisms*, Reports of the Church of Scotland General Assembly (Edinburgh, 22 May 1997).

[5] The original EECCS working group comprised mainly Protestant churches and ecumenical groups in seven countries in Western Europe. The CEC group was expanded to ten, including members from Eastern European and Orthodox churches.

[6] European Union, *Directive 98/44/EC of the European Parliament and the Council, on the Legal Protection of Biotechnological Inventions* (Brussels, 6 July 1998).

2   What is patenting?

Patenting began several centuries ago as a means to protect inventors from commercial abuse. A patent gives an inventor a limited time, typically twenty years, during which other people are forbidden from making commercial gain from the invention. In exchange, the inventor makes the information public, rather than keeping it as a trade secret. It is complex and often counter-intuitive. Although called 'intellectual property' a patent does not give ownership rights in the normal sense. It does not give the inventor any right to make or market the invention as such. To do that, the inventor must also go through all the other relevant laws of the country. A patent is a purely negative right which gives the inventor the right to stop others marketing the invention without paying royalties.

In Europe, one cannot patent a mere discovery, which one found in nature or isolated from it. It has to involve something inventive. To obtain a patent, one must prove to the satisfaction of the relevant patent office that what one proposes to make has an inventive step, that it was not simply obvious to anyone else 'skilled in the art', and also that it has a specified industrial application. Once the patent application has been published, others have a limited time in which to challenge it on any of these grounds, before the examiner then decides to award the patent or not. The patent is expressed as a series of clauses making claims which begin quite specifically and become progressively broader. A patent lawyer will typically advise the organization to make claims for as wide-ranging a scope of protection as it thinks it can get away with. A good examiner may then rein back some of the more speculative or outrageous claims, allowing only certain clauses and not others. Thus a claim for a pesticide-resistant genetically modified cotton was granted, but clauses that sought to extend the patent protection to any type of GM cotton were rightly rejected. Examiners have sometimes mistakenly allowed patent claims which should never have granted, including, on at least one occasion, claims for genes with no known function.

Generally, inventors have to apply separately in each country where they want protection. A UK inventor may thus have to apply for protection in each of the USA, Canada, Japan, Korea, Australia, etc. Patents can, however, be issued by the European

Patent Office (EPO) which cover most Western European countries. It is an expensive and lengthy process, which nowadays is promoted mainly by companies, universities and research institutes rather than individuals. It has become a fiercely litigious field, subject to claim and counter-claim between large biotechnology companies which can afford to pay patent lawyers handsomely to maximize the benefits of an invention for their organization. From humble beginnings, patenting has turned into a major piece in the chess game of corporate competitivity, with high stakes involved.

As originally conceived, patenting is ethically based on a compromise between two societal goods. The first is the open access to information for the widest benefit of society. The second is the presumed right of any individual or group in society to benefit financially from their inventiveness. Patenting invokes a principle of justice in granting a limited term monopoly to exploit the invention commercially, in exchange for making the knowledge of the invention freely available for basic (as opposed to commercial) research.

3   Biotechnology patenting

Over the years the character of patenting has changed, however, especially with the development of industrial biotechnology. One factor is that a very long time scale and a huge financial investment are typically involved between making an initial invention and bringing the product to market. For a mainline pharmaceutical these can be as much as fifteen years and half a billion pounds, respectively. Thus for the bio-industry, the filing of a patent serves more a function of investment insurance for research expenditure than it does the protection of an existing product. In lobbying for gene patents, companies make the pragmatic claim that if such patents are not allowed then genetic research will be inhibited. They assume a moral position that this holds back knowledge about serious diseases and thus treatments. This has found common cause with support groups for patients with particular various genetic diseases, but by no means all such groups.

This argument is a half-truth. It is based on an idealized view of the patenting process to enable open publication while protecting   the   holder   from   commercial   predation.

Unfortunately this is not always borne out in practice. The genetic research community has itself begun to express some concerns that patents may sometimes impede research instead of enhancing it.

The main reason which companies cite that gene patents are essential is that they would not do costly research unless there was the prospect of gaining intellectual property protection. By the same token, however, another company is unlikely to invest in research in an area where the first company now holds a patent. Patenting may thus be done for strategic purposes, to try to block a competitor's research in a different field from one's own, but on a potentially rival product. Such factors are being examined by the European Commission.

In principle, a patent ought not to prevent pure research on the subject, but again it may sometimes act as a constraint. This is especially so where patents are very broad or where they control key steps in a technique. A Swiss university research team, led by Professor Ingo Potrykus, invented a GM vitamin A rice variety for potential use with the poor in developing countries. He spent two years obtaining releases from various institutions and companies of the many patents and materials transfer agreements upon which his invention relied. The testing of a potentially important humanitarian application was thereby delayed.

In the political trend of the last thirty years to reduce public funding for research, academic institutions are under pressure from governments to obtain patents, both to raise their research assessment rating and to prove their worth for their next round of funding applications. The commercial pressure which this places on scientific information sits awkwardly with the long-established academic conventions of peer-reviewed publication and the open exchange of information among colleagues.

It is, however, the ethical dimension which biotechnology patenting has most aroused concern. Patenting is a compromise which seeks to reconcile two conflicting ethical principles. One is that knowledge of how to make the invention should be the common property of humankind. The other is that an inventor, who wishes to gain a livelihood from selling something he or she has invented, should be protected from someone else selling the invention as if it was theirs. This was relatively uncontroversial while dealing with inanimate objects or chemical processes. Disputes concerned the largely technical criteria of the inventive step, novelty and industrial application. Ethical issues were raised only at the extremes where antisocial inventions might be involved. A design for a letter bomb was cited as a theoretical example, for which there would be no conceivable benefit either from publishing the information or granting anyone monopoly rights.

Substantial new ethical problems were posed, however, when intellectual property was applied to the living world, biological material, cells, human genes and even life forms. The patent offices made the presumption of merely extending the assumptions of inanimate objects and processes. It was seen simply as an extension of the logic from patenting chemicals to biochemicals, and thence to proteins, microbes, and to other living organisms. If an invention involving any of these was novel, inventive and had industrial application, it was seen as quite wrong to deny a patent. Patent lawyers, many of whom were formerly scientists, have tended to regard the patenting process in a reductionist way as a purely technical, legal procedure, almost a scientific exercise. Although an *ad hoc* ethical committee was set up at the EPO, it was generally considered that if there were ethical issues, these were for wider society to consider, not patent agents.

4   The churches and the EU Biotechnology Patenting Directive

In the early 1990s an EC Directive was proposed which sought to harmonize European patent legislation and to enshrine the concepts of gene patenting in law. It embodied a technical and reductionist logic which was roundly opposed by many groups in civil society, including the churches. A lengthy and acrimonious debate lasted for over a decade. In 1995 it prompted an unprecedented rejection of the original Directive by the European Parliament, after a lobbying campaign by various environmental groups. This was the first time the Parliament had used its power of veto. While this caused much disturbance within the corridors of the EU it had little effect on patents, because the EPO continued to issue these under the European Patent Convention of 1976.

When a new draft was issued the European churches bioethics working group decided to enter into the discussions in September 1996 by making a critique of the proposals.[7] The group objected first to the fact that the Directive primarily viewed biotechnology in a narrow commercial light, and therefore failed to take into account wider ethical issues within European society. In its view the Directive continued to enshrine a basic flaw in the thinking of the patent profession, the biotechnology industry and their supporters, namely the assumption of the supremacy of commercial criteria over all considerations. The basic philosophy was that literally anything biological should be patentable, as a product of human invention, if it could be isolated, identified and found a use. The purpose was to have a Directive which would enable competition with the large number of North American patents on genes and biological material. A few *ad hoc* ethical exceptions were made, such as cloning and germ-line genetic modification, but without giving a proper ethical rationale. These were selected primarily to overcome certain objections expressed by MEPs in voting against the previous draft.

Indeed, a basic concern of the churches' group was that the Directive did not identify or justify its ethical presuppositions at all. Without a proper ethical case it had no suitable basis for legislation. In particular, the churches objected to the patenting of living organisms and of human genetic material. It was also heavily critical of the use of the so-called 'copy gene' argument with which the Directive sought to justify gene patenting. This claimed that isolated human genes could be classed as inventions simply because they had been copied in the laboratory from the original genes in the human body.

Finally, the working group highlighted the fact that no proper mechanism existed to consider the ethical dimension of biotechnology patents. At present an illogical situation arises if a patent is refused on ethical grounds. The EPO rejected a patent claim by the Upjohn company for using a hairless mouse for baldness treatment, because it was too trivial an application to justify such use of the animals. However, as noted above, patenting is only a negative right to stop others doing

---

[7] European Ecumenical Commission for Church and Society, *Critique of the Draft EC Patenting Directive* (Strasbourg, September 1996).

something. Hence, the refusal of the patent did not mean that the invention itself was banned. It merely meant that Upjohn was not given any monopoly rights. Ironically, instead of preventing the mouse from being used in an ethically unacceptable way, the outcome was that *anyone* could now market the mouse as a test for baldness treatments.

If a patent is refused on ethical grounds, no mechanism currently exists to require the production of the invention to be banned. The EECCS working group therefore called for an ethical body to be set up which would operate in parallel to the patenting process to give an ethical judgement on any controversial invention. To obtain the approval of such a body would be conditional on the granting of a patent. An amendment calling for a separate ethics committee for patents was eventually proposed by the European Parliament, but it was then rejected by the European Commission. Explaining the reason, Commissioner Monti later wrote to the churches to say that 'such a group could only seriously disturb the patent procedure'.[8] This remarkable attitude exemplifies the narrow commercial philosophy behind the Directive and its proposers, and their disdain for wider societal considerations. This exchange prefigured the crisis which would soon occur over GM food in Europe.

Thus the EC responded formally to the churches' first submission in a letter with a statement that

> the ethical perspective must not a priori interfere with the objective approach of patent law by introducing elements which are alien to it. In other words, one must not invent an emotional evaluation of patenting conditions related to the system of belief to which one adheres.[9]

The EECCS group replied by critiquing the EC's rhetoric of 'emotional evaluation' and the notion of the objectivity of the patent procedure. It pointed out the ways in which ethics is already centrally implied in patenting. The group then met with the senior European Commission officials, including the author

[8] M. Monti, Letter from European Commissioner for Internal Market to the General Secretary of European Ecumenical Commission for Church and Society, 3 March 1998.

[9] D. Vanderghenyst, Letter to the General Secretary of European Ecumenical Commission for Church and Society, English trans. 28 October 1996.

of the Directive, to clarify and underline its position, and to have a frank discussion of the principal issues.

Meanwhile the churches' position became used, in opposite senses, by the opposing sides in the debate. Bio-industry lobbyists sought to discredit the church group to MEPs. It portrayed the churches' position as being against biotech-nology research and opposed to cures for genetic disabilities. It even claimed that the group was being disbanded. Meanwhile some green groups claimed the churches were supporting anti-biotechnology positions. The group therefore issued a further clarification position.[10] It stated that it was not opposed to biotechnology research, nor genetic modification as such, nor patenting in itself, nor even the patenting of novel gene constructs as genuine inventions. It reiterated its objection to the patenting of transgenic organisms and human genes as such as unethical.

The Directive was heavily amended by the European Parliament, making several improvements that the churches had suggested. Most of these amendments were then cancelled by the Commission, to the annoyance of many MEPs. In the view of the Churches' working group, the resulting text remained almost as flawed as the original. The group thus made a final submission to the Commission and Parliament, and also addressed MEPs at a special meeting of non-aligned groups.[11] Meanwhile both sides of the debate continued intense advocacy. MEPs were put under pressure from the Parliament's rapporteur and the bio-industry lobbyists, who successfully persuaded many parliamentarians to accept the text with the fear of being singled out as being opposed to cures for genetic diseases. MEPs were greeted with wheelchair patients and the slogan 'no patents, no cures'. Late in the day several prominent patients' support groups came out in opposition to the Directive. They considered it to be against their members' best interests, for example, that it might make treatments more expensive and less widely available. By then, however, the die

---

[10] European Ecumenical Commission for Church and Society, *Clarification of the Submission on the EC Draft Patenting Directive from the European Ecumenical Commission for Church and Society* (Strasbourg, 5 November 1996).

[11] European Ecumenical Commission for Church and Society, *Submission to the European Parliament on the 'Common Position' of the Draft Directive on the Patenting of Biotechnological Inventions* (Strasbourg, 28 March 1998).

was largely cast for the European Parliament to accept the Directive.

A further factor was the strong desire of the UK government, which held the EU Presidency during this period, to push the Directive through to support its own biotechnology industry. It called for a three-line whip of all its Labour MEPs. The vote for the largely unamended Directive was duly passed in July 1998, amid a sense of a deep democratic failure among some MEPs and many others who had been observing the process.

Widespread doubts have continued to be expressed about gene patenting at many levels in Europe, however. The Dutch Parliament unsuccessfully took the EC to the European Court to have the Directive overturned on both substantive and proce-dural grounds. The French National Ethics Committee has called for the patenting of human genes to be made illegal, with the churches' support. Several other countries seem to have had second thoughts about aspects of the Directive. By the official deadline of July 2000 for enshrining the Directive in national law only three member states out of fifteen had ratified it. The European churches working group has continued its involvement and recently produced a statement in opposition to the patenting of human stem cells. [12]

5   Why the churches objected to gene patents

There are four basic theological or ethical points behind the European Churches working group's opposition to parts of the Directive. There are intrinsic ethical discussions centred on two important distinctions – between things that are alive and things that are not, and between discoveries of nature and inventions of humankind. There is also the consequential aspect of the ethical social responsibility laid upon the monopoly holder. Finally, questions of justice are posed by the failure of the patenting system to reflect the wider concerns and views of society at large, in that it focuses primarily on patenting as a technical discussion involving only industry and the legal profession. These points are now considered briefly in turn.

---

[12] Conference of European Churches (CEC) Working Group on Bioethics, *Human Stem Cell Patents would be Unethical* (Strasbourg, 2001).

(a) The life–non-life distinction

When human genes and living organisms are involved additional ethical criteria become important, compared with mechanical or chemical inventions. These may restrict what can be patented. This became enshrined in the slogan 'no patents on life'. This was a misnomer, because life itself is not an invention, but it did serve to highlight the question whether life forms and components of their bodies should be regarded as human inventions, and might therefore be subject to intellectual property rights. The EECCS group pointed out that the EC and the patenting authorities made an implicit assumption that patenting could be extended from complex chemicals to living things without ambiguity. A leading patent lawyer expressed this assumption as follows.

> Historically, the patent system came to birth to meet industrial needs. Industry was perceived as activities carried on inside factories ... Manufacture was the key word. Agriculture was felt to be outside the realm of patent law. Living things were also assumed to be excluded as being products of nature rather than products of manufacture ... This restricted view no longer persists in most industrialised countries. Thus the European Patent Convention of 1973 declares agriculture to be a kind of industry. Nevertheless vestiges of the old idea can still be found ... From the point of view of industrial and social policy, the application of technology to living organisms as industrial tools or products should raise no objection in principle. [13]

The EECCS group disagreed and concluded, 'Boundaries need to be drawn to make this distinction clear, to avoid reducing life conceptually to being merely an economic commodity, and then treating it as such. Living organisms have an inherent significance which sets them apart as "products of nature" from all "products of industry".' To do otherwise would reduce them to an equivalent status to mechanical parts in a machine.

The Society, Religion and Technology Project of the Church of Scotland was working closely with the EECCS group. In a report to the Kirk's General Assembly it developed the argument further. Subjects of the life that God has given them

---

[13] R.S. Crespi, *Patents in Biotechnology: The Legal Background*, Proceedings of an International Conference on Patenting Life Forms in Europe, Brussels, 7–8 February 1989, p. 7.

are owed a duty of respect which humans do not give to inanimate objects, and this precludes applying intellectual property to them.

> Living organisms themselves should therefore not be patentable, whether genetically modified or not. It is wrong in principle. An animal, plant or micro-organism owes its creation ultimately to God, not human endeavour. It cannot be interpreted as an invention or a process, in the normal sense of either word. It has a life of its own, which inanimate matter does not. In genetic engineering, moreover, only a tiny fraction of the makeup of the organism can be said to be a product of the scientists. The organism is still essentially a living entity, not an invention. A genetically modified mouse is in a completely different category from a mouse trap. [14]

(b) Genes, discoveries and inventions

The second point is perhaps more logical than theological. As noted above, in European patent law mere discoveries are normally unpatentable. There has to be an inventive step. The EECCS group argued that genes, animals and plants are discoveries of nature and therefore unpatentable. The major genetics and pharmaceutical company SmithKline Beecham claimed that the intellectual effort to decipher a gene and identify its function 'elevate them beyond the status of mere discoveries. In this sense, DNA molecules are inventions that can legitimately be patented.'[15] This was regarded as special pleading for their own case. Since all discovery entails a measure of intellectual effort, on this logic there would be no end to patenting. Mendelev might justifiably have claimed that he could patent the then unknown element germanium, because his elucidation of the periodic table of the elements required innovative thinking. The mere identification of a gene's function does not provide an ethical ground to claim exclusive rights. The intellectual effort involves the discovery of what is there in nature as a common heritage of all, be it a chemical element or a gene. Neither of these is in itself something which human ingenuity has created or adapted.

---

[14] Op. cit., Church of Scotland, *Ethical Concerns*.
[15] SmithKline Beecham, *What is the Case for Patenting DNA?*, a promotional brochure (1996).

The US patent system nonetheless allows patents on intellectual effort and discoveries. To keep a competitive edge, the EU wanted to find a premise in its own system to patent the discovery of any part of the human genome. It cited an argument that, while genes in their natural state in the body are unpatentable, in practice genes have to be isolated and copied. The act of copying, it argued, turns them from discoveries into inventions, so that they become patentable, provided a use is specified. This has been widely criticized, and few outside patenting and the biotechnology community appear to agree with it.

There are several basic flaws. First, the act of gene copying is a routine laboratory procedure and not a novel or inventive act. Second, the key point is not where the atoms of the gene came from, but that its information is that of a human gene. If the information is the same, it is not an invention. As the Society, Religion and Technology Project's report observed, 'Many people would regard a copy gene of human origin as remaining "human" because of the way they understand the notion of identity – that it is primarily to do with connections and relationships, not atomised entities.' The church thus rejected the reductionist view of the role of the gene in an organism, which the Directive implicitly upholds, in which its location and context is of little significance. A more holistic concept of the nature of an organism is argued to accord better with a Christian world view.

Despite this critique, the EECCS group argued that patents might be allowed on applications of genetics that were truly inventive, and were not mere discoveries. These might include a novel gene construct or the use of a human or animal gene for a particular purpose, provided this was not seen to constitute a claim to monopoly over all other uses of that gene which might be discovered by someone else. The key factor was that one should not claim monopoly rights over what is part of the common heritage of all people. It was important to maintain a clear distinction between this and genuine human invention.

(c) *Social justice and the responsibility of the patent holder*

The notion of gene patents raises important questions of justice and social responsibility. Patenting itself has a basis in social ethics. The theological approach of the EECCS group recognized that a fallen human nature has a tendency towards selfishness. One example of this is where some would sell the inventions of others, and claim them as their own. The group thus supported the general ethical case for intellectual property rights, insofar as it offers a practical remedy for what amounts to a failure of relational justice. This tends to generate an individualistic view of property, however, which may not relate well to the concept of genes as a common good. Moreover, in biotechnology, property rights are expressed increasingly in terms of corporate bodies, as quasi-individuals. This presents significant problems in the relative lack of corporate accountability of the patent holder to the community. This deficit in international corporate responsibility was one of the key themes to emerge from the 2002 World Summit on Sustainable Development in Johannesburg.[16]

The desire of companies and institutions to claim intellectual property over genes themselves has two main drives. The first is to gain as much financial return from an investment in genetics as the system will allow. The second is that it is easier to defend a patent on a product – the gene – rather than a process – the use of the gene. The first is the profit motive, which needs ethical restraint to prevent it from being reduced to basic greed. The second is merely a legal convenience. The EECCS group considered that neither of these provided adequate ethical ground for allowing genes to become the exclusive intellectual property of a few, instead of the common inheritance of all people. The EECCS's experience of the EU patenting Directive suggests that the drive for patents as a due recompense for biotechnology companies for expensive genetic research has been taken too far, resulting in an undue private control over a universal public good. The maximum claims sought by companies or patent lawyers to obtain as much monopoly as possible from a given invention for the private benefit of the patent holder may be seen to conflict with wider goods. Restrictions on biotechnology patenting should therefore be applied, for example, if an exclusive claim may

---

[16] United Nations, *Plan of Implementation on Sustainable Development of the World Summit on Sustainable Development, Johannesburg, 26 August–4 September 2002* (New York: United Nations, 2002).

result in diminution of a general good, or a violation of some ethical principle about the thing invented.

Thus the CEC working group paper argued that the grant of a US patent on human stem cells and the differentiated cells derived from them represents a monopoly which was not in society's best interests.[17] Given the medical potential for treating so many diseases and the early stage of research, such wide-ranging aspects should remain in the public domain, in the same way as the human genome. In this case there is also the fundamental objection, that cells are integral parts of the human body and therefore are not the right of anyone to claim as intellectual property. The EC's ethical advisory group agreed, but was equivocal about cells which have been modified in some way. While technically valid, if these are the crucial cells on which the progress of research depends, then to allow patents on them could also be against the wider public interest.[18]

This raises the question of what legitimate goods patents should protect and whether ownership is the right conceptual model. At a time when modern liberal concepts of individual autonomy and private property are failing to facilitate an adequate ethic of law and genetics, what resources does the Christian tradition offer? Esther Reed's following paper explores these questions more fully.

(d) How patenting should relate to ethics in practice

Although ethics is implicit in the very notion of patenting and is explicit in its application to biological matter and living organisms, the ethical dimension of patenting has not been welcomed by the profession. Patent lawyers and governments set on securing protection for nascent industries have tended to regard the patenting process in a reductionist way as a technical, legal procedure, in a rather objective almost scientific exercise. Ethics was recognized to a limited extent in the European Patent Convention in the concept that a patent could be refused if the production of the invention or its publication would be contrary to *ordre publique* and morality. In practice, this

---

[17] Op. cit., CEC Working Group on Bioethics, *Human Stem Cell Patents*.
[18] European Commission, *Opinion on Stem Cell Patents*, European Ethical Group on Science and New Technologies (April 2002).

was seldom cited until modern biotechnology was involved. The EC's Ethical Group argued that when biological material was involved the ethical dimension becomes central,[19] but, as observed above, the patent process is not the best place to examine the issues. Patent agents are also under a professional obligation to patent unless there is a technical reason not to do so. Their culture does not consider ethics, and examiners are not trained in ethics nor easily held accountable to civil society. There is a need for a separate system for an ethical review of the more sensitive inventions. This should take place in parallel with the patent process and could take wider issues and implications into account. This point has recently been belatedly acknowledged by the EC's Ethical Group in their opinion on stem cell patents, but there is little sign of support from governments.[20]

6   Endpiece: public accountability

The notion of the ethical assessment of patent applications is feared by the industry and its promoters as an inhibition to the commercial advancement of biotechnology, as M. Monti's comment made clear. But the churches argue that this is a fundamental part of the social responsibility of biotechnology. It has been suggested that biotechnology has an invisible social contract with its culture.[21] Society may be prepared to accept novel inventions only provided certain conditions are fulfilled. If significant public issues are marginalized by the policy, regulatory, or patenting processes, there is a risk that public hostility will reject the technology. In March 1998, the Church of Scotland raised this potential problem with the then UK Science Minister. If more account was not made of wider public concerns, in the name of commercial drives, the risk was that the public would not want the products and that the market which patenting was intended to create would be lost. A year

---

[19] European Commission, *Ethical Aspects of Patenting Inventions Involving Elements of Human Origin*, Opinion of the Group of Advisors on Ethical Implications of Biotechnology of the European Commission (25 September 1996).

[20] Op. cit., European Commission, *Opinion on Stem Cell Patents*.

[21] D.M. Bruce, 'A Social Contract for Biotechnology: Shared Visions for Risky Technologies?', *Journal of Agricultural and Environmental Ethics* 15 (2002), pp.279–89.

later precisely this happened, in the public revolt over geneti-cally modified food.

Although the GM food crisis had many features of its own, certain of its roots lay in the notion of gene patenting and the EC Directive. This was where the underlying mindset that the experts know best had first established itself. In 1998, the tide of official attitudes on biotechnology might have been turned, had the concerns on patents been taken seriously, instead of commerce being seen as the only relevant public virtue. It might be said that this is an expression of the fact that one cannot love God and money. Ultimately, the full set of public values must be taken into account, in the assessment of the ethical acceptability, or otherwise, both of biotechnological inventions and of applying patents to them. Without this, mistakes like the importing of unlabelled GM produce into the UK, and failures of accountability like the EU Patenting Directive in its present form, will probably continue. The practi-calities of doing this represent one of the most difficult but most important issues of our times.

Bibliography

Bruce, D.M., 'Patenting Human Genes: A Christian View', *Bulletin of Medical Ethics* (January 1997), pp.18–20.

Bruce, D. and A. Bruce (eds), *Engineering Genesis* (London: Earthscan, 1998).

Church of Scotland, *Ethical Concerns about Patenting in Relation to Living Organisms*, Reports of the Church of Scotland General Assembly, 22 May 1997 (Edinburgh: Church of Scotland, 1997).

European Union, *Directive 98/44/EC of the European Parliament and the Council, on the Legal Protection of Biotechnological Inventions*, 6 July 1998 (Brussels: European Commission, 1998).

Reiss, M.J., 'Is It Right to Patent DNA?', *Bulletin of Medical Ethics* (January 1997), pp. 21–4.

12

Thinking Liturgically

Esther D. Reed

The previous chapter by Donald Bruce has ably recounted the history and thinking of the Working Groups on Bioethics attached to the European Ecumenical Commission for Church and Society (EECCS) and the Church and Society Commission of the Conference of European Churches (CSC–CEC).[1] This chapter looks in more detail at one submission by CSC–CEC to the Council of Ministers of the European Union, examining some of its theological arguments and offering further support for its conclusions. Briefly, we are interested in *why* the human body should not be made the subject of trade and *why* the products of nature should not be patented. These points might seem too basic and obvious to warrant discussion but it is sometimes the seemingly obvious that repays investigation. Theological intuition may tell us that neither of these things should happen, but good moral reasoning requires attention to the empirical features of the situation and careful analysis in the light of Christian tradition. EECCS and CSC–CEC did both, and were ready at the appropriate moments to submit clear and persuasive arguments to policy-makers. In writing this chapter, I want to give due acknowledgement to their work and mark the service that the various Working Groups give to the

[1] The European Ecumenical Commission for Church and Society (EECCS) merged with the Conference of European Churches' Church and Society Commission (CSC–CEC) in a process that was completed on 1 January 1999.

churches. I also want to bring some of their work into dialogue, so to speak, with the liturgy.

The Working Groups on Bioethics attached to EECCS and later to CSC–CEC were ecumenical, and so I adopt a broad definition of 'liturgy' as the shape and content of worship as conducted in most churches that adopt a prescribed order for public worship, often involving the use of authoritative texts.[2] Our intention is to test and illuminate the rationale and conclusions of one CSC–CEC submission to the Council of Ministers of the European Union by subjecting it to the ethical discipline of the liturgy – in the general sense of following the structure of the liturgy and attempting to conceive of present-day issues in light of its theological witness. The Working Groups developed an ethico-theological statement entitled *A Theological Framework for Bioethics*, in which members of Lutheran, Reformed, Orthodox and Evangelical churches articulated an agreed way of looking at the world as the theatre of God's glory.[3] This statement was developed over the course of several years as new members joined the Group and is well worth a read. It speaks of seeking the wisdom of the Bible and the Holy Spirit, and the vocation to responsible stewardship in light of recent technological advances and the Gospel. It also reflects on the brokenness of creation and the moral limits (Fr. *conscience des limites*) that should constrain scientists, industrial managers, politicians, and such like. Its influence can be discerned in the letter that we shall consider, namely that sent by Keith Jenkins of CSC–CEC to Hubert Vedrine of the European Parliament on 28 June 2000. The letter condemns the EC Directive on the Legal Protection of Biotechnological Inventions (98/44/EC). The text of this letter is as follows.[4]

---

[2] There are, of course, many non-liturgical churches that still have habits of worship and also many liturgical texts that could have been chosen for special study. For present purposes, we draw on the *Orthodox liturgy of St Chrysostom and St Basil the Great*, and the Holy Communion during Ordinary Seasons (Second Service) in *The Methodist Worship Book* (Peterborough: Methodist Publishing House, 1999), pp. 198–210.

[3] Available at <http://www.cec-kek.org/English/Bioethictheol.htm> (accessed 28 April 2002).

[4] Available at <http://www.cec-kek.org/English/genomeE.htm> (accessed 20 May 2002). See <http://www.cec-kek.org/Francais/genomeF.htm> for the original French version of the text.

Mr. Hubert Vedrine,
President in office of the Council of Ministers of the European Union
Ministère des Affaires Etrangères
37, quai d'Orsay
75007 PARIS

Strasbourg, 28 June 2000

Original in French

Subject: Patentability of the human genome

Mr. President,

Under directive no. 98/44/CE of 6 July 1998, the European Parliament and the Council provided that the European Community would allow the patenting of human genes under certain conditions.

Recently a number of opinions have been expressed asking for the abandonment or modification of this provision and allowing free access to the human genome (1). The Church and Society Commission of the Conference of European Churches, covering almost all the Anglican, Orthodox and Protestant Churches of the European continent, fully associates itself with this initiative and opposes any attempt to establish ownership of what must be regarded as a common good of all humanity.

Although we start from a particular theological perspective, we are aware that our ethical conclusion will be shared by many who start from other religious and philosophical perspectives.

From our perspective, the world and humanity in particular are the creation and creature of the God who confers on humanity the management of his work without abandoning it.

On this basis, the human body cannot be the subject of trade. Making genes patentable opens the door to this, seriously injuring human dignity.

Furthermore, knowledge is the common good of all. The discovery of genes cannot be compared to an invention and cannot be the subject of a patent.

Finally, we cannot ignore the serious problems of social justice and equity at the global level which the ownership and commercial exploitation by a part of humanity would inevitably bring about.

Certainly, we positively welcome biotechnological progress and genetic engineering (2) but clearly this progress must benefit equitably the greatest number.

The Church and Society Commission of the Conference of European Churches wishes to ask you to profit from the French presidency of the European Union to propose the re-opening of the debate, to extend it if possible to the global level, and to arrive at ethically acceptable proposals.

Signed on behalf of Keith Jenkins,

Director of the Church and Society Commission of the Conference of European Churches.

by Rev. Richard Fischer,

Executive Secretary (Strasbourg)

Copies to: Mr. Jacques Chirac, President of the French Republic; Mr. Pierre Moscovici, Minister; The governments of the other 14 member states of the European Union; The European Commission; The European Parliament; The Council of Europe; The member churches of the Conference of European Churches

NOTES

1. e.g. Universal declaration on the human genome of Unesco in 1998, meeting of the Research Ministers of the G8 countries (June 2000), opinion of the French National Consultative Committee on Ethics, Madame Elisabeth Guigou, French Minister of Justice, before the National Assembly (June 2000), position of the Parliamentary Assembly of the Council of Europe (June 2000), declaration of Prime Minister Blair and President Clinton (March 2000), initiative of Members of Parliament Jean-François Mattei (France) and Wolfgang Wodarg (Germany).

2. In September and November 1996 the predecessor of our Commission, the European Ecumenical Commission for Church and Society, presented its position in the two attached documents on the draft directive of the European Community relating to the legal protection of biotechnological inventions. It specified that it had no objection to the patenting of a specific application using genetic information but that it was opposed to the patenting of a gene sequence as such.

Three issues present themselves for comment: (i) the limitations inherent in the concept of ownership when applied to the human genome; (ii) the link between a belief in God as creator and affirmations of human dignity; (iii) the apparently self-evident distinction between 'discovery' and 'invention' and the limit it places on patentability. These issues touch on different aspects of the patenting debate, but each gives rise in some way to the questions: How does thinking theologically help the Christian community to recognize moral limits relevant to the human genome and patent law? Can the liturgy guide our thinking about such complex issues?

(i) We turn first to issues of ownership and property. As Donald Bruce has explained in Chapter 11, a patent does not convey full rights of ownership but is an exclusionary right that should, in principle, allow the balancing of legitimate interests. Patents are not *prima facie* claims to ownership but to a different kind of social contract between inventor, investor and society. Their several justifications include the protection of the interests of those who have invested time, energy and money; the creation of motivation and incentive for new research; and the publication of useful knowledge. Why, then, does CSC–CEC find it necessary to oppose 'any attempt to establish ownership of what must be regarded as a common good of all humanity'? Does gene patenting amount to holding something as property in ways that differ from the patenting of other 'inventions'? The CSC–CEC answer is found in their references to the peculiar nature of the human genome and to the 'serious problems of social justice and equity at the global level'. Because the genome is a 'common good of all humanity' it should not be subject to proprietary patent rights that could be used to prevent others from publishing research or marketing tests based on DNA as it occurs in the body. The ethical significance of the human genome, as that which instructs for proteins that provide for normal human development and function, means that benefits accruing from the genetic knowledge should be shared: 'biotechnological progress and genetic engineering ... must benefit equitably the greatest number'. This last claim is especially startling and exceeds the recommendation in the April 2000 Human Genome Organisation (HUGO) Ethics Committee Statement on Benefit-Sharing that 1–3 per cent of net profits from commercial projects should go to a healthcare infrastructure project and/or humanitarian effort.[5] Is their suggestion unrealistic and naive? Or did the CSC–CEC letter offer timely witness to the economic implications of the gospel?

[5] HUGO Ethics Committee, Statement on Benefit-Sharing, 9 April 2000. Available at <http://www.gene.ucl.ac.uk/hugo/benefit.html> (accessed 19 May 2002).

If one of the goals of liturgical living is to show what divine justice and love might look like in the economic affairs of everyday life, then the letter sent by CSC–CEC to the European Parliament is refreshingly bold and direct. Genetic knowledge should, it claims, be shared in ways that benefit equitably the greatest number. An operative distinction implicit in this claim is between 'knowledge for use' and 'knowledge for profit'. In the former case, genetic knowledge is the material basis of an ordered, purposeful biotechnology industry, in which need plays a large part in determining the meaning of justice. In the latter, it is monopolistic control of patent rights on sequence data that prevents others from publishing research or marketing tests based on DNA as it occurs in the body. The problem of reconciling the genome as 'a common good of all humanity' with the necessities of patenting is arguably one of the major moral challenges of our day. The CSC–CEC witness to the gospel priority of social justice over profit, and of justice as equity, is a stark reminder that all judgement belongs to the God who holds individuals and also nations to account for their stewardship of the created order.

The CSC–CEC letter draws conclusions with confidence from a Christian way of handling biotechnological advances in which substantive notions of good exceed procedural conditions of fairness. In contrast to liberal conceptions of formal equality that centre around the principle of consistency – likes must be treated alike – it suggests that legal instruments should be employed to ensure a particular type of outcome: knowledge must benefit equitably the greatest number. The letter does not go into details and so it is not possible to know exactly what the Working Groups had in mind. Clearly, however, they do not ask for equality of outcome in the sense that all should receive exactly the same share in the distribution of benefits. They lobby instead for a broad value-driven approach that emphasizes values central to Christian thinking. Central to this approach is the commitment that the human genome 'must be regarded as a common good of all humanity'. One of the big questions facing the EECCS and CSC–CEC Working Groups was whether Article 5(2) would, in effect, facilitate forms of stealing and carelessness with regard to social justice. They concluded that it would, because God-given obligations to 'manage' creation should not entail attempts to establish ownership. Our questions concern the theological arguments that might underlie this conclusion.

(ii) This brings us to the subject of human dignity and the claim that making the human body the subject of trade is incompatible with Christian faith. At a time when secular ethical theory centres around Lockean-influenced arguments for self-ownership and Kantian-influenced arguments against reifying the bodies of rational persons, it is worth pausing to consider the rationale in Christian thinking.[6] Note, for example, how G.A. Cohen, a political philosopher at Oxford, claims that a theory of self-ownership is a necessary and useful protection against exploitation and abuse. He argues that each person is the moral and rightful owner of him/herself and is entitled, morally speaking, to dispose of her/himself as s/he chooses.[7] As owner of him/herself, each person would be entitled to sell body parts, reproductive tissue, etc., but would also have a legal claim against their body being made the subject of trade if they did not wish it. Donna Dickenson argues from a liberal, feminist perspective that Western society should accept and recognize 'property in the person'. Women, she argues, have been disadvantaged historically from gaining legal ownership of property and thereby excluded from a positive social good. This good should be reclaimed within a reconstructed view of property as that which entails a 'set of relationships' rather than as 'a set of objects'.[8] In light of these types of argument, our question is whether thinking theologically and liturgically encourages a different conception of human dignity, with possibly different implications for making the human body the subject of trade.

[6] See John Locke, *The Second Treatise of Government* (Indianapolis, IN: Hackett, 1980), ch. 5, 'Of Property'. See also 'Moral Philosophy: Collins' Lecture Notes', in Immanuel Kant, *Lectures on Ethics*, The Cambridge Edition of the Works of Immanuel Kant, ed. Peter Heath and J.B. Schneewind (Cambridge: Cambridge University Press,(1997), p. 127.

[7] G.A. Cohen, *Self-Ownership, Freedom and Equality* (Cambridge: Cambridge University Press, 1995), p. 215. See also G.A. Cohen, 'Self-Ownership, World-Ownership and Equality', in F. Lucash (ed.), *Justice and Equality Here and Now* (Ithaca: Cornell University Press, 1986), p. 109.

[8] Donna Dickenson, *Property, Women and Politics* (Cambridge: Polity Press, 1997), *passim*.

The CSC–CEC letter appeals to the doctrine of creation as grounds for its claims with respect to the human body. 'From our perspective', it says, 'the world and humanity in particular are the creation and creature of the God who confers on humanity the management of his work without abandoning it. On this basis, the human body cannot be the subject of trade.' God is the Author of all creation and respect is due to the human body for this reason alone. Something is lacking, however, because it's not clear why God's creation of the human body excludes its becoming the subject of trade. God created other things that are legitimately the subject of trade. What's different about the human body as compared to other creatures? Does the difference lie in the fact that humans are persons not things, and only things can be owned? Immanuel Kant advanced this argument, claiming that humans are persons and only things can be owned or sold. His conclusions have subsequently been challenged by theorists like G.A. Cohen who claim that Kant failed to demonstrate that only things can be owned.[9] In light of this kind of challenge, it's not clear from the CSC–CEC letter why making the human body the subject of trade is ethically unacceptable. What's wrong, for instance, with Cohen's claim regarding the right of self-ownership? Perhaps he claims correctly that the concept of self-ownership, which might permit a person to make their body the subject of trade if they so chose, is precisely what's needed to prevent abuses of the kind feared by CSC–CEC.

A letter to the President of the Council of Ministers of the European Union is not the place for lengthy theological treatise. Hence the comments that follow should not be read as a criticism of the letter but as an opening of the topic for further exploration. More is needed than just an argument from creation, however, to establish that the human body should not be the subject of trade. We need further theological and more fully Trinitarian reasons to justify the claim that making the human body the subject of trade is unethical.

Thinking liturgically suggests that it is unethical because it violates the properly sacramental character of human living. Making the human body the subject of trade is an inappropriate

---

[9] Immanuel Kant, *Lectures on Ethics*, trans. Louis Infield (New York: Harper and Row, 1963), p. 165; Cohen, *Self-Ownership*, p. 215.

response to the divine invitation to receive freely of abundant
life; a 'non-eucharistic-like' response to the divine gift of life
and invitation to participate in the life of Christ. The liturgy says
little about human dignity *per se* but much about the worthiness
of Christ and our participation in him. In the Orthodox liturgy,
the deacon moves to stand before an icon of Christ just after the
opening anthems and before the litanies or prayers of suppli-
cation, summoning the people to praise the God revealed in
Jesus Christ. Human dignity (meaning the quality or state of
being worthy, honoured or esteemed) follows from human
integrity (meaning the state of having been made entire and
complete, sound and incorruptible in Christ). This could be
developed to yield the following propositions:

Proposition 1:   Redemption is the internal basis for Christian
                   confession of the doctrine of creation.
Proposition 2:   We know the true character of God and the
                   extent of his commitment to humankind only
                   in Christ; here alone do we have a reliable
                   measure of human worth.
Proposition 3:   Christian affirmation of human dignity follows
                   from confession of redemption and integrity/
                   recreation in Christ.

Whatever Christians say about human dignity follows from the
saving works of God in Christ. The Church's eucharistic
offering of the world and ourselves to God in Christ anticipates
the world to come in which the need for private property and
trade is removed. Private property and trade are an integral part
of human existence before the eschaton. Until that time, the
liturgy of the Church is an *anaphora*, a lifting up, an offering
and consecration to God of what he has given us. This will have
implications for trade and business dealings. Our question is
whether it precludes making the human body the subject of
trade.

Neither scripture nor the liturgy are alone sufficient to guide
the conscience in these matters. More is required by way of
moral reasoning to complete the integrity of conscience. Yet
many Gospel passages shed light on the question, and one
presents itself as especially relevant because it combines our
interest in worship with Jesus's own involvement in the socio-
political issues of his day. Consider the account in John's Gospel
of Jesus's cleansing of the temple. It tells how Jesus 'forcibly

interrupted' usual commercial activity in an act of overt rebellion against inappropriate financial transactions.[10] John does not spell out the implications of this act in ways that give direct answers to our questions. Nevertheless, his placing of this account early in his material, as compared to the chronology of the synoptic tradition (Matthew 11.15–18; 21.12–17; Luke 19.45f.), suggests that it contains important theological considerations. First, the temple is an inappropriate place of trade. The synoptic allusion to Jeremiah 7.11 is absent in John's Gospel but there is little doubt that the trading itself is regarded by Jesus as wrong, even if conducted fairly and honestly. Second, Jesus's body is the true temple where God and human nature are mystically conjoined: '"Destroy this temple, and in three days I will raise it up." ... he was speaking of the temple of his body' (John 2.19, 21). John does not imply that Jesus's body was a kind of shrine, a possible further implication being the quasi-sacralization of all human bodies. He speaks instead of Jesus's body as the 'unique manifestation' of God in human form; the Word of God made flesh who is the new place where God and humanity meet.[11] Third, Jesus's words foretell the resurrection by which he gives to all who believe the power to become 'children of God' (John 1.11). God will raise up Jesus's body and with it the church that is to live in witness to the new life that all may have in his name (John 20.31). This supplies the following argument:

Proposition 1:	The temple is an inappropriate place of trade.
Proposition 2:	Jesus Christ's body is the new temple that God raises from the dead.
Proposition 3:	All are called to share in Christ's resurrection and become members of his body, the Church.
Conclusion:	The human body is an inappropriate place of trade because it dishonours what is rightly God's and abuses that which, in Christ, is properly dedicated to prayer.[12]

[10] C.K. Barrett, *The Gospel According to John* (London: SPCK, 1955), p. 162.

[11] Barrett, *The Gospel According to John*, p. 167.

[12] Absolutes are rarely useful in Christian moral reasoning and, while I hold that this conclusion should direct and guide our thinking, there might be circumstances in which exceptions are warranted. For instance, it might be deemed acceptable to grow tissue-cultures in research work that later have commercial applications. The matter is complex and needs fuller investigation than is possible here. It is worth noting, however, that a recent UK government research paper pertaining

This established, if only in general terms, the next question is whether patenting genes or partial gene-sequences isolated from the body equates to making the human body a place of trade. It requires a related but different kind of reasoning. Careful scrutiny of the empirical features of the topic is required before decisions can be made with respect to the moral significance of what happens when genes are isolated from the body. Defenders of the European Directive, and Article 5(2) in particular which allows a gene sequence isolated from the human body to constitute a patentable invention, cite arguments such as that maintained by the American Medical Association (AMA) with respect to patenting regulations in the USA:

> The argument that naturally occurring substances are not patentable has been upheld. However, if a naturally occurring substance is isolated or manipulated from nature it may be patentable. Naked nucleic acids do not occur in nature. DNA molecules within a cell are organized as part of a chromosome or within a plasmid such as mitochondria.[13]

The AMA maintains that a genetic sequence will encode for a particular protein in identical fashion to that of the naturally

---

to *The Transplant of Human Organs Bill* 2000/01 <www.parliament.uk/commons/lib/research/rp2001/rp01-023.pdf> states in paragraph 2:
> To what extent if at all we possess any property rights over bodily products is an issue of increasing importance at a time when it is possible for certain bodily products to be used to produce substances of commercial value.
> The issue of 'possession' is an area where the law is described as 'unclear'. A decision of the Court of Appeal in Dobson v North Tyneside Health Authority (1996) 33 BMLR 146 held that the claimant had no right to possess the brain of her adult daughter for evidential purposes in order to bring a claim for clinical negligence, but lawyers acting for parents in the Alder Hey case (see Part IV, below) are believed to be preparing legal action against the hospital. This may possibly raise the issue of parental interest in the preservation and use of body parts from a deceased minor.

Also, the Nuffield Council on Bioethics recognizes growing public concern about 'commercialization of the body' and especially trafficking in human organs. It writes in *Human Tissue: Legal and Ethical Concerns* as follows: 'There is a growing body of international regulation and guidance prohibiting commercial dealings in organs and other human tissue (paragraph 2.21) ... Our conclusion is that there are strong reasons against organising the procurement of human tissue along commercial lines' (London: Nuffield Council on Bioethics, April 1995, para. 13.24, p. 13).

[13] Report 9 of the Council on Scientific Affairs (I-00) Patenting of Genes and their Mutations <http://www.ama-assn.org/ama/pub/article/2036-3603.html> (accessed 9 May 2002).

occurring sequence but that the isolated sequence has been designed to be relevant for a commercial context and will not be found in the patentable form within a living organism. In other words, a gene patent does not (and should not) give rights over a gene as it is found to occur naturally, but the isolated gene is sufficiently different from that occurring naturally in the body to render it eligible for patent. By contrast, opponents of the Directive maintain that this difference is morally indifferent and that a human gene-sequence should not constitute a patentable invention, even if isolated from the body. Donald Bruce has explained above that this is the CSC–CEC position. And they are not alone. Consider the statement issued in September 2001 by the *Institut Curie* in Paris and the French Ministry of Health which challenged the two Myriad European patents in a Resolution to the European Parliament. It expressed 'dismay at the possible consequences of the granting by the European Patent Office of a patent on a human gene'.[14]

There is no disguising that the matter is contentious. In such situations of disagreement, meditation on the liturgy must be supplemented with expert scrutiny of the arguments and evidence. Christian moralists can only seek the best available medical and scientific advice and base their decision on it. Working Groups such as those associated with the Conference of European Churches must be interdisciplinary if Christian contribution to public debate is to be intelligently aware of, and responsive to, the complexity of contemporary life, and to engage with the forces that shape human existence today.[15] Drawing on the advice of expert members, the EECCS and CSC–CEC concluded that isolated genes and partial-gene sequences are not sufficiently different to those found naturally to warrant patentability. Patenting a nucleic acid – produced in a laboratory using genetic information about a human genetic sequence and chemically identical to it – amounts to patenting a part of the human body. Hence their opposition to the European

---

[14] Available at <http://www.cptech.org/ip/health/biotech/eu-brca.html> (accessed 5 April 2002).
[15] I am indebted to an unpublished paper by Daniel W. Hardy, 'Interdisciplinarity and the "Coherence" of Theology', delivered to the Center for Theological Inquiry, Princeton, 1995.

Directive with respect to the patenting of human genes. At a time when the contemporary academic scene too often allows a gap to open between Christian ethics and moral reasoning, between articulation of the Gospel and engagement with particular 'cases of conscience' or moral dilemmas, we have good reason to be grateful for the integrity that characterizes their work.

(iii) We turn thirdly to the distinction between 'discovery' and 'invention' and the limit it places on patentability. As Donald Bruce has explained, long-established conventions in patent law exclude products of nature from patentability.[16] But, in the now-famous Chakrabarty ruling, the majority decided that Chakrabarty's bacterium was not found in nature before the application of his genetic engineering techniques. It is now widely acknowledged that the bacterium he 'invented' resulted from naturally occurring bacteria and by naturally occurring processes.[17] The ruling was as follows:

> [Chakrabarty's] microorganism plainly qualifies as patentable subject matter. His claim is not to a hitherto unknown natural phenomenon, but to a nonnaturally occurring manufacture or composition of matter – a product of human ingenuity 'having a distinctive name, character [and] use.' (*Hartranft v. Wiegmann*, 121 US 609, 615 (1887)) ... [T]he patentee has produced a new bacterium with markedly different characteristics from any found in nature and one having the potential for significant utility. His discovery is not nature's handiwork, but his own; accordingly it is patentable subject matter under §101.[18]

---

[16] In America, the Patent Act of 1952 specified four basic statutory requirements that must be met to obtain a patent: (1) the claimed invention must be statutory subject matter and have utility; (2) it must be novel; (3) it must not have been obvious to a person having ordinary skill in the art at the time the invention was made; and (4) it must be fully and unambiguously disclosed in the text of the patent application, so that the skilled practitioner would be able to practise the claimed invention. In 2001, new utility guidelines required patent applicants to identify explicitly, unless already well established, a specific, substantial and credible utility for all inventions; the US Patent and Trademark Office Guidelines for Determining Utility of Gene-Related Inventions (4 January, 2001) raised the utility threshold.

[17] This is argued by Mark Sagoff in 'DNA Patents: Making Ends Meet', in Audrey Chapman (ed.), *Perspectives on Genetic Patenting: Religion, Science and Industry in Dialogue* (Washington, DC: American Association for the Advancement of Science, 1999), pp. 254–7.

[18] I have deliberately cited this information from the statement of Dennis J. Henner,

Hailed as a landmark decision, the Chakrabarty case opened the way for phenomenal growth of the biotechnology industry in America. In its wake, the American Patent Office issued patents on other genetically engineered plants and animals, including the now-famous Harvard 'onco mouse'.[19] Despite the consequences of the ruling, there is widespread consensus among religious leaders, Christian ethicists and environmental campaigners that it blurred the distinction between discovery and invention and crossed an established ethical boundary.[20] But why is this boundary especially significant? Why should the boundary not be sentience or some other capacity? Is an absolutist position necessary from a Christian perspective, such that nothing animate should be patented? Might a moral case not also be made to the effect that the level of legal protection appropriate to plants and animals should be decided according to the level of life that each species enjoys?[21]

Arguably the best philosophical approach to these questions to date is Martha Nussbaum's 'capacity approach' adapted from work in collaboration with Amartya Sen on international human development. Regarding international development, their central moral question is: 'What are individuals actually able to do or to be?' the idea being that development policy should be linked to the most significant human capacities (e.g. for life, bodily health, bodily integrity, thought, imagination, affiliation and play).[22] When adapted to animals and patent law,

---

Senior Vice President, Research, Genentech, Inc., before the Subcommittee on Courts and Intellectual Property of the Committee on the Judiciary House of Representatives 13 July 2000. Available at <http://www.house.gov/judiciary/henn0713.htm> (accessed 10 February 2002).

[19] I cite the statement of Q. Todd Dickinson, Under Secretary of Commerce for Intellectual Property and Director of the US Patent and Trademark Office, before the Subcommittee on Courts and Intellectual Property Committee on the Judiciary US House of Representatives, 13 July 2000. Note his wording re: the granting of patents on plants and animals <http://www.house.gov/judiciary/dick0713.htm> NB the 'onco mouse' was genetically engineered to be more susceptible to tumour growth.

[20] Audrey Chapman provides a useful summary in Chapman, *Perspectives on Genetic Patenting*, pp. 17–21.

[21] On this, see Martha Nussbaum, Book Review: 'Animal Rights: The Need for a Theoretical Basis', review of Steven M. Wise, *Rattling the Cage: Toward Legal Rights for Animals* (Cambridge, MA: Perseus Books, 2000), *Harvard Law Review* 114 (2001), pp. 1506–47.

[22] Martha C. Nussbaum, *Sex and Social Justice* (Oxford: Oxford University Press, 1999), pp. 41–2.

this question becomes: 'What level of life does it enjoy?', the implication being that the legal protection due to animate things should be linked to its significant capacities. Legal protection should be increased as significant capacities (e.g. for pain and communication) increase. The protection due to animate things should increase according to the level of life that they enjoy – so that, for example, it might be deemed morally acceptable to grant patents on a bacterium but not on a higher primate. The approach has much to commend it and differs significantly from Chief Justice Burger's citation of the Congressional Report accompanying the 1952 Patent Act which noted that Congress intended statutory subject matter to 'include anything under the sun that is made by man'. A 'capacity' approach would put limits to current patenting practices because much more discrimination between animate things would be required than is implied by this comment. 'Real world' utility, and the additional criteria currently employed in Europe and America, would not be the only considerations to be taken into account because the level of life enjoyed by the animate thing worked on by researchers would also be significant. Unfortunately, it is notoriously difficult to differentiate morally between animals of different species. Evidence suggests that cold-blooded animals such as fish, snakes and frogs suffer pain, and that cephalopods (such as octopus and squid) can learn complex tasks and appear to form social bonds. Recent advances in genetic science render the issues even more complex as biologists tell us that there may be very few genes expressing proteins that are unique to human beings. Most genes we use are also used in one form or another by other organisms but are regulated differently.[23] Nevertheless, according to a 'capacity approach', a morally coherent argument could probably be made to the effect that some products of nature may be deemed patentable while others are not.

In contrast, the EECCS and CSC–CEC Working Groups were of the opinion that no products of nature should be patentable. The CSC–CEC letter states: 'The discovery of genes cannot be compared to an invention and cannot be the subject of a patent.' As Donald Bruce has explained, the essential factor in

---

[23] I am indebted at this point to Mr Dan Wood.

the argument was the distinction between 'what is a genuine human invention' and 'what is the common heritage of all'.

The liturgy says little, if anything, about 'nature' – in the sense of the genetically controlled qualities of an organism – or about how we should value it. It says a lot, however, about our offering back to God all that he created, sustains, and has given for our benefit. In the Orthodox liturgy, the priest says: 'Thy gifts of what is Thine, do we offer to Thee, in all we do and for all Thy Blessings.' Similarly, in the Methodist Service of Holy Communion during Ordinary Seasons (First Service), bread and wine are brought to the table (or uncovered) and the minister says:

> Lord and Giver of every good thing, we bring to you bread and wine for our communion, lives and gifts for your kingdom, all for transformation through your grace and love, made known in Jesus Christ our Saviour. Amen.

Both services include a paradoxical offering to God of what is not really ours; presenting to God what is already his. Creation does not merely exist. Its being is not neutral or bad but good, and human relations to the non-human created order should affirm and not deny this. But what further ethical significance attaches to the Church's paradoxical offering of bread and wine to God? Many Gospel passages could be called upon to aid our interpretation, but consider especially Jesus's words when going up to Jerusalem. Some of the Pharisees in the crowd tell him to order his disciples to stop singing: 'Blessed is the king who comes in the name of the Lord! Peace in heaven, and glory in the highest heaven!' Jesus replies: 'I tell you, if these [the disciples] were silent, the stones would shout out' (Luke 19.37–40). Not only the disciples but every created thing has its own special way of giving glory to its Father in heaven. All humanly derived valuations of life are thereby relativized, the implication being that all creation is valued for God's sake and not ours. As Karl Barth observes, 'The creature [meaning nonhuman animals] precedes man in a self-evident praise of its Creator, in the natural fulfilment of the destiny given to it at creation.' [24]

---

[24] Karl Barth, 'Creation as the External Basis of the Covenant', in *Church Dogmatics* III/1 (Edinburgh: T and T Clark, 1958), §41, p. 177.

Arguably, this means that, while Christians may share the same material ethical goals as advocates of the 'capacity approach', they do not necessarily share formal similarities in terms of ethical reasoning. Ethically prior to any measuring of capacities entailed in levels of life enjoyed by diverse species is the recognition that stones, bacteria, and all inanimate and animate things are capable of giving glory to God.

These rather general-sounding comments become more focused and meaningful as we return to the specifics of the Chakrabarty case. In delivering the opinion of the Court, Chief Justice Burger cited the Congressional Report accompanying the 1952 Patent Act which noted that Congress intended statutory subject matter to 'include anything under the sun that is made by man'. In a dissenting opinion, however, Mr Justice Brennan, together with three other judges in the '5 to 4' split decision, said:

> Patents on the processes by which he has produced and employed the new living organism are not contested. The only question we need decide is whether Congress, exercising its authority under Art. I, §8, of the Constitution, intended that he be able to secure a monopoly on the living organism itself, no matter how produced or how used. Because I believe the Court has misread the applicable legislation, I dissent.[25]

Mr Justice Brennan argued that Congress had never before intended to extend the scope of patenting legislation to living organisms, and that it was the role of Congress and not the Court to broaden or narrow the reach of the patent laws. He recognized the legitimacy of process patents in biotechnology but challenged the extension of patent law to living organisms.

This dissenting judgement is similar to the EECCS and CSC–CEC claim that simply extending the rules for inorganic materials to the biological sphere can encourage inappropriate attitudes to nature. But can we, or should we, go the next step and condemn the patenting of all living organisms, regardless of the level of 'capacity' they enjoy? Brennan argued from the intention of Congress. Christian ethicists need to talk with professionals and practitioners who are close enough to the

---

[25] Mr Justice Brennan's ruling is available at <http://www2.law.cornell.edu/cg> (accessed 12 April 2002).

'coal face' to make practically informed judgements. What theological arguments might we employ in dialogue with them?

Arguably, the logic of the liturgy as studied so far can be expressed as follows:

Proposition 1: Every created thing is capable of giving glory to God and benefiting creation.

Proposition 2: Humans have the peculiarly priestly responsibility of commending the world to God and praying for justice and peace.

Proposition 3: Human stewardship of the created order must not violate the destiny given by God to any creature or thing.

Conclusion: Whether or not the patenting of genetically modified organisms constitutes an inappropriate attitude to nature will depend upon its facilitation or otherwise of the destiny given by God to it.

Perhaps disappointingly, the propositions advanced here do not translate immediately into an argument to the effect that no patents should at any time be granted on animate things. Proposition 3 could be interpreted strongly or weakly. A strong interpretation might be that humans should not interfere at all in the destiny given by God to any creature or thing. But this would be more or less impracticable in any form of human society and might not take account of the responsibilities of stewardship. A weak interpretation might accept human interventions in, for example, a cow's life-experience with respect to the change entailed in moving from life in the wild to life in a dairy-herd, but not accept the modification of an animal's genes to make it more susceptible to tumours. The logic of the liturgy does not yield any moral absolutes on this point. The skills of the casuist are required to decide individual cases.

Donald Bruce hit the nail on the head when he said that the essential factor is to identify 'what is a genuine human invention'. Claiming for ourselves what belongs entirely to God was the sin of Adam and Eve in paradise. Christians confess in the liturgy that creation has no being of its own but exists in the hand of God, and its proper attitude towards God is one of praise. Where patent rights over a product of nature are concerned, we must at least stop and ask whether we know our limit before God. Is this another forbidden fruit that denotes the limit of humankind? As noted above, human creativity, inventiveness and legitimate trade may, in a fallen world, be ways of praising God and giving him honour. The issue here, however, is not the expression but the limits of human creatureliness. Thus, in agreement with the CSC–CEC letter, we are concerned about injury done to human dignity. We must also be concerned about whether the action constitutes an affront to God.

In multi-cultural and multi-faith settings, we do not necessarily expect all dialogue partners to agree with our stance or argumentation. What matters is that public theology is explicit about its argumentation and ready to give biblically and liturgically informed reasons for the positions taken, even if situations sometimes demand that arguments are implicit rather than explicit. Recent Protestant ethics has tended to downplay the task of casuistry, concentrating instead on virtue, character-formation, and living as the body of Christ. There is nothing wrong with any of these! The big challenge, however, is for Christian moral reasoning that does not accommodate itself to dominant liberal philosophies but is publicly available and able to enter into dialogue with policy-makers, and such like, in life's different spheres. To this end, we need to submit ourselves to the ethical discipline of the Bible and the liturgy, endeavouring to conceive of present-day issues in light of their theological witness. We also need to reinvigorate methods of moral reasoning familiar to the Church in previous centuries and talk again about conscience in relation to our actions and God's law. In this chapter, we have attempted this in modest fashion and have learned that study of the liturgy helps in at least two ways. First, its structure highlights connections between what God has done in Christ and the tasks of Christian ethics and moral reasoning. Second, its participative and dialogic nature reminds us of the dynamic integrity that properly characterizes Christian ethics and moral reasoning. It still helps us expound what Ambrose of Milan called the intercourse between what is virtuous and what is useful.[26]

---

[26] Ambrose, 'Duties of the Clergy', in Philip Schaff and Henry Wace (eds), *Nicene and Post-Nicene Fathers,* Second Series (Edinburgh: T & T Clark, 1950), vol. x, Bk II, ch. VII, §28.

Bibliography

Ambrose, 'Duties of the Clergy', in Philip Schaff and Henry Wace (eds), *Nicene and Post-Nicene Fathers*, Second Series (Edinburgh: T & T Clark, 1956).

Barrett, C.K., *The Gospel According to John* (London: SPCK, 1955).

Barth, K., 'Creation as the External Basis of the Covenant', in *Church Dogmatics* III.1 (Edinburgh: T & T Clark, 1958).

Chapman, A. (ed.), *Perspectives on Genetic Patenting: Religion, Science and Industry in Dialogue* (Washington, DC: American Association for the Advancement of Science, 1999).

Cohen, G.A., 'Self-Ownership, World-Ownership and Equality', in F. Lucash (ed.), *Justice and Equality Here and Now* (Ithaca: Cornell University Press, 1986).

Dickenson, D., *Property, Women and Politics* (Cambridge: Polity Press, 1997).

Hardy, D.W., 'Interdisciplinary and the "Coherence" of Theology', delivered to the Center for Theological Inquiry, Princeton, 1995. Unpublished paper.

Kant, Immanuel, *Lectures on Ethics*, ed. P. Heath and J.B. Schneewind, The Cambridge Edition of the works of Immanuel Kant (Cambridge: Cambridge University Press, 1997).

Locke, J., *The Second Treatise of Government* (Indianapolis, IN: Hackett, 1980).

Nuffield Council on Bioethics, *Human Tissue: Legal and Ethical Concerns* (London: Nuffield Council on Bioethics, 1995).

Nussbaum, M.C., *Sex and Social Justice* (Oxford: Oxford University Press, 1999).

Nussbaum, M.C., Book Review: 'Animal Rights: The Need for a Theoretical Basis', review of Steven M. Wise, *Rattling the Cage: Towards Legal Rights for Animals* (Cambridge, MA: Perseus Books, 2000), *Harvard Law Review* 114 (2001), pp. 1506–47.

Sagoff, M., 'DNA Patents: Making Ends Meet', in Audrey Chapman (ed.), *Perspectives on Genetic Patenting: Religion, Science and Industry in Dialogue* (Washington, DC: American Association for the Advancement of Science, 1999), pp. 254–7.

13

Is the Goodness of God Good Enough? The Human Genome Project in Theological and Political Perspective

Peter Scott

1 On being fearful

So numerous are the issues raised by the Human Genome Project (HGP) that perhaps it should be renamed 'Legion'. Jesus's response to the demonic phenomenon, Legion, was to permit it/them to escape by inhabiting some pigs (poor things!).[1] What should a theological response be to a contemporary Legion: exorcism, or something else? It is difficult to frame a theological answer to this question, for two reasons.

First, the primary level at which Christianity engages the matter of identity is not the genomic but the sacramental. In other words, it is through the rites of baptism and eucharist that the Christian acquires and learns anew of her identity. Such an identity cannot be discerned or practised without reference to Christ and the Church. By participation in these rites, the Christian is placed 'in Christ' and learns to be 'in Christ'. These rites are practised only in the social context of the Church and are intelligible only there. The core movement is not that of mapping, but instead of *rescue*.[2] To speak of Christian identity is

---

[1] Mark 5.1; 20; Matthew 8.28-34; Luke 8.26–39.
[2] Rowan Williams, *On Christian Theology* (Oxford: Blackwell, 2000), p. 210; cf. pp. 214–15.

thereby to speak of an identity forged through God's rescuing of the embodied self by Christ. Through such rescuing, the Christian acquires an identity in Christ through social participation in the Church's basic sacraments, baptism and eucharist, in the Spirit. In other words, the Christian is rescued into the community of the Church.[3]

Admittedly, this is a very curious account of identity: not an identity won but an identity received; an identity bestowed in which the Christian is delivered or liberated from a false, opposed-to-God, identity. Of course, what the Christian is rescued from, and thereby what Christian identity is, must be discerned ever anew according to prevailing circumstance, here genetics. I am not arguing that Christian identity may be gleaned only by attention to a sacramental theology. Plainly, to be rescued is to be rescued *from* something or someone. In the present context, I am claiming that we need to be rescued from the sin of mapping, which is in turn part of a larger modern project that 'has as its goal the elimination of contingency, by wilful human manipulation'.[4] Through this essay, then, I shall argue that the Christian Gospel invites our emancipation from such false desiring. For, as Hauerwas and Shuman summarize, 'it is our baptism and our discipleship as members of that body [of Christ], and not the information encoded in our genes, that finally determines our lives'.[5]

Second, a theological response is difficult because of the problem of teleological and non-teleological accounts of genetic order. An important Christian affirmation understands creation's complexity and change as having its source and destiny in an ordering by God. In other words, the created order is a teleological order, and the *telos* of that order is given by the purposes of God. However, as Janet Radcliffe Richards

---

[3] I thank Joel Shuman for this point, in personal correspondence.

[4] Joel Shuman, 'Desperately Seeking Perfection: Christian Discipleship and Medical Genetics', *Christian Bioethics* 5:2 (1999), pp. 139–53 (p. 145, italics removed). Cf. Bronislaw Szerszynski, Chapter 7, this volume.

[5] Stanley Hauerwas and Joel Shuman, 'Cloning the Human Body', in Ronald Cole-Turner, (ed.), *Human Cloning: Religious Responses* (Louisville, KY: Westminster/John Knox Press), pp. 58–65 (p. 60). I am not suggesting that we need to be rescued from genetics but rather from the modern desire of mapping. For a careful account of the ways in which Christian communities might respond positively – from a prior sceptical stance – to genetic manipulation, see Shuman, 'Desperately Seeking Perfection', pp. 150–1.

has conclusively shown, for such an account of teleological order neo-Darwinian biology can find no place.[6] Neo-Darwinism promotes an evolutionary materialism in which the complex is to be understood as emerging out of the simpler, and the former is to be explained by reference to the latter. The identification of genes has tended to confirm this evolutionary hypothesis (most human genes are shared by chimpanzees) and thereby to affirm *non*-teleological forms of naturalistic explanation. That the complex is to be explained by the simpler runs through the popular presentation of genetic science: specific human behavioural traits may be sourced, for example, to a gene for homosexuality (the 'gay gene') or for a predisposition to violence. So an important theological question emerges: how is genetic science as a non-teleological explanation to be related to the *telos* of the will of God?

Through this chapter, I shall be exploring the interaction between this identity and order by consideration of the goodness of the *deus Christianorum*. The phrase 'the goodness of God' indicates the way in which Christian theology acknowledges that 'all human life searches for a way forward, and thus seems wedded to the prospect of a good outcome from history'.[7] In my view, the goodness of God as it emerges in human life both rescues and socializes, and in that movement bestows identity and an ordering. Unless we are content to say that the notions of identity and order to be found in the HGP are convergent with Christian understandings, we cannot begin in direct fashion with the HGP. Instead, my argument begins from an account of goodness in the interaction between the body of Christ (the Church), the social body and the body of evidence that is the HGP. A theological perspective on the HGP will thereby be hard-won. Only through an exercise of interpretative cunning will the HGP's cartographic body be displayed and its relations to the goodness of God discerned.

Powerful forces are unleashed in the Human Genome Project. Are these powers inimical to human flourishing and opposed to the goodness of God? Should we be fearful of the

---

[6] Janet Radcliffe Richards, *Human Nature after Darwin: A Philosophical Introduction* (London and New York: Routledge, 2000), pp. 11–23.

[7] Daniel W. Hardy, 'Eschatology as a Challenge for Theology', in David Fergusson and Marcel Sarot (eds), *The Future as God's Gift* (Edinburgh: T & T Clark, 2000), pp. 151–8 (p. 153).

HGP? The aim of this chapter is to explore the sacramental dynamics of the goodness of God and to enquire whether the HGP impedes or advances this goodness. By such a formulation, I do not intend to essentialize God's goodness. Such sacramental goodness is worked out through the movements of human and non-human life and in concentrated form in the operation of the sacraments, here especially the eucharist. Such goodness should not be understood as somehow behind these movements in the manner of a soteriological 'shadow'. Rather, goodness inheres, if it does, in these human practices and orients these practices on their fullness and completion in the triune God.

In the next section, I briefly set out the theological context in which I propose to engage the HGP. This context is that of Christian politics, to which an account of the eucharist – as the visibility of the body of Christ – is central. From such a perspective, the genomic body and various theological interpretations of the HGP will be interrogated. In section 3, I enquire after the sorts of goodness and dis-goodness that the Human Genome Project promotes. A brief formulation of the goodness of God and how that informs a sacramental theology of technology – with special attention to the eucharist – follows in section 4. In a final section, under the rubric of the de-restricting of God's goodness, I comment on how such a sacramental construal of God's goodness operates in criticism of the Human Genome Project.

2   Theologies of the genome

I begin with a basic question: Why does the HGP call forth theological comment? Part of the answer lies in one aspect of the rationale of the HGP: the identification, and perhaps overcoming, of specific sorts of *suffering* through an identification of their genetic sources. In a comment on the ubiquity of suffering, US Catholic theologian M. Shawn Copeland writes, 'Suffering is universal, an inescapable fact of the human condition; it defies immunities of all kinds.'[8] The religions offer

---

[8] M. Shawn Copeland, '"Wading Through Many Sorrows": Toward a Theology of Suffering in Womanist Perspective', in Emilie M. Townes (ed.), *A Troubling in my Soul: Womanist Perspectives on Evil and Suffering* (Maryknoll, NY: Orbis, 1993), pp. 109–29 (p. 109).

responses to suffering: Copeland's essay presents some of the ways in which black women in the USA during formal slavery drew strength from their appropriation of a Christian inheritance. Suffering is no respecter of persons and thereby for theistic perspectives appears to call into question the just ordering of the world by a good God. If technologies, such as the HGP, are developed to counter suffering – physical, social and cultural – it is not surprising that these technologies should call forth theological comment. If technologies are thought to enhance life by overcoming certain types of suffering, or in other ways to improve our 'quality of life' through the domination of nature, these technologies demand theological critique.

Copeland's comment, however, repays careful study: suffering, she argues, defies immunities. An important question now emerges: How should we respond to that against which we shall not be able to secure immunity? How shall we think of an ordering that includes suffering that cannot be overcome? A eucharistic perspective does not avoid the issue of suffering: soteriologically, the suffering of the crucified Jesus is central to the drama of the rite; anthropologically, as liberation theologians tirelessly insist, the Christian sacraments require and support acts of justice against suffering. A eucharistic perspective, furthermore, speaks of a transition of rescue in which the goodness of God is specified and the identity of a community secured. Such a eucharistic perspective, however, does not permit the scope of theological attention to be construed narrowly. To participate in a eucharist is to invoke a place, a history and a society. That place is the actual 'environs' of the eucharist, the history is that of Israel and the Church, and the society is the Church. This is not a confined, ecclesiastical perspective: the renditions of place, history and society in the eucharist have reference *ad extra*, as we shall see.

I shall return to the matter of the eucharist in the last two sections of this chapter. For the moment, I want to review the ways in which theologians engage the Human Genome Project. Here I do not wish to comment on the moral judgements that are made about the Project but instead I want to pay attention to the ways in which the Human Genome Project is approached theologically. What is remarkable about many of the theological commentaries on the HGP is how positive they are about genetic mapping. Are the theological roots of such warmth discernible?

In a review of ecumenical responses to the HGP, Roger L. Shinn notes that responses to genetic engineering have on occasion come from those theologians interested in 'social justice' rather than 'technical matters'. The occasion of this comment is a report on the WCC's 'World Conference on Faith, Science and the Future' (1979) at which two speakers from the 'political Left' raised issues of money and power in the consideration of genetic engineering. Shinn concludes: 'Most delegates, more comfortable discussing social than technical issues, welcomed the two addresses.'[9] What technical issues are being referred to here? On this, the text is silent. There are of course many technical issues in the mapping and sequencing of the Human Genome. For example, how is a stable DNA fragment to be secured to permit its mapping? One development, as R. David Cole explains, enables longer sequences of human DNA (up to 1,000 Kbp) to be inserted into a yeast artificial chromosome. As the yeast bacterium is easily grown, large numbers of fragments can be prepared in this way to facilitate mapping.[10] Is this the sort of 'technical issue' that Shinn has in mind? It is not clear to me, however, that Christian theology has much to contribute regarding such technical matters.

It is interesting at this point to ponder whether much of the theological discussion of the HGP is premised upon a distinction between the technical and the social, with ethical attention focused on the 'consequences' of certain techniques. Certainly, federal funding in the USA was secured for the HGP by the making of a distinction along these lines. Deeply anxious that the funding of the HGP might be held up while ethical issues were attended to, pro-HGP scientists and bureaucrats proposed a twin-track approach. Thus genome scientists, suggests Alice Domurat Dreger, agreed:

> that research into ELSI [ethical, legal and social implications of the HGP] should be funded, so long as it did not delay or detract

[9] Roger L. Shinn, 'Genetics, Ethics and Theology: The Ecumenical Discussion', in Ted Peters (ed.), *Genetics: Issues of Social Justice* (Cleveland, OH: Pilgrim Press, 1998), pp. 122–43 (p. 127).
[10] R. David Cole, 'The Genome and the Human Genome Project', in Peters, *Genetics*, pp. 49–70 (p. 59).

from the business of mapping and sequencing. HGP proponents advocated a division of labor whereby ethical concerns would be handled by other 'sub-cultures' of the nation. In fact, the portion of the budget dedicated to ELSI research ... has tended to keep analyses focused on the potential applications of genetic research rather than on the nature, meaning, and propriety of the research itself.[11]

Given this judgement, the distinction made by Shinn between the technical and the social appears less persuasive: 'ethical' discussion of the HGP is pre-structured along a division between 'pure science' and 'moral problems of application'. In this fashion, reference to social justice appears as a type of after-thought that can make no contribution to the science itself. That is, technical issues refer us to the place of the human body. Historical and social perspectives are, however, to be considered separately from the cartographic construal of the genetic body. The mapping of the human body is presented as an issue to which neither history nor society are relevant. There are of course moral 'problems', but these must then be handled by ethicists and specialists in jurisprudence.

Moral problems are construed technically: the body is mapped, moral problems are fixed. Or, better, the language of frontier is pertinent here. The centrality of the metaphor of the 'myth of the frontier' in winning cultural and financial support for the HGP, 'the genetic frontier', has been highlighted by Dreger.[12] By extension, the frontier of genome mapping is also an ethical frontier which can be pushed back only by the brave. (Fearful religionists, moaning from the perspectives of their wisdom traditions, must perforce be sidelined; only modernized religions are welcome at this frontier.) Reductionism is at work here: not the reductionism that claims that 'we are our genes' but the sort of reduction that relocates questions of historical direction and social equality as questions of technique. That is, the range of enquiries needed to engage the whole of the HGP could be reduced to one: the technical part. If other matters emerge in consequence, these must be addressed; if the

---

[11] Alice Domurat Dreger, 'Metaphors of Morality in the Human Genome Project', in Phillip R. Sloan (ed.), *Controlling Our Destinies: Historical, Philosophical, Ethical and Theological Perspectives on the Human Genome Project* (Notre Dame, IN: University of Notre Dame Press, 2000), pp. 155–84 (p. 171).

[12] Dreger, 'Metaphors of Morality in the Human Genome Project', pp. 159f.

matters are moral, ethical 'solutions' must be sought. Moreover, just as failure in the mapping is not contemplated, neither is failure in the area of moral fixing to be entertained. In other words, the reduction to technique does not *deny* the reality of the moral problems raised by the HGP. However, a reductive shift is executed in which a *diversity* of approaches shaped to engage the whole that is the HGP is denied. Theological approaches are welcomed only to the extent that such ontological restriction in diversity is accepted.[13]

In noting this ontological restriction in diversity, a critical space is opened up: because of the eucharistic perspective being developed here, we may refuse the disjunction between the technical and the social. 'The heated controversies over the hazards of ... recombinant DNA', Murray Bookchin rightly argues, 'are evidence that science is thoroughly entangled in debates that deal with its claims not just to technical compe- tence but to moral maturity as well.'[14] What requires attention, then, is the ways in which the mapping and sequencing of the human genome form an historical and social project that throws forward an account of goodness. In addition, that account of goodness will be deeply marked by the history and society out of which it emerges. Deficiencies in practice, and the interpretation of that practice, that pertain through this society may also be present in the HGP. The HGP is not some free- floating project, nor is it a development that can be traced back to a science interested only in that rare artefact, knowledge. (The fact that the US Department of Energy was one of the co-sponsors of the HGP indicates that the military interests of the United States post-Hiroshima and Nagasaki are present in the HGP.[15])

From this critical space, with its identification of a reductive move, some of the theological assessments of the HGP are rendered intelligible, if not persuasive. In other words, we may appreciate that these theological judgements proceed because

[13] In these comments on reductionism, I am drawing on Ernan McMullin, 'Biology and the Theology of the Human', in Sloan, *Controlling Our Destinies*, pp. 367– 93 (pp. 371f.).

[14] Murray Bookchin, *The Ecology of Freedom*, rev. edn (Montreal/New York: Black Rose Books, 1991), p. 281.

[15] See John Beatty, 'Origins of the U.S. Human Genome Project: Changing Relationships between Genetics and National Security', in Sloan, *Controlling our Destinies*, pp. 131–53, esp. pp. 133f.

of the separation between the technical and the social. Consider the following judgement made in a report on genetic engineering from a WCC consultation, with a gloss by Shinn: 'On genetic therapy, [the report] said, "In principle there is no ethical difference between treatment at the level of the gene and treatment at the level of symptoms as in ordinary medicine." Thus, it regarded the prospective replacement of a defective gene, via a carrier virus, as ethically comparable to an inoculation.'[16] Why is there no ethical difference? The suggestion seems to be that there is no ethical difference because there is no medical difference: gene replacement and inoculation occur at the same physiological level, the molecular.[17] If we come to a positive ethical judgement on inoculation, we may come with certainty to an identical judgement on gene replacement therapy. Such a conclusion is only secure, however, if the historical and social pressures that inform the HGP are the same as those that inform the procedure of inoculation; or, if not identical, are equally benign. In other words, in the perspective that I am developing here, the ethical aspects and status of the HGP cannot be determined only by attention to its self-presentation as technique.

Such acceptance of the HGP as technical informs some theological judgements. Consider the following conclusion to be found in the WCC Report, *Human Life and the New Genetics* (1980): 'Theologically understood, God may work as truly through intentionally human genetic acts as through the humanly unintended genetic processes that have made humanity genetically what it is now.'[18] A reductive shift is again evident here, the movement of which I shall try to identify. First, we should note that with minor amendment the statement is, indeed, theologically true: God may work through human acts as well as the natural processes that brought human beings to

[16] Shinn, 'Genetics, Ethics and Theology: The Ecumenical Discussion', pp. 124–5.
[17] There is a medical difference of course: genetic therapy turns upon the interface between phenotype and genotype in a way that inoculation does not. Whether this medical difference makes an ethical difference, I am not sure. If it does make an ethical difference, such a conclusion would of course weaken the analogy between gene therapy and inoculation in a fashion that weakens the case made by the theological supporters of the HGP.
[18] Cited in Shinn, 'Genetics, Ethics and Theology: The Ecumenical Discussion', p. 133.

be. If this were not true, we should note, the status of Jesus Christ in the Christian drama would be in question! Second, it is of course also true that human intervention in natural processes is not to be denied. We have here an ecological truism: there can be no truly human life without the alteration by the human of its habitat. That God works through human acts and that human beings must transform their situation to make a habitable environment are conclusions to be affirmed.

However, third, nothing follows from this claim for the legitimacy of 'genetic activity' or 'genetic practice'. All that is legitimated thereby is transformation of human circumstance. The character of that transformation is not identified nor its zone located. Just because God acts through certain processes beyond the intention of human beings does not require the conclusion that human beings have moral warrant to act in the same processes. Even if those processes are the processes by which human beings come to be, this does not invite the conclusion that human beings may act in them. Indeed, I think that you could make a case that human beings may transform their environment but may not alter that which causes their environment to be. If genes are a 'cause' of the human environment, intervention in these genes would then be ruled out.

That God may act as truly through human genetic practice as through gene-based natural processes is thereby a false claim. I agree that for there to be a human world there must be active human life, brought to be by certain processes, including gene-based processes, in which the world is humanized. However, to argue for the transformation of an environment is not thereby to argue for the transformation of the *conditions* of that environment.[19] God of course may work through the

---

[19] In *What is Nature? Culture, Politics and the Non-Human* (Oxford: Blackwell, 1995), pp. 155–6, Kate Soper distinguishes various meanings of nature: one is environmental; another indicates the 'structures, processes and causal powers within the physical world'. Arguably, the WCC judgement confuses these two levels: to transform an environment does not carry the same meaning as altering fundamental structures and processes. Any organism must transform its environment to live but no organism – until now – has altered fundamental structures, the conditions of its environment (here, the human body). Once this difference between environment on the one hand and condition of the environment on the other is identified, the onus is on the proponents of genetic manipulation to show why we should fail to respect this difference.

environment *and* its conditions. From that judgement, however, we learn nothing about the scope of human action, at least not without further argument. Indeed, such further argument would need to be teleological: to show how intervention in human genes contributes to the purposes of God, and is informed by the will of God in the economy of salvation. That we have here a 'technicization' of the argument is evident: the environment is construed as the site of the operation of the technical even to the extent that technical interventions in its causes are considered appropriate. A reductive account of nature is presented as amenable to the operations of human technical reason, and this reduction is justified – although not conceptually secured – by reference to God.

There are other emphases and perspectives in the theological consideration of the HGP. On these, I shall be drawing in the next section. I conclude this section by reporting the judgement of three religious representatives – a Jew, a Catholic and a Protestant – made in a hearing at the USA's House of Representatives. In answer to the question, 'Does genetic research get a green light?' the three representatives agreed on the reply: 'A yellow light: proceed with caution.'[20] Through this section, I have been exploring the rationale for such an affirmation. In my view, this affirmation turns upon a distinction between technique and social justice. If we refuse this distinction, what sorts of goodness may the HGP be understood as offering?

3   Not good enough: the Human Genome Project as technology

Although accurate diagnosis and screening and health-giving therapies are important goods and may be understood as one aspect of the goodness mediated by the HGP, through this section I do not focus on these medical benefits. Instead, I investigate the account of technology invoked by theological considerations of the HGP in order to make problematic again the distinction between the technical and the social. At the

---

[20] Cited in Shinn, 'Genetics, Ethics and Theology: The Ecumenical Discussion', p. 137.

conclusion of this section, I shall consider the sorts of goodness implied by such an account of technology.

To begin, we should note that theological supporters of genetic engineering and the mapping of the human genome do not consider the nature of technology. Again, we see operative the distinction between the technical and the social in which 'the nature, meaning and purposes' of the HGP are pushed out of the discussion. One way of trying to get a purchase on its nature and meaning, and thereby on its purpose, is to ask after the meanings of technology in theological affirmations of genetic manipulation. Elsewhere I have argued that the understanding of nature and technology on which such affirmations depend may be described as *modern*.[21] In this modern tendency, nature (including the nature of the human body) is regarded as other, and technology is understood to be a value-free set of instruments for the manipulation of that otherness. Such an optimistic assessment by theology of genetic manipulation draws heavily – if implicitly – on a theological reading of temporality.[22] The drive towards the instrumentalization of nature, technology and, finally, Christian commitments, draws on gradualist notions of the unfolding of medical therapies as part of the co-creative work of human beings in relation to God.[23] The actions of technological humanity follow God's redeeming actions towards creation and thereby contribute to the fulfilment of the purposes of the redeeming God. Just such a view can of course be discerned in the theological judgement that I reported earlier: 'Theologically understood, God may work as truly through intentionally human genetic acts as through the humanly unintended genetic processes that have made humanity genetically what it is now.' Human genetic acts are associated with God's redemptive will. The implication here is that the human genome is insufficiently productive.

---

[21] See Peter Scott, 'The Technological Factor: Redemption, Nature and the Image of God', *Zygon: Journal of Religion and Science* 35.2 (June 2000), pp. 371–384 (pp. 375f.).

[22] Here I am treating the work of Ronald Cole-Turner, *The New Genesis: Theology and Genetic Revolution* (Louisville, KY: Westminster/John Knox Press, 1993) and Ted Peters, *Playing God? Genetic Determinism and Human Freedom* (New York and London: Routledge, 1997).

[23] For the concept of created co-creator see Philip Hefner, *The Human Factor: Evolution, Culture, and Religion* (Minneapolis: Augsburg, 1993), *passim*.

Genetic technology, aligned with the will of God, fixes that deficiency.

It is important to note that technology is here ascribed a redemptive status. As I have argued elsewhere, in the association of redemption and a genetic technology the providential ordering of the world is presented. The goodness of God is mediated by such technology and theology thereby legitimates the technology of genetic engineering. To support this technology is to participate in this goodness. If I may be permitted the liberty of self-quotation: 'The circle is complete: God, genetic engineering and the medical well being of western humanity are linked together in a seamless loop.'[24]

Notice also the connection between this view and some of the commitments of a liberal polity. Technology is regarded as neutral and a 'natural' feature of human life. By such commitments a complicity is evident in the much-announced promise of technology in which technology itself is regarded 'as an essentially uninteresting if powerful tool, neutral in its relation to cultural values and subservient to political goals'.[25] This view of technology is deeply consonant with a liberal democratic polity in which the principle of self-realization, understood as a certain equality of all individuals in the development of their talents, requires the 'neutral' instrument of technology to secure such self-realization.[26] Furthermore, the agent whose function it is to ensure 'equality of all' is the state. The HGP thereby requires the activities of the state, that ancient foe of the Church, if its mediation of goodness is to be efficacious, for the state is the agency charged with securing an equality of treatment for all. In this connection, the German Catholic theologian Karl Rahner has argued that, 'To pursue the practical possibility of genetically manipulating man is to threaten and encroach upon this free area [of human personal life]. For it offers incalculable opportunities of man's manipulation – reaching to the very

---

[24] Peter Scott, 'Nature, Technology and the Rule of God: (En)countering the Disgracing of Nature', in C. Deane-Drummond *et al.* (eds), *Re-ordering Nature: Theology, Society and the New Genetics* (Edinburgh: T & T Clark, 2002), pp. 275–92 (p. 285)

[25] Albert Borgmann, *Technology and the Character of Contemporary Life: A Philosophical Inquiry* (Chicago: University of Chicago Press, 1984), pp. 35.

[26] Borgmann, *Technology and the Character of Contemporary Life*, pp. 85ff.

roots of his existence – *by organized society*, i.e., the state.'[27] The HGP thereby supports and requires the actions of the liberal state: such genetic technology supports political rule being expressed through the agency of a levelling state. However, it remains doubtful whether such a distribution of goodness is closely related to Christian construals of the social nature of goodness. Indeed, the appropriate theological question – How does the Western state embody and fall short of God's purposes for human life? – is not raised. The goodness of God, we may conclude with regret, is here associated with certain troublesome features of a liberal polity. Investment in a liberal polity requires that God's goodness be associated with a 'neutral' technology and its manifestation in an individualistic self-seeking. In a further irony, Christian support is offered to the contemporary form of the state in Western democracies, thereby contributing to the reproduction of present society.

To oppose such a modern theological construal of technology is not to affirm a Christian conservatism in the face of technological innovation. One sort of Christian piety – which I am calling Christian conservatism – might object to the manipulation of nature that genetic engineering appears to require. Such conservatism is criticized by the US Lutheran theologian Ted Peters – correctly – as one in which Christians hide behind a static view of creation.[28] Peters quotes Rahner approvingly: resistance to technological development is 'symptomatic of a cowardly and comfortable conservatism hiding behind misunderstood Christian ideals'. By this, Rahner means that creation cannot be regarded as static, and somehow opposed to human history. Part of being human is the trans-formation of the material world; humans are, strangely, the subject who is also an object: we transform our bodies as object, thereby becoming our own creator.[29] To reject such a view, to argue that technological development is 'playing God', is to hide behind a view of the created order as given by God and therefore as unalterable. A different way of commending such Christian conservatism would be to appeal to traditions of

---

[27] Karl Rahner, cited in Thomas A. Shannon, 'Genetics, Ethics, and Theology: The Roman Catholic Discussion', in Peters, *Genetics, Issues of Justice*, pp. 144–79 (p. 158).

[28] Peters, *Playing God?*, p. 156.

[29] Ibid., p. 143.

'custom and practice' to which technological innovation is
alien. That is, to insist that what is humanly important occurs
within cultural traditions in which the operations of technology
have little impact. At the back of this view is an account of
society as organic. From the perspective of such organicism,
technological development is not central to the construal of
human intercourse.

Such a perspective can also claim that forms of technological
manipulation may be dubbed 'playing God'. We can see why:
from the perspective of this conservative position, the reconstruction of matter effective in some technologies presupposes
a new type of society – perhaps a society understood as mechanistic, or as socially engineered (as in eugenics), or as entirely
artificial and thereby contingent. Such views of society are
deeply opposed to an organic view. As, on this conservative view,
the goodness of God is associated in some providential manner
with an organic society, any operation of technological means
that presupposes or requires a different type of society seems to
be opposed to the will of God. Hence the charge: playing God.

To oppose the 'modern' theological affirmation of the HGP
is not, in my view, to affirm such conservative accounts of God's
goodness. Resistance to technology in such conservative
Christian commitments supports the privatization of
Christianity: the technological realm is overlooked and the
transcendence of God domesticated. Such a Christian
perspective on technology cannot affirm living in and towards
the unrestricted goodness of God for all creation. Neither the
refusal of the technological realm nor the investment in a
liberal polity fit easily with an unrestricted account of the
goodness of God.

4   The goodness of God: a sacramental theology of technology

If living under God's unrestricted goodness requires seeking
the good in history and working towards the overcoming of
suffering, how is this unrestricted goodness of God to be
thought of? What is the goodness of God in the context of a
theology of technology?

The unrestricted goodness of the rule of God for all creation
is articulated and enacted by the sacraments whose medium is

water, bread and wine. In a discussion of the eucharist, Rowan Williams has characterized this unrestricted goodness as God's 'guarantee of hospitality'. God's care, renewed and guaranteed through the resurrection of Jesus Christ, is unbounded in its hospitality. Moreover, such a view is traceable back to the Gospels' testimony to the table-fellowship (including the Last Supper) of Jesus himself. The Church in its social form, and through its concrete 'political' actions as social form, seeks to serve the regeneration of society towards such sacramental substance. 'A Christian practice of the political is embodied in the Eucharist,' argues William Cavanaugh.[30] He is right, and that practice is sacramental. This means, in turn, that the Church's sacramental labour *ad extra* is towards a God-given social identity that enacts hospitality for all. The eucharist invokes a world that cannot be fully grasped except by reference to Jesus Christ. That is, a world in which change cannot be thought theologically except in terms of the overcoming of suffering in justice towards goodness: hospitality for all. That is, only if eucharist is accompanied by concrete acts of justice is the ritual itself not an 'empty action'.[31] If eucharist is not to be an 'empty action', it must be directed outside the Church towards the overcoming of suffering.[32]

However, such an offer of hospitality puts into question the actual configuration of a society in its distribution of material goods. Such an offer of hospitality thereby requires the militant, sacramental labour of the Church's witness, in its own life and outward testimony and practice. Such militant impartiality, as I call it, draws into the daylight the ways in which the rich refuse the poor access to material goods and the ways in which the rich refuse or do not acknowledge the gifts of the poor. It is the poor, of course, who are likely to be most familiar with the failures in any society's hospitality. Therefore, the following question is immediately raised by a sacramental perspective: How do the present configurations of society deny people access to all kinds of materials? The militant impartiality of the

---

[30] William T. Cavanaugh, *Torture and Eucharist: Theology, Politics and the Body of Christ* (Oxford: Blackwell, 1998), p. 2.

[31] Gustavo Gutiérrez, *A Theology of Liberation* (London: SCM Press, 1974), pp. 262–5.

[32] This paragraph from Peter Scott, 'A Eucharistic Theology of Place: Pilgrimage as Sacramental', in C. Bartholomew and F. Hughes (eds), *Explorations in a Christian Theology of Pilgrimage* (Aldershot: Ashgate, forthcoming).

eucharistic 'guarantee of hospitality' is a criterion of Christian
judgement in the technological realm.

Technological development is then to be tested against this
sacramental perspective: God's guarantee of hospitality. A
Christian, theological perspective on technology does not
require the invocation of a static creation in order to deny
changes and new possibilities offered by technological development. Nor does it require that God's goodness be associated
with particular technological developments. Technology is
thereby not to be understood as playing God, or as providential.
Instead, a sacramental theology of technology understands
technological development as *ambiguous.* If technology blocks
democratic extension and renewal, it should be opposed. If it is
used to control access to the meeting of basic human needs, it
is to be opposed. If its harmful or negative effects are experienced disproportionately by clearly identifiable sections of the
population (technology as racist, classist, misogynist),
technology is to be opposed.

To enquire after technology, we may conclude, is always to
ask about God's goodness as hospitality and the disbenefits of
technology. To participate in a eucharistic rite is to declare
one's allegiance to this commitment of God to all creatures
towards goodness and against suffering; and to invite the
construction of that goodness in the world.

5   De-restricting God's goodness

In other words, the task of a sacramental theology of technology
is to discern and work in society for God's unrestricted
goodness that has the form of the guarantee of hospitality for
all. The Christian task is to show that to say the name of the
triune God is always also to declare hospitality, and that hospitality's guarantee in Jesus Christ.

If we are to consider more fully its de-restricting, some
account of God's goodness is required. How is this goodness to
be understood? According to the account of Christian identity
with which I began this chapter, the goodness of the triune God
has the form of rescue. This rescuing, I argued, socializes and
thereby confers identity and blessing. Its movement is always
'ex-centric'. The goodness of God always refers to movements
in sociality. Expansive movements in sociality may be ascribed

to the actions of the Spirit of God; restrictive movements may be understood as incursions into the freedom of the Spirit of God. A central indicator here will be the shapes and qualities of freedom operative in any society.

The emphasis on sociality may be traced to the origins of Christianity. Of the depiction of the social in Scripture, Daniel W. Hardy has written: '[T]he person of Jesus Christ as "sent" by God – and his work – are intrinsically social. In continuity with Israel, he and his associates are called to be the people of God, not only to teach and transform individuals one to one, but many to many, and in doing so to be their representative before God. He with them is, so to speak, the concentration of society and its responsibility beyond itself to God, in their fullest form.'[33] The sacrament of the eucharist is one of the ways in which the Church learns doxologically of the social, in its relation to the triune God and its purposes in the eschatological fulfilment of social life. The eucharistic 'guarantee of hospitality' insists on the social character of the movement of the triune God in and with the world (it is hospitable to all, impartially); and on the Church's doxological mandate to practise and foster such hospitality militantly. In being shaped by this guarantee of hospitality, the Church desires both to live as a society from God and to witness to the eschatological completion of the social in God. The goodness of God as hospitality is both a matter of the Church's internal constitution as worshipping community and its external witness as the primary sign of God's kin-dom.[34] The Church's orientation is both doxological and practical: it embodies and witnesses to the claim that true human sociality is from God and, furthermore, demands and seeks to practise the enactment of that fuller sociality in the world.[35]

De-restricting God's goodness cannot thereby be thought and practised without reference to the form and movement of the social: that is, its impartiality and its tendency towards militancy. What, however, has this to do with the genetics of

---

[33] Daniel W. Hardy, *Finding the Church: The Dynamic Truth of Anglicanism* (London: SCM Press, 2001), p. 26.

[34] The term 'kin-dom' is from Ada Maria Isasi-Diaz, 'Solidarity', in S.B. Thistlethwaite and M.P. Engel (eds), *Lift Every Voice: Constructing Christian Theologies from the Underside* (Maryknoll, NY: Orbis, 1998), pp. 30–9.

[35] Hardy, *Finding the Church*, p. 39.

bodies? The shape and direction of the social are not something that we are outside as if the goodness of God in social life somehow precedes the individual. Indeed, our histories and our bodies are only active in sociality, and are truly good only in their relation to the economic being of the triune God. Such a view is supported by the refusal to separate the technical from the social and the criticism of modern construals of technology in which nature is regarded as the manipulable other. It is not that human sociality is one thing and human embodiment another. Instead, our bodies are always social bodies and our sociality is always embodied. Human beings are embodied, relational and historical beings: *qua* human, human genes are only fully grasped as embodied, relational and historical.

Human genes are therefore *human* genes only *in sociality*. It is only as genes inform and are informed by social forms and processes through histories that these genes are operative in the *human* sphere. This is in contrast to the modern view that stresses the otherness of nature as manipulable or the separation of the social from the technical. In theological perspective, genes are to be understood as interacting with a historical and social environment. It is only from within such a human context that genetic interventionism can be related to the goodness of God. To repeat: Human genes are *human* genes only *in sociality*.

At this point, I must stress that – in my view – from such a perspective alone is it possible to speak truly of bodies. In other words, the human 'medical body' is graspable only as 'constituted by an extraordinary web of contingencies on a multitude of levels'.[36] If we are to speak of the transcendence of a particular human body, the sphere of that transcendence is into the social. As Robert Song argues, 'our culture increasingly sees the body as something which is to be transcended, to be manipulated in accordance with desire'.[37] The distinctive social space of the sacraments offers a different sort of transcendence and a different desire.

It follows from such a position that the 'humanness' of genes

---

[36] Hauerwas and Shuman, 'Cloning the Human Body', p. 63, following Wendell Berry.

[37] Robert Song, *Human Genetics: Fabricating the Future* (London: Darton, Longman & Todd, 2002), p. 127.

is always relative to the social order in which genetic science is undertaken. Moreover, as any social order is always relative to God, and relative to its end in God, the extent of the humanness of genes is relative to the economic being of God. If, for example, genetic science is undertaken in a society 'designed for no other purpose but survival on any terms',[38] then genetic science will be framed by that social purpose. In addition, if survival can be had only in competition with other societies, we should expect that genetic science will also be shaped by a *telos* of competitiveness. (It is well known that one of the arguments made in support of the HGP was that it offered one way for the USA to beat the Japanese in the – commercial and potentially financially lucrative – area of genetic screening and the development of therapies.[39])

Furthermore, where you are placed in any social order will affect your view of, and your relations to, the findings of the HGP. The Human Genome Project may present itself as an exercise in value-neutral biological science and as a venture of a liberal polity: without gender, race, class or nationality. However, such a judgement is true only if the social order in which the genome is being mapped does not discriminate by gender, race, class and nationality. Should such distortions in sociality exist, then the HGP's capacity for humanization is threatened in that the findings of the project emerge in and through a distorted social context in which human freedom is restricted. In the restriction of human freedom is the restriction of God's freedom to be God in the ways of the world.[40]

What is true about the HGP lies in its attempt to provide a bridge between gene-based suffering and therapeutic relief. Such an attempt is over-determined, however, by the pressures of a hierarchical society in which a fully social humanity is distorted, and the conferral of the blessing of social life by the triune God is inhibited, by the separation of technique from justice. In this perspective, it is not clear that the HGP can be trusted to provide the benefits ascribed to it. By no means can we be sure that its findings will be available medically to all nor

---

[38] Murray Bookchin, *Toward an Ecological Society* (Montreal: Black Rose Books, 1980), p. 279.
[39] Beatty, 'Origins of the U.S. Human Genome Project', pp. 131–53, esp. pp. 141f.
[40] Daniel W. Hardy, 'The God Who Is with the World', in F. Watts (ed.), *Science meets Faith* (London: SPCK, 1998), pp. 136–53 (pp. 149–53).

that its findings will escape being used in support of eugenic programmes (even if of the less malevolent sort).[41] Yet the eucharistic guarantee of hospitality requires 'the vision of a society in which almost the only thing we can know about the good we are to seek is that it is no one's possession, the triumph of no party's interest. The search for my or our good becomes the search for a good that does not violently dispossess any other ... because of a conviction that the creative regard calling and sustaining myself is precisely what sustains all.'[42] The political point here is needle-sharp: a sacramental identity of rescue and sociality calls for a social order in which the expansion of freedom is to the benefit of all, and not to some group with medical insurance; and where those who are least able to articulate their interests – the unborn – are not sacrificed to prevailing cultural or economic mores. The polity required is not that of a meritocracy in which individuals are granted an abstract equal standing but one in which the dispossessed may trust that the social processes for the distribution of goods (economic, environmental and cultural) work in their favour and thereby find ways of allowing the same dispossessed to make a social contribution. In this perspective, the burden of proof – which cannot be split between the technical and the social – is on the HGP.

Epilogue as prologue

The human genome is now mapped, the Project is now projectile. To whose benefit is it aimed? I frame the matter as a question to acknowledge that the first phase of the Project has now been completed. It would have been preferable if it had not begun. That is not where we are, however, and I am sure that the HGP's findings will be used in medical care, if only in

---

[41] In the consideration of eugenics, it is important to distinguish between negative and positive, and between voluntary and involuntary eugenic practices, and the level – individual or social – of those practices. Aborting a foetus because of a confirmed genetic test result for, say, cystic fibrosis is a voluntary, negative, individual-based eugenic practice; forced sterilization of a group because of their ethnicity is an involuntary, negative, population-based eugenic practice. Positive eugenics offers incentives to particular groups to encourage greater numbers of offspring. Cf. Arthur L. Caplan, 'What's Morally Wrong with Eugenics?', in Sloan, *Controlling our Destinies*, pp. 209–22 (pp. 210f.).

[42] Williams, *On Christian Theology*, p. 219.

genetic screening. (Some commentators on genetic 'engineering' caution whether many positive genetic therapies will in fact emerge from the mapping and sequencing of the human genome.[43])

It is the task of the Church in such circumstances to argue persistently that it is time to switch metaphors: from abstractive maps to actual bodies. Moreover, in turning attention to bodies, the Church will enquire after their identity and ordering. As the goodness of God emerges in social forms, it will be the role of the Church stubbornly to enquire of every development in genetic engineering: what social form is presupposed by this development? Does this social form enable or inhibit the conferral of goodness from one group to another? Are these social relations reciprocal, and are they mutual? In what ways have they been tested against the Christian conviction that the triune God is the giver of sociality, its origin, form and movement? As the mapping task is completed, the sacramental toil begins. To eat the body and drink the blood of a son of Mary and Joseph means no less.

Bibliography

Beatty, John, 'Origins of the U.S. Human Genome Project: Changing Relationships between Genetics and National Security', in Phillip R. Sloan (ed.), *Controlling our Destinies: Historical, Philosophical, Ethical and Theological Perspectives on the Human Genome Project* (Notre Dame, IN: University of Notre Dame Press, 2000), pp. 131–53.

Bookchin, Murray, *Toward an Ecological Society* (Montreal: Black Rose Books, 1980).

Bookchin, Murray, *The Ecology of Freedom*, rev. edn (Montreal and New York: Black Rose Books, 1991).

Borgmann, Albert, *Technology and the Character of Contemporary Life: A Philosophical Inquiry* (Chicago: University of Chicago Press, 1984).

Caplan, Arthur L., 'What's Morally Wrong with Eugenics?', in Phillip R. Sloan (ed.), *Controlling our Destinies: Historical,*

---

[43] See Philip Kitcher, 'Utopian Genetics and Social Inequality', in Sloan, *Controlling our Destinies*, pp. 229–62 (pp. 234–5).

Philosophical, Ethical and Theological Perspectives on the Human Genome Project (Notre Dame, IN: University of Notre Dame Press, 2000), pp. 209–22.

Cavanaugh, William T., *Torture and Eucharist: Theology, Politics and the Body of Christ* (Oxford: Blackwell, 1998).

Cole, R. David, 'The Genome and the Human Genome Project', in Ted Peters (ed.), *Genetics: Issues of Justice* (Cleveland, OH: Pilgrim Press, 1998), pp. 49–70.

Cole-Turner, Ronald, *The New Genesis: Theology and Genetic Revolution* (Louisville, KY: Westminster/John Knox Press, 1993).

Copeland, M. Shawn, '"Wading through Many Sorrows": Toward a Theology of Suffering in Womanist Perspective', in Emilie M. Townes (ed.), *A Troubling in my Soul: Womanist Perspectives on Evil and Suffering* (Maryknoll, NY: Orbis, 1993), pp. 109–29.

Dreger, Alice Domurat, 'Metaphors of Morality in the Human Genome Project', in Phillip R. Sloan (ed.), *Controlling Our Destinies: Historical, Philosophical, Ethical and Theological Perspectives on the Human Genome Project* (Notre Dame, IN: University of Notre Dame Press, 2000), pp. 155-84.

Gutiérrez, Gustavo, *A Theology of Liberation* (London: SCM Press, 1974).

Hardy, Daniel W., 'The God Who Is With the World', in Fraser Watts (ed.), *Science Meets Faith* (London: SPCK, 1998), pp. 136–53.

Hardy, Daniel W., 'Eschatology as a Challenge for Theology', in David Fergusson and Marcel Sarot (eds), *The Future as God's Gift* (Edinburgh: T & T Clark, 2000), pp. 151–8.

Hardy, Daniel W., *Finding the Church: The Dynamic Truth of Anglicanism* (London: SCM Press, 2001).

Hauerwas, Stanley and Shuman, Joel, 'Cloning the Human Body', in Ronald Cole-Turner (ed.), *Human Cloning: Religious Responses* (Louisville, KY: Westminster/John Knox Press), pp. 58–65.

Hefner, Philip, *The Human Factor: Evolution, Culture, and Religion* (Minneapolis: Augsburg, 1993).

Isasi-Diaz, Ada Maria, 'Solidarity', in S.B. Thistlethwaite and

M.P. Engel (eds), *Lift Every Voice: Constructing Christian Theologies from the Underside* (Maryknoll, NY: Orbis, 1998), pp. 30–9.

Kitcher, Philip, 'Utopian Genetics and Social Inequality', in Phillip R. Sloan (ed.), *Controlling our Destinies: Historical, Philosophical, Ethical and Theological Perspectives on the Human Genome Project* (Notre Dame, IN: University of Notre Dame Press, 2000), pp. 229–62.

McMullin, Ernan, 'Biology and the Theology of the Human', in Phillip R. Sloan (ed.), *Controlling Our Destinies: Historical, Philosophical, Ethical and Theological Perspectives on the Human Genome Project* (Notre Dame, IN: University of Notre Dame Press, 2000), pp. 367–93.

Peters, Ted, *Playing God? Genetic Determinism and Human Freedom* (New York and London: Routledge, 1997).

Peters, Ted (ed.), *Genetics: Issues of Social Justice* (Cleveland, OH: Pilgrim Press, 1998).

Richards, Janet Radcliffe, *Human Nature after Darwin: A Philosophical Introduction* (London and New York: Routledge, 2000).

Scott, Peter, 'The Technological Factor: Redemption, Nature and the Image of God', *Zygon: Journal of Religion and Science* 35.2 (June 2000), pp. 371–84.

Scott, Peter, 'Nature, Technology and the Rule of God: (En)countering the Disgracing of Nature', in C. Deane-Drummond *et al.* (eds), *Re-Ordering Nature: Theology, Society and the New Genetics* (Edinburgh: T & T Clark, 2002).

Scott, Peter, 'A Eucharistic Theology of Place: Pilgrimage as Sacramental', in C. Bartholomew and F. Hughes (eds), *Explorations in a Christian Theology of Pilgrimage* (Aldershot: Ashgate, forthcoming 2003).

Shannon, Thomas A., 'Genetics, Ethics, and Theology: The Roman Catholic Discussion', in Ted Peters (ed.), *Genetics: Issues of Justice* (Cleveland, OH: Pilgrim Press, 1998), pp. 144–79.

Shinn, Roger L., 'Genetics, Ethics and Theology: The Ecumenical Discussion', in Ted Peters (ed.), *Genetics: Issues of Social Justice* (Cleveland, OH: Pilgrim Press, 1998), pp. 122–43.

Shuman, Joel, 'Desperately Seeking Perfection: Christian Discipleship and Medical Genetics', *Christian Bioethics* 5.2 (1999), pp. 139–53.

Song, Robert, *Human Genetics: Fabricating the Future* (London: Darton, Longman & Todd, 2002).

Soper, Kate, *What is Nature? Culture, Politics and the Non-Human* (Oxford: Blackwell, 1995).

Szerszynski, Bronislaw 'That Deep Surface: The Human Genome Project and the Death of the Human', in Celia Deane-Drummond (ed.), *Brave New World? Theology, Ethics and the Human Genome* (Edinburgh: T & T Clark, 2003), pp. 145–63.

Williams, Rowan, *On Christian Theology* (Oxford: Blackwell, 2000).

Postscript

Celia Deane-Drummond

Those readers who have diligently read the full text of this book will have become aware of the diversity of the viewpoints expressed here in relation to the prospects offered by the Human Genome Project, even while being couched in such a way that there is mutual respect for alternative positions. Yet in spite of these differences, key trends and concepts surface in such a way that it is possible to discern common areas of concern, even if the evaluation of the significance of such trends is different. The purpose of these concluding remarks is to draw out some common threads that have appeared in different ways in the argumentation offered by different authors, as a way of pointing to further discussion and deliberation. I do not attempt to disguise the differences in view, but rather offer this synopsis as a stimulus for further discussion.

Science as socially situated

The appreciation of the way societal values inform and shape the practice of science, including the emergence of the Human Genome Project, is echoed in different ways by different authors. Robert Song, for example, argues that reductionist forms of science could only have taken root once they were couched in societal and moral claims about health and disease, with such a desire for freedom from disease going back to the earlier understanding pioneered by Bacon of the purpose of science. Science, in this sense, takes on a wider 'salvific' role in society, one that theologians would not necessarily wish to endorse, unless it is explicitly linked with global societal issues of justice. Peter Scott situates the Human Genome Project less in the historical social trajectory of early modern science, than in the development of modern technology as such, arguing that the severance of the technical from social analysis has hidden the political dimensions running beneath the surface. Instead, he develops the theme of socially informed reflection on the merits (or otherwise) of mapping the human genome, concluding, sharply perhaps, that we would have been better off without it. Maureen Junker-Kenny looks instead to the consequences of a socially aware analysis, arguing for the development of an institutional ethics. Behind all such discourse is the belief that the analyses of the specific techniques of genetic science do not open up discourse in theology and ethics sufficiently clearly in order to come to an appropriate analysis of the underlying processes inherent in contemporary medicine and genetics. Indeed, implicit here is the assumption that such analysis of techniques themselves might even be *unhelpful* in framing such discussion. Yet this need not imply hostility towards science as such and genetic engineering in particular. Rather, the suggestion is made that a greater awareness of the social context of science can serve to contextualize its particular claim for social priority.

Language and liturgy

Of course, one of the threads picked up by the authors of this volume is how far the claims made for the possible benefits of genetic applications are realistic. Bronislaw Szerszynski's chapter considers how the language of the Human Genome Project might contribute to a shift in understanding of what it is to be human. He draws a parallel, somewhat provocatively, between the 'death' of God-language in post-medieval discourse, and the prospect of the 'death' of the human, understood in terms of its limitation to reductionist language, purified of ambiguity in search of the 'deep surface' of DNA. Scientists themselves might not recognize such implicit implications of the way they think about the human person. However, it is the authority of science, or lack of it, in the public sphere that is important to note in this context. Even while there is more public distrust of scientific endeavours, paradoxically perhaps, the potency of genetics as a cultural symbol in the Western world is immediately apparent in the relative attention paid to it in media discourse. It is in this sense that Szerszynski suggests, as does Song, that genetics is a theological project, insofar as it acculturates a particular interpretation of the human.

Given such a trend it becomes less surprising that some theologians in this volume have looked to the language and liturgical practice of the Church as a way of evaluating the language of genomics. Esther Reed draws on particular liturgical rites in order to consider how to evaluate issues associated with the patenting of parts of the human genome, arguably the culmination of a particular instrumental attitude towards the natural world in general and the human person in particular. She is also concerned to use particular biblical themes as a way of measuring the validity of detailed practices, revisiting an ancient theme of casuistry from a biblical point of view. Not all the theologians in this volume would adhere to the deontological approach that she presents. Junker-Kenny, for example, while accepting that 'Christian inspiration' is appropriate, prefers an ethics that draws on philosophical anthropology and the ideal of autonomy. Peter Scott's view is intermediate, suggestive of an ethic that uses the theme of eucharistic hospitality in order to critique the wider social implications of genomic science. Neil Messer also draws on ecclesiastical humanitarianism developed in Hauerwas's writing, and such a view is also implicit in my own chapter on virtue ethics. However, Junker-Kenny is wary of such moves towards more specifically Christian understandings of ethics as being unable to provide an adequate bridge into secular philosophy, even while she remains highly critical of the implicit norms in the Human Genome Project. The potential (or otherwise) of eucharistic forms of ethical reflection, and their value to the Christian and/or secular community, remain unresolved and reflect, perhaps, the ambiguity in theological and ethical reflection of which Ruth Page has so cogently reminded us.

Health and disease

One of the themes that is particularly strong in the chapters written by practising scientists is the focus on the particular aims of the genetic projects in terms of combating genetic disease. It is worth noting that in the early history of genetic research such goals were less restricted. Soon after James Watson's and Francis Crick's discovery of the structure of DNA in 1953 genetic scientists began to speculate about the possibility for the future genetic transformation of the human race. Scientists then were worried about what they saw as the potential disaster facing humanity, that the ability of medicine to keep those with genetic defects alive would in effect increase the deleterious genetic load on human evolution. In the late 1950s the American geneticist Professor H.J. Muller predicted a future genetic apocalypse, so that 'the then existing germ cells of what were once human beings would be a lot of hopeless, utterly diverse genetic monstrosities'.[1] For the scientists there were two ways of tackling such a problem. The first was genetic surgery of deleterious genes or insertion of desirable genes through 'germ-line' therapy. The second was preventative measures through social change, i.e. parental choice. Yet greater awareness of the spectre of eugenics of the kind practised in the Nazi era has made most geneticists wary of any enforced political implementation of genetic control of humans. Hence even Muller is insistent that genetic change is achieved through *voluntary* means, rather than coercion.

It is worth noting that there has been a shift in attitude among genetic scientists. Textbooks in human genetic science today are more likely to be far more cautious about making *any* social recommendations for the human race. Even the idea of preventative measures through social change does not square well with contemporary understanding of population genetics, so that 'the simplest equations of population genetics show that preventing people with rare genetic disorders from reproducing will not significantly reduce the frequency of these detrimental genes'.[2]

If we ask contemporary geneticists what the possibilities are for genetic science, the reply is more often than not in terms of specific medical applications, rather than any grand plan for

[1] H.J. Muller, 'The Guidance of Human Evolution', in *Perspectives in Biology and Medicine* (Chicago: University of Chicago Press, 1959), vol. iii, p. 11.

[2] Arthur P. Mange and Elaine Johnson, *Genetics: Human Aspects* (London: Sinauer, 1990), p. 10.

eugenics. By focusing on particular instances of genetic disease, the possibility of medical treatment of severe conditions such as cystic fibrosis or Huntington's disease comes closer to reality. Even the susceptibility to more general diseases, such as some cancers, various forms of heart disease and a host of other medical conditions, has a genetic component. The idea that genetic science could alleviate an individual's suffering is one that has particular appeal. It is in this context that the geneticist Duncan Shaw suggests that 'we can look forward to a new era in molecular medicine, where intervention at the level of the gene will provide new opportunities for conquering some of the most intractable conditions known to medicine'.[3]

The Human Genome Project boosted this optimism further. More important, as far as geneticists are concerned, we would be irresponsible not to use genetics to improve the human condition. While there is some fear expressed, there is consciousness that a power has fallen into human hands. For: 'Until now we had no control over this random distribution. The genetic material we have been awarded is the result of a lottery, the lottery of life. Today we have the power to manipulate the genetic material at will, to modify what it took Nature 4.5 billion years to create. These are exciting, but scary times.'[4] James Watson, co-discoverer of the structure of DNA, is one of the most outspoken geneticists in support of the prospect of using genetic technology to alter human genetics. The moral consequences of *not* using the knowledge is, for him, just as significant as focusing on the possible risks and dangers.

Given this background, it is appropriate that Robert Song identifies the treatment of disease as the prime motivation of genetic scientists. Nonetheless, such a claim also needs to be qualified by the realization that scientists working on the HGP were well aware that unless such a claim was made, funding would not be forthcoming. In other words, it was a necessary formulation in order to win public support. Yet while we might doubt the genuineness or otherwise of some of the claims made for funding, it becomes clear that a particular understanding of what health means is implicit in genetics research. Michael

---

[3] Duncan Shaw, *Molecular Genetics of Human Inherited Disease* (London: John Wiley, 1995), p. 4.
[4] Philippe Frossard, *The Lottery of Life: The New Genetics and the Future of Mankind* (Bantam Press, 1991), p. 13.

Reiss asks us to stretch the ideal of science further in suggesting that science might not just limit itself to a discussion of disease prevention, but include, perhaps as a 'side-effect', increased longevity. Neil Messer gives us an analysis of contemporary notions of health and disease and asks what a Christian response might be, drawing as it does on the fragility of life and theological interpretation of suffering (as exemplified in Paul's thorn in the flesh). Implicit in his discussion are the contrasting norms underlying genetic science and philosophical/theological visions of reality helpfully spelt out by Junker-Kenny. In addition, due account needs to be taken of the way medical practitioners themselves understand their own practice in terms of key principles that have dominated medical bioethics discussions. Julie Clague asks us to consider how such principles have tended to reduce the account of what it is to be human to one focused on personal autonomy, rather than on a wider notion of human dignity.

Theology and ethics

Questions about the possible role of theology and ethics emerge from this discussion of health. Could, for example, the idea of the common good identified by Clague replace the more static alternatives of divine ordering as opposed to genetic mastery? While divine ordering, when understood in terms of fixity of created beings, leads to a more fearful response towards genetics, the theme of genetic mastery leads to a much more cavalier approach, one that could even be endorsed theologically by the concept of humanity as co-creator. None of the contributors to this volume argue for either of these extremes, though there is a spectrum of interpretation as to how far theological insights might take priority in ethical analysis. Reed, Messer and to some extent Scott argue for a robust theological approach that begins unashamedly in biblical and liturgical principles. Junker-Kenny and Reiss are less convinced that such language will help in secular debate. To some extent my own approach is intermediate in making a claim for a strong notion of the good in terms of the theological notion of Wisdom, while at the same time recognizing the appropriateness of drawing on philosophical reflection through the Aristotelian notion of prudence. In a similar way, Clague argues for a recovery of the common good that draws on theological insights, while not being restricted to them. Scott also emphasizes the importance of perceiving more clearly what the goodness of God might mean, expressed in a communal way through the notion of hospitality. Many authors (especially Messer, Clague, myself and Scott) put emphasis on the communitarian aspects of seeking out the good, rather than more individualistic interpretations. Most of the authors in this volume would also resist an outright rejection of genetic manipulation or endorsement, though Reiss perhaps comes closest to theological affirmation, while Song and Scott possibly come closest to theological resistance. The subtleties in the discussion are not lost in any of the accounts, which calls to mind once more Page's insistence on ambiguity in the way we approach how to understand persons. Her suggestion that we need to widen our concept of the image of God so that it includes other members of the planet Earth is a salutary reminder that the context in which discussions of the human Genome Project need to take place are not just social, but also environmental. The temptation towards a narrowly defined anthropocentrism is all too clear in the realization that germ-line changes in non-humans are accepted almost as a matter of course. In other words, we need to be aware of the ecological consequences, if any, of the concentration on human genetic research. I am not arguing that human dignity and uniqueness does not exist, rather that justice issues are not just confined to the human community, but arise in relation to the wider community of life as well. Reed illustrates this beautifully in her discussion of the value of all life forms in their relation to the possibility of their giving glory to God. Hence the discussion points not just to the narrowly defined issues around human genetic science, but more generally in terms of the reordering of nature and its implications for our own sense of human identity and purpose.[5]

Conclusions

What are the tentative conclusions arising from this conversation between different perspectives on human genetic

---

[5] For further discussion see C. Deane-Drummond and B. Szerszynski, *Re-Ordering Nature: Theology, Society and the New Genetics* (Edinburgh: T & T Clark, 2002).

science? The following are indicative areas for further discussion:

1. The social, cultural, political and historical embeddedness of genetic science needs to be appreciated fully in making any theological and ethical recommendations.
2. Following from this it is insufficient to explore ethical issues in terms of the application or development of technology, rather the philosophical, historical, social and political basis and nature of such technology needs to be explored.
3. Theologians may choose to be explicit in advocating principles drawing from liturgical life in Christian community, and/or align their thinking with philosophical analysis, such as philosophical anthropology.
4. Specific theological ideas, such as image-bearing, are ambiguous reference points in view of the variety of interpretations through history. Theologians, as much as scientists, need to be sensitive to the social and historical context in which their ideas take shape.
5. Theological discussion can offer approaches to genetics that avoid the extremes of hostility on the one hand or blanket endorsement on the other.
6. The language of such reflection is exemplified in that of the common good, or more specifically, virtue ethics.
7. While both virtue ethics and the common good can be theorized in a secular way, particular approaches from a Christian perspective can form the basis for dialogue with secular traditions.
8. Such an understanding necessarily includes specifically Christian notions of justice, hence the concept of the good is not just individual, but social, political and environmental.
9. Theological discussion on genetics is also inclusive of eschatological and salvific themes of redemption and immortality, so that the clash (if any) with visions from genetic science becomes an arena for further debate and dialogue.

Overall, much of this book has been concerned about the urgent need to locate the HGP in a larger picture, not just as an isolated technological initiative, but as something embedded in history, culture, symbol, ideas of human purpose and flourishing, justice, the common good and so on. Hence, there is an urgent need for dialogue between different disciplines, and also the opportunity for theological reflection to contribute to the debate and to discuss the prospects for human genetics in its own terms, that is from the point of view of its own intellectual resources. The HGP and associated emerging technologies cannot claim to be outside the normal domain of such debate in some purely technical space. Indeed, the recognition by scientists that public debate and wider reflection is necessary displays a wisdom that sees the only way science is going to progress is through being embedded in a shared ownership of its aims and initiatives. While those outside scientific endeavour cannot claim expert knowledge, the outcomes of such initiatives are of public, social and political importance.

The social and political importance of the HGP becomes more transparent once one sees it as a project in the way discussed by Robert Song in this volume. Of course the implications of the HGP are much wider than the project itself, but the theme of project had the effect of uniting effort in a particular way in a given direction. Politics in the post-Reformation tradition can also be seen in terms of a project to change society, and in this sense the HGP fits into a political agenda. Michael Walzer traces such a tradition in politics to Puritan sects, the idea 'that there were goals quite apart from the preservation and health of the body politic, goals that made men into instruments and changed politics itself from a self sufficient organic existence into a means, method and purposive discipline'.[6] Given this scenario it becomes even more urgent to ask particular ethical and theological questions about the Human Genome Project, not just in terms of its role in the reordering of nature, but also in terms of its wider impact on social and political life. The way such questions could even begin to be answered requires sensitivity and listening to the other in a way that is difficult for those used to considering issues simply from within their own discipline. The nature of the problems arising are such that not only is a multidisciplinary approach necessary, it is also vital if some movement towards a shared ownership of change is going to be achieved. Fragmented knowledge is necessarily partial; we need those

---

[6] M. Walzer, *The Revolution of the Saints: A Study in the Origins of Radical Politics* (New York: Atheneum Press, 1968), p. 182. I am grateful to Bronislaw Szerszynski for giving me this reference.

who are prepared to see both the limitations in specialist areas and the possibilities in reconnecting different areas of knowledge. It reflects a return to understanding wisdom as integrated knowledge, where mutual respect and cooperation are fostered and developed.

My hope is that this book has contributed in a small way to raising such issues for further discussion. We are at a critical point in history where many of the promises and prospects offered by genetic scientists have yet to be realized. Hence theological and ethical reflection need not simply be an *a posteriori* exercise; rather, in helping to inform public debate about science it can serve to inform policy-making and ultimately scientific practice.

The Edifice of the Genome

(after Umberto Eco)

[*Eco's novel* The Name of the Rose *is set in an imaginary mediaeval monastery, possessed of a great library, the Aedificium, laid out in the form of a labyrinthine map of the world.*]

Sometimes it seems as though
After long wanderings looking for the key
We are at last possessed of a map
Of the labyrinth. We roam there freely
By day and night. We take down books
At will. Some are a surprise –
Recipes overlap, or are bound strangely,
As though by a logic long since lost.
Some are ancient, nearly as old
As life itself – and have passed into
The common syntax of things.
A few paragraphs, here and there,
Are distinctively human – they power
The learning of babies, the mind of the priest,
The poet, the woman of science.

Are we then already in the hidden sanctuary
With the book of books in our hands?
It is not to be thought so.
There are no ideas in the manuals we read,
Only hints behind wiring diagrams.
These are not holy texts – we call
Much of them junk.
Yet we cannot banish a fear
That all this decipherment
Means more than appears,
That it may carry some curse.
We cannot fail to doubt ourselves,
To wonder if we are after all cast out
Among the ruins of our wisdom,
Leafing through fragments.

By some quantum tunnelling of the spirit
Our predicament is all of these –
Onlookers, explorers, initiates of the sanctum,
Refugees from the terrible power
Of our own ingenuity.
We trade phrases – image of God,
Playing God, humanity coming of age –
None is able to edge out the others.
It is as well. May we not be too eager
To know the name of our desire.

Christopher Southgate

Index